Mental Health among Higher Education Faculty, Administrators, and Graduate Students

Lexington Studies in Health Communication

Series Editors: Leandra H. Hernández and Kari Nixon

National and international governments have recognized the importance of widespread, timely, and effective health communication, as research shows that accurate, patient-centered, and culturally competent health communication can improve patient and community health care outcomes. This interdisciplinary series examines the role of health communication in society and is receptive to manuscripts and edited volumes that use a variety of theoretical, methodological, interdisciplinary, and intersectional approaches. We invite contributions on a variety of health communication topics including but not limited to health communication in a digital age; race, gender, ethnicity, class, physical abilities, and health communication; critical approaches to health communication; feminisms and health communication; LGBTQIA health; interpersonal health communication perspectives; rhetorical approaches to health communication; organizational approaches to health communication; health campaigns, media effects, and health communication; multicultural approaches to health communication; and international health communication. This series is open to contributions from scholars representing communication, women's and gender studies, public health, health education, discursive analyses of medical rhetoric, and other disciplines whose work interrogates and explores these topics. Successful proposals will be accessible to an interdisciplinary audience, advance our understanding of contemporary approaches to health communication, and enrich our conversations about the importance of health communication in today's health landscape.

Recent Titles in This Series

Mental Health among Higher Education Faculty, Administrators, and Graduate Students: A Critical Perspective
By Teresa Heinz Housel
Communicating With, About, and Through Self-Harm: Scarred Discourse
By Warren J. Bareiss
The Ethos of Black Motherhood in America: Only White Women Get Pregnant
By Kimberly C. Harper
Medical Humanism, Chronic Illness, and the Body in Pain: An Ecology of Wholeness
By Vinita Agarwal
Social Support and Health in the Digital Age
By Nichole Egbert and Kevin B. Wright
Narrative Journeys of Young Black Women with Eating Disorders: A Hidden Community among Us
By Stephanie Hawthorne
Unintended Consequences of Electronic Medical Records: An Emergency Room Ethnography
By Barbara Cook Overton
eMessaging and the Physician/Patient Dynamic: Practices in Transition
By Susan Wieczorek
Communicating Mental Health: History, Contexts, and Perspectives
By Lance R. Lippert, Robert D. Hall, Aimee E. Miller-Ott, and Daniel Cochece Davis

CTE, Media, and the NFL: Framing of a Public Health Crisis as a Football Epidemic
By Travis R. Bell, Janelle Applequist, and Christian Dotson-Pierson
*Challenging Reproductive Control and Gendered Violence in the Americas:
   Intersectionality, Power, and Struggles for Rights*
By Leandra Hinojosa Hernández and Sarah De Los Santos Upton
*Politics, Propaganda, and Public Health: A Case Study in Health Communication and
   Public Trust*
By Laura Crosswell and Lance Porter
Communication and Feminist Perspectives on Ovarian Cancer
By Dinah Tetteh

Mental Health among Higher Education Faculty, Administrators, and Graduate Students

A Critical Perspective

Edited by
Teresa Heinz Housel

Foreword by
Katie Rose Guest Pryal

LEXINGTON BOOKS
Lanham • Boulder • New York • London

Published by Lexington Books
An imprint of The Rowman & Littlefield Publishing Group, Inc.
4501 Forbes Boulevard, Suite 200, Lanham, Maryland 20706
www.rowman.com

86-90 Paul Street, London EC2A 4NE

Copyright © 2021 by The Rowman & Littlefield Publishing Group, Inc.

All rights reserved. No part of this book may be reproduced in any form or by any electronic or mechanical means, including information storage and retrieval systems, without written permission from the publisher, except by a reviewer who may quote passages in a review.

British Library Cataloging in Publication Information Available

Library of Congress Cataloging-in-Publication Data

Names: Housel, Teresa Heinz, 1972- editor.
Title: Mental health among higher education faculty, administrators, and graduate students : a critical perspective / edited by Teresa Heinz Housel.
Description: Lanham, Maryland : Lexington Books, 2021. | Series: Lexington studies in health communication | Includes bibliographical references and index. | Summary: "Mental Health among Higher Education Faculty, Administrators, and Graduate Students argues that mental illness stigma surrounds not being able to cope with the rigors of academia is viewed as personal weakness. It examines the complex mental health issues in higher education and offers best practices for institutions from a communication approach"— Provided by publisher.
Identifiers: LCCN 2021030862 (print) | LCCN 2021030863 (ebook) | ISBN 9781793630247 (cloth) | ISBN 9781793630261 (paperback) | ISBN 9781793630254 (epub)
Subjects: LCSH: Graduate students—Mental health—United States. | Graduate students—Mental health services—United States. | College teachers—Mental health—United States. | College teachers—Mental health services—United States. | College administrators—Mental health—United States. | College administrators—Mental health services—United States. | Education, Higher—Psychological aspects.
Classification: LCC RC451.4.S7 M42 2021 (print) | LCC RC451.4.S7 (ebook) | DDC 616.8900835—dc23
LC record available at https://lccn.loc.gov/2021030862
LC ebook record available at https://lccn.loc.gov/2021030863

This book is dedicated to all those whose voices, courage, and strength are represented in this book's chapters.

Contents

Foreword   xi
Katie Rose Guest Pryal

Preface   xvii
Teresa Heinz Housel

Acknowledgments   xxv

PART 1: MENTAL DISTRESS AND MENTAL ILLNESS IN ACADEMIC CULTURE   1

1. The Perfect Storm of Mental Health Issues in Academia and the Need for Critical Research and Policies   3
Teresa Heinz Housel

2. Anxiety in Academia: An Autoethnographic Account   35
Andrea L. Meluch

3. Structuration of U.S. Communication Graduate Students' Stress   53
Rahul Mitra, Nubia Brewster, Patrice M. Buzzanell, Julia Grzywinski, Elizabeth-Ann Pandzich

4. "Burn It Down": The Graduate Student Burnout Experience   69
Victoria McDermott and Nike Bahr

PART 2: INTERSECTIONS OF MENTAL HEALTH AND MARGINALIZED ACADEMIC POPULATIONS   103

5 Effects of Chronic Exposure to Invalidation on People of Color in Academia: An Exploratory Study   105
Juan S. Muhamad, Jessica Wendorf Muhamad, and Maria Elena Villar

6 First-Generation Graduate and Professional Students in the United States: A Critical Narrative Review   121
Erinn C. Cameron

7 Give and Take: Exploring the Role of Confidants When Friends Disclose Chronic and/or Mental Health–Related Information   139
Robert D. Hall

8 The Academic Amygdala: Tropes of PTSD in Higher Education News Coverage   169
Alena Amato Ruggerio and Erica Knotts

PART 3: INSTITUTIONAL POLICIES ON MENTAL HEALTH AND RECOMMENDATIONS FOR BEST PRACTICES   187

9 Culturally Sensitive Mental Health Support for Higher Education Employees   189
Lukasz Swiatek and Ursula Edgington

10 Having Emotional Support Animals at College   207
Susan Hafen

11 Navigating Boundaries while Creating Safe Spaces for Faculty and Students   227
Sandra Smeltzer, David M. Walton, Nicole Campbell

12 The Mental Health Impacts of Making a Workers' Compensation Claim for a Mental Injury   245
Philip Dearman and Beth Edmondson

Appendix: Mental Health–Related Resources for the Communication Classroom   277
Teresa Heinz Housel, Andrea L. Meluch, Vanessa R. Sperduti, Sandra Smeltzer, Rahul Mitra

Index   289

About the Editor and Contributors   297

Foreword
Katie Rose Guest Pryal

Many years ago, in a warm December, I received a promotion at my institution. After seven years of work, I was promoted from Clinical Assistant Professor to Clinical Associate Professor. A few weeks later, I quit.

After nearly fifteen years of working in higher education at three different institutions, teaching with no job security and little possibility of advancement, I had mentally and physically burned out. I might have finally earned a promotion, but the "clinical" in my title meant I was non-tenurable. Worse, my promotion did not even merit a raise. I earned half of that which my colleagues without the "clinical" designation earned. To compound the situation, I didn't even have the job security of tenure. I would always and forever feel insecure, at the mercy of student course evaluations and the fifty tenured professors and deans whose opinions about my retention were the only ones that mattered.

As I look back on this experience now, my story might sound like that of every higher ed worker who has walked away from academia—except that it isn't. The stress I was under as a contingent faculty member took a unique toll. My fear about job security had a special twist.

In short, I was working in higher education while also hiding an invisible disability. I lived in constant fear that someone would find out that I was disabled and that the knowledge would be used against me.

There were also the working conditions that included not only endless hours of teaching first-year legal writing and evaluating hundreds of pages of work, but also endless hours of grueling student support work. I taught nervous first-year students who needed emotional support and often could only find it from me. That emotional support work was not in my job description, but the students turned to me anyway because I was the only professor who knew them well. Where else would they go? To their professors who taught lectures with hundreds of students? Not likely.

If I didn't provide the emotional support, my students burned me on my precious course evaluations. After all, female professors are supposed to nurture our students. But the fact is, I only had the spoons to be a great professor (Miserandino 2003).[1] I didn't have the spoons (let alone the training) to be a counselor or therapist. Thus, I lived a double-bind during all the years I worked: I would expend my reserves caring for my students, or take the risk of losing my job if I didn't. Asking for help was out of the question because it could reveal that I was disabled and needed accommodations.

I would rather quit, I thought.

And so, in that January, after I received what amounted to a fake promotion with no raise, I did.

Not everyone has the luxury of quitting that I had. I am a white woman with invisible disabilities; I have a doctorate and law degree. I am also married to a person who has a job. Therefore, I had more options than most people. For example, some higher ed workers are first-generation academics with extended families to financially support. Some are single parents. Some are from marginalized communities and feel an obligation to stay and advise students. The point is, many do not have the freedom to quit that I had.

Shortly after I quit, I pitched a monthly column to *The Chronicle of Higher Education,* called "Life of the Mind Interrupted," about mental health and disability in higher education. In the first column in the series, titled "Disclosure Blues," I wrote about whether one should disclose one's mental illness if one works in higher education (Pryal 2014). I weighed the pros and cons, and I came out somewhere in the middle. If you have job security, fine; you get the benefit of unburdening yourself of your secret.

What if you do not have this security? As I wrote in my column, "It's hard for me to suggest that graduate students, contingent faculty, or pre-tenure faculty disclose their mental illnesses to their academic colleagues. We are, in academia, often still devoted to the mythos of the good man speaking well, the professor as bastion of reason, the *cogito ergo sum*" (Pryal 2014). Although it might be nice to not have to carry a secret like I did, the risks of disclosure were too great.

Let's face it: Neurodivergent faculty are hardly encouraged to speak up in a place where we're supposed to be living the life of the mind. If your job is on the line, the risks outweigh the benefits. However, the burdens of secrecy are real. I told lies my colleagues and supervisors about "feeling under the weather" when I felt depressed or anxious and couldn't hide it completely. I constantly worried that my behavior did not match the social expectations of colleagues, especially at large gatherings where I felt uncomfortable. I tried to fake it: I often failed. As a result, I worked even harder to make sure that my work record was impeccable; I had to make up for the fact that my *social* record was not.

I have a long list of disabilities—so many that I called them a *bouquet*. When I was still in college I was diagnosed with bipolar disorder, a diagnosis that has only been confirmed as I've got older. It is a diagnosis that I treat with respect; meaning, I see my doctor, I take my medicine, I exercise, and I get enough sleep. I have a family, including two small children who count on me, and I refuse to put my life at risk.

I also have anxiety disorder, which is frankly wrecking me as I write these words during the COVID-19 pandemic. Lastly, I am autistic, which makes it hard for me to make friends and sometimes makes it hard for me to say the right thing in the moment (which is probably why I prefer writing). In fact, autism makes it hard for me to do a lot of things that other people find easy.

On the other hand, autism also makes it easier for me to do things that other people find hard. For example, it was easy for me to see that leaving higher education was the right thing to do. The pieces fell into place so clearly as I weighed the good and bad, the pros and cons. I could make the decision without emotions getting in the way. Not because I don't have emotions, but because I do, and I know how to put them aside. It is easier for me to step back and observe things from a distance when the chaos gets too much. I received the promotion, and the clarity was so striking as to be the clanging of a bell. To survive, I had to leave.

My departure caught most of my colleagues by surprise. As I noted earlier in this foreword, I did so much to make sure that my record was impeccable. I heard from one person on the inside that my promotion vote was unanimous. Perhaps they understand now. In fact, I teach a course now, at the same institution, as an adjunct, on my terms, one of my own design for which I even wrote the book.

Even though others were surprised at my sudden departure from my institution, no one came to me and asked, "What could we have done better? What could we have done to make you stay?" Workers like me shouldn't feel like we have to leave higher education. We shouldn't feel alienated and afraid. But we do, and that's a loss to everyone. That's why a book like this one is so very important.

I also point out that this book is important for a second reason (and more than that, besides): Yes, there are those of us who enter higher ed as neurodivergent workers who are often afraid to disclose. However, the academic culture of overwork, of bullying, of insecure employment so often drives us to leave. We suffer, or we quit. Or, in very rare cases, I suppose, we do get tenure and write books about it (Saks 2007; Jamison 1995).

It is imperative to openly discuss another mental health problem that haunts higher education: those who are normate (Garland-Thomson 1997),[2] but because the circumstances of higher education are so grueling and unhealthy, they develop mental illness. The unhealthy culture of academia creates a large population of workers that will inevitably develop burnout (Lackritz 2004), anxiety, depression (Pain 2017), addiction, and more. And conditions in higher education are worsening under COVID-19, as workloads get heavier, and as institution rely even more on contingent workers. Higher ed workers have few resources available to help them. However, this book is part of a growing movement of academics who seek to change this trend by offering adequate support; institutional programming around mental health and mental illness; and the eradication of the culture of shameful silence around mental health–related issues in academia.

Five years ago, I published my mental health and higher education book, *Life of the Mind Interrupted: Essays on Mental Health and Disability in Higher Education* (Pryal 2017a). Five years later, we still need these books. The need remains acute for all higher ed workers: faculty, administrators, and graduate students. Now, at this particular moment, we face the COVID-19 pandemic and a reckoning with police and other culturally sanctioned violence against Black people. We also face issues that universities must deal with administratively and that their workers encounter as well, on a much more personal level, sometimes with devastating consequences. Too often, institutions are not prepared to support their faculty even at the best of times. Institutions most certainly on not prepared to do so in a crisis of these proportions.

Disability Studies Professor Margaret Price, from Ohio State University, was a lead author of a recent large-scale study of faculty with mental illness and resource guide (Price 2017). I interviewed Price about the guide, titled *Promoting Supportive Academic Environments for Faculty with Mental Illnesses: Resource Guide and Suggestions for Practice*. When I asked her about how institutions can ready themselves to support faculty, how they can make their spaces more accessible, Price replied, "The thing is, you can have the most thorough resource guide in the world"—and, having read it, I can tell you that Price's guide comes close—"and you can dutifully implement every recommendation it makes," but, as Price notes, this implementation isn't enough (Pryal 2017b). No, you must do more: your institution's *culture* must change as well. Price notes, "Unless the culture of your institution includes a sense of shared accountability—basically, of giving a crap about those you work with and share space with, of noticing when you might need to intervene, of when you need to take an extra moment to listen or care or try something new on another person's behalf—then access just won't work."

My work over the past decade has been to push for a change of culture, one of understanding and acceptance of disabled people. Clearly, there is still more work to do. That is why I am so pleased to see this book come to print.

This book pushes against the culture of silence that has surrounded mental health in academia. It pushes against the idea that walking away from unhealthy *rigorous* research, teaching, and service is a sign of personal or professional weakness. I am pleased to play a small part in endorsing this collection, and I hope that the chapters here make the world more humane for all of us.

Katie Rose Guest Pryal, JD, PhD
October 26, 2020

NOTES

1. In "The Spoon Theory," disability activist Christine Miserandino, notes that "the difference in being sick and being healthy is having to make choices or to consciously think about things when the rest of the world doesn't have to" and refers to the rationing of energy as "spoons."

2. The term "normate," as used to refer to a non-disabled person, was coined by Rosemarie Garland-Thomson in her book *Extraordinary Bodies: Figuring Physical Disability in American Culture and Literature*.

REFERENCES

Garland-Thomson, Rosemarie. 1997. *Extraordinary Bodies: Figuring Physical Disability in American Culture and Literature*. New York: Columbia University Press.

Jamison, Kay Redfield. 1995. *An Unquiet Mind: A Memoir of Moods and Madness*. New York: Knopf.

Lackritz, James R. 2004. "Exploring Burnout Among University Faculty: Incidence, Performance, and Demographic Issues." *Teaching and Teacher Education*, 20, no. 7: 713–729.

Miserandino, Christine. 2003. "The Spoon Theory." *But You Don't Look Sick*. https://butyoudontlooksick.com/articles/written-by-christine/the-spoon-theory/.

Pain, Elisabeth. 2017. "Ph.D. Students Face Significant Mental Health Challenges." *Science Magazine*, Apr. 4, 2017. https://www.sciencemag.org/careers/2017/04/phd-students-face-significant-mental-health-challenges.

Price, Margaret, and Stephanie L. Kerschbaum. 2017. "Promoting Supportive Academic Environments for Faculty with Mental Illnesses: Resource Guide and Suggestions for Practice." Philadelphia, PA: Temple University Collaborative on Community Inclusion. http://www.tucollaborative.org/sdm_downloads/supportive-academic-environments-for-faculty-with-mental-illnesses/.

Pryal, Katie Rose Guest. 1997a. *Life of the Mind Interrupted: Essays on Mental Health and Disability in Higher Education*. Chapel Hill, NC: Blue Crow Books.

Pryal, Katie Rose Guest. 1997b. "On Faculty and Mental Illness." *The Chronicle of Higher Education*. Dec. 18, 2017. https://www.chronicle.com/article/on-faculty-and-mental-illness/.

Pryal, Katie Rose Guest. 2014. "Disclosure Blues: Should You Tell Colleagues About Your Mental Illness?" *The Chronicle of Higher Education*. June 13, 2014. https://community.chronicle.com/news/546-disclosure-blues-should-you-tell-colleagues-about-your-mental-illness.

Saks, Elyn. 2007. *The Center Cannot Hold: My Journey Through Madness*. New York: Hachette Books.

Preface

Teresa Heinz Housel

In late 2010, I planned my sabbatical for the 2011–2012 academic year after what I expected would be a successful tenure application process at my American institution. I was more than ready for a change. Although I had traveled internationally throughout my twenties, my long-held dream to eventually live overseas was shelved as I sprinted on the professional treadmill as a full-time faculty member in communication studies.

I enjoyed teaching courses in my specialty but, over the ensuing years, found it increasingly difficult to ignore that I needed to move on. Though I certainly met caring colleagues as friends, I was weary of the institution's polite outward performances of religiosity that belied a passive aggressive internal environment. A gentle, free spirit at heart, I was trying to make life work in the wrong place.

As I planned my sabbatical, I decided that New Zealand would be the target location. I have been drawn to New Zealand ever since reading Keri Hulme's (1983) *The Bone People* in an undergraduate English literature class at Oberlin College. I have always loved geographically remote areas with dark landscapes and unpredictable weather. Having universities with journalism and communication studies courses was a plus.

My New Zealand plan was, in part, guided by my previous experience in Western Australia. In the late 1990s, I spent several happy, productive years on a postgraduate Rotary fellowship in cultural studies at Murdoch University in Perth. Everything about the experience was strong and life-giving. I loved our intense classroom discussions across courses ranging from social semiotics to critical food studies. Often, those discussions spilled into the university library's courtyard café, where we discussed our research papers over coffees and meat pies.

The Perth area's landscape matched the fierce intellectual environment. Even now, I can close my eyes and experience the place all over again: the white-gold dirt and plants, the endless sun that caused me to squint and shield my eyes, and the winds that crashed like waves against my Fremantle flat every afternoon. I felt fearless, ready to conquer any challenge. It might seem obvious that I would choose Australia for my sabbatical site, but I wanted to experience New Zealand with its own history and cultural variances from Australia. I was also thrilled to return to this general part of the world.

Now, as I write this preface in early 2021, my home study looks out onto our neighbor's garden with native trees in a valley north of Wellington. Within a week after arriving in Wellington on my sabbatical in early 2012, I decided to leave my job and pursue toward my dream to move overseas. My husband and I immigrated to New Zealand in 2013. My goal to live in a place that I love so much is an amazing reality, but the path was marked by acute anxiety. Anxiety, and its intersection with my academic work, is the inspiration for this book.

THE SHOCK OF PANIC

I did not realize how inadvertently insular my life had become until my sabbatical. My first month in Wellington in April 2012 was a culture-shock blur after living for seven years in a conservative region of the United States. At the same time, I experienced cultural-professional transition between my home institution, in a city structured around church connections, and a public urban university in a capital city. I acclimated by joining a local hiking (tramping) group, reading New Zealand cultural and social history, making new friends, and enjoying all the foods I remembered from Perth, as well as new local ones.

I resumed academic work shortly after my arrival. Soon thereafter, a faculty member at my guest institution invited me to present a lecture to a postgraduate class. Excitedly, I wrote the lecture on general differences between American and New Zealand journalism.

Several weeks later in the classroom, I started the guest lecture accompanied by a visual slide presentation. Coming from a family of storytellers, I enjoy weaving everyday anecdotes into lectures to explain complex theories. Many students have told me that they often learn without realizing it in my classes because I seamlessly interweave narratives with the theories that they demonstrate. I once again drew from this familiar well of stories as I shared experiences from various journalism jobs against a visual background of photos and maps.

After a few minutes, I shifted the focus from myself to the students as I asked them about their career interests. As I responded to their contributions, I slowly noticed that my breathing had quickened. I brushed sweat from my forehead as I joked about being in a heated room, which is not common in New Zealand. We all laughed.

Alarmingly, my attempt to dissipate the sudden anxiety through humor didn't work. Looking down at my carefully typed and highlighted notes, I noted that my breathing was now so rapid and shallow that I could not catch my breath. No longer able to speak, I paused for a terrifying few seconds and forced myself to recompose. The odd physical episode passed a moment later and I resumed the lecture while pretending nothing had happened.

An hour later, I returned to my borrowed office, furious at myself for bungling this opportunity to shine. After all, public speaking had always been easy for me, an introvert who enjoys the rush of performance energy. I had delivered many lectures, sometimes in front of hundreds of people, in many different contexts. Never did I become unusually anxious, other than typical pre-performance nerves.

I hoped the incident was a fluke, just a weird by-product somehow of speaking in front of unfamiliar people in a new situation. However, a month after the guest lecture, I delivered a lunchtime presentation to a Wellington-area Rotary Club about my postgraduate fellowship in Perth, a topic I can usually discuss effortlessly. I was startled to find the same symptoms returning a few minutes into my talk. Catching my breath, I managed to finish the presentation. I feared that something was wrong, but cautiously assumed that the odd symptoms would disappear once I returned to my American institution for the new semester.

AN EPIPHANY THROUGH COURAGE

I don't remember much of the 2012–2013 academic year back in the United States. By this time, my husband and I had decided to immigrate to New Zealand under the Skilled Migrant Scheme. The application process took an entire year, but we could not say a word to anyone other than immediate family.

At first glance, it seems completely contradictory, even illogical, that someone with anxiety and panic attacks would make the stressful and seismic shift to quit a tenured job and move to the other side of the world, all the while hardly telling anyone. I can only attribute my decision to an epiphany in which I concluded that I needed to do what I felt was morally right. Shortly before my sabbatical in New Zealand, I attended an emotionally wrought city council meeting in the small city where we were living. The councilors and local residents debated if the city should pass a measure that would protect LGBT people from discrimination from employers and landlords when applying for jobs or finding housing. The meeting lasted into the late hours as many local residents tearfully shared either their pain or their children's experiences of being marginalized based on sexual identity in this city.

After the city's mayor (who would cast the deciding vote and had political aspirations) read a pre-prepared response about why he could not support the proposed measure, something powerful shifted within me. I told my husband after the meeting that it was over for me in this place. It took me great courage to admit that I had this epiphany because we were set for life with our professional jobs in our respective fields, beautiful home, and the friends we had made there. However, living there as a full person was no longer tenable for me. I could no longer live in a city, or work at an institution, where such discrimination openly occurred, or where it was even a question to consider someone's sexual identity in the workplace or housing. I also wanted to live and work in a place where religion was not used to justify discrimination or any form of incivility.

Realizing the emotional reasons for moving to New Zealand would come later, after I had fully comprehended the traumatic impact of a bullying incident that I experienced at the hands of some colleagues. I realize now that my anxious behaviors (not making eye contact during conversations, stumbling over my words when talking with others, and beginning to avoid social events) that I exhibited during my last year on the job reflected the underlying trauma.

A DIFFERENT ROOM, BUT STILL ME

With the decision made to emigrate, I dutifully taught my assigned full load of courses, advised students, and completed college service requirements. I listened vaguely when an administrator approached me in early 2013 about being the new department chair at some point in the near future. At home, propelled by adrenaline and resolution to move, I steadily sold household items and mentally prepared to live elsewhere. The year felt hollow somehow. Outwardly, we fulfilled our work and community duties, but internally I had already left.

Meanwhile, much to my dismay, the panicked loss of breath now appeared at the start of almost every class session, including courses I had written in my specialist subject areas of journalism and cultural studies. I never dismissed a class, but the unsettling symptoms deeply rattled me. Still, I remained hopeful. Our upcoming move to New Zealand was a chance to start anew, a fresh start away from a life that felt increasingly claustrophobic.

Not surprisingly, I did not become a different person after we moved to New Zealand. I just entered a new room as a person with increasing anxiety that had now turned into panic attacks. When I could no longer go to my local mall without nearly fainting from panic, I contacted the Anxiety New Zealand Trust for help.

MENTAL HEALTH ISSUES IN ACADEMIA

This volume's contributors discuss the complex issues of mental health in academia. As the chapters collectively point out, academic roles, including those of graduate students, faculty, and administrators, are fertile ground for common mental health challenges such as anxiety and depression. Increasingly, academics are presenting with other mental illnesses such as schizophrenia and post-traumatic stress disorder (PTSD).

As this volume's research demonstrates, many academics with mental illnesses and mental distress have quite successful careers. At the same time, faculty, administrators, and graduate students with mental distress and illnesses are increasingly speaking out about their struggles to manage their conditions in a demanding career. However, the stigma around mental illness and distress in academia is real and silencing, as many of this volume's contributors point out from their research and personal experiences. An academic who speaks out about their condition must weigh the often-isolating stigma around mental illness and distress in a profession that is based on the mind.

While working at my American institution, I occasionally consulted a local counselor and my family doctor about feeling on-edge. However, it was only when working with an anxiety specialist in New Zealand that I truly began to understand my condition. The specialist taught me about the causes of anxiety, how anxiety impacts the brain, and how to manage its triggers and symptoms. My anxiety is a likely combination of genetics (anxious behaviors are prevalent in my family), personality predispositions (perfectionism in my case), and adverse childhood experiences.

I characterize my anxiety as both a helper and intruder. Though my family jokingly referred to me as a "worry wort," my talents and anxiety actually helped me achieve many goals. I have always prided myself on being a highly resilient person, able to take on any challenge and come out strong on the other side. I did not realize it when I was younger, but anxiety helped fuel my relentless drive to complete projects at a meticulously perfectionist level. I sailed through various academic degrees, traveled to many countries, made friends around the world, and won awards for my teaching and writing. The praise that I received only reinforced my focused drive. My personal standards of work were often almost impossible to maintain, but I liked the thrill of reaching them. Moreover, my strategies of perfectionism and overwork gave me the control and confidence to keep anxiety at bay, at least for a little while.

WHEN TALENT AND PERFECTIONISM AREN'T ENOUGH

My first panic attack during my sabbatical in New Zealand shattered my calm confidence. For the first time ever, painstaking preparation and sheer talent were not enough. Through working with my anxiety specialist, I realized how a workplace bullying incident triggered panic disorder more than a year later, during my sabbatical.

As I briefly describe my workplace bullying experience, I readily acknowledge that many people endure much worse, and even ongoing harassment and bullying in their workplaces. My current research of workplace bullying in academia indicates the severity of many cases across countries.

In my own case, the bullying incident occurred at the end of what had been a successful tenure application and pre-tenure probationary period. My only warning was a colleague dropping by my office at the end of the previous work day to mention that an administrator wanted to meet with me. During this hastily called meeting about sudden "problems" in my application, the administrator rifled through files from my first semesters and read out selected critical comments that students had made. I had been given no agenda for the meeting beforehand.

I sat, stunned. The meeting confused me because my annual pre-tenure reports praised my work. My department endorsed my tenure. Any potential problems would have been raised long before, not shortly before the college committee's tenure decision. Sure, I struggled sometimes as I taught courses in a highly demanding teaching environment, but I was a deeply committed teacher with consistently solid evaluations and a student following. As I quickly weighed these facts, others present at the meeting sat silently while the colleague who led the meeting read out the "problems" with my teaching.

Being ambushed at the meeting was my first outright experience with workplace bullying. With the hindsight of more life experience, I would have ended the meeting and secured legal advice. I wondered if the meeting had violated institutional policy (only more recent semesters' evaluations were supposed to be considered for tenure applications). However, I had been a first-generation college student and naively trusted my colleagues with whom I thought I had good relationships. I assumed that their goodwill and my genuine love for the job would clear up any misunderstandings.

After I moved to New Zealand, I internally questioned if the idea for the meeting had originated from somewhere else in the school's hierarchy. I wondered if the silent colleagues followed along out of reticence, or perhaps in hope of advancing up the academic chain of command. I will probably never know the truth. What I *did* know at the time was that the school's environment was now toxic for me. When the school's president and provost hand-delivered my tenure award letter to my faculty office a few weeks later, I already knew I was quitting.

BREAKING THE SILENCE AROUND MENTAL HEALTH IN ACADEMIC WORKPLACES

Though the meeting greatly upset and confused me at the time, I arrived at work the next day as if nothing had happened. After all, this strategy had always worked for me: Work cheerfully and well, be friendly, and eventually I would calmly surmount the newest obstacle or uncomfortable situation. I did not confront my colleagues because I just wanted to forget about the bad memory. I was also afraid that I would be the target of further bullying and also rumors in the small community if I spoke out. As a former first-generation college student, I even wondered if my tenure approval could somehow be reversed if I made waves. Remarkably, I bounced back to complete one of my strongest semesters ever in the spring of 2012.

I now know that the body stores trauma memory. Nearly a year later, while delivering a guest lecture in a situation where I had pressured myself to shine, the traumatic experience from the meeting, and its unspoken communication to me that I was not good at my job, manifested as a panic attack. One of my New Zealand anxiety specialist's treatments is Eye Moment Desensitization and Reprocessing (EMDR) therapy (a psychotherapy that helps people heal from distress related to traumatic memories) (EMDR Institute 2020). Through EMDR I mentally reprocessed and reduced the emotional trauma from the experience. Today, I remember the meeting as a disappointment, rather than with anxiety and panic symptoms.

This is the first time that I have publicly shared my experiences of workplace bullying, anxiety, and panic disorder. I share these experiences for a few reasons. First, I speak from a motivation of social justice. My theoretical training in critical cultural studies and pedagogy has taught me that speaking truth to power can shine light on injustices such as workplace bullying. The research on mental health in academia indicates that workplace bullying and harassment are several primary triggers of employees' mental health distress.

Second, I share these experiences to give my readers guidance and encouragement. As I write this preface, I emphasize this book's goal to provide the most up-to-date research on mental health in academia. I hope that the collective knowledge shared in the chapters can help readers, their colleagues, students, and institutions better understand the current crisis around mental health in higher education and to develop institutional policies, best practices, and empathic communication around mental health support.

Third, as many of this volume's chapters indicate, there is a strong silencing stigma around mental health and illness in academia. In a career that relies so profoundly on the mind, it is both ironic and saddening that mental health problems are often viewed in academia as being signs that someone is not able to cope with the professional rigors. This volume seeks to help break this silence through its chapters that discuss the complex intersection of mental health with the career's cultural, institutional, and structural facets.

The timing for this book in addressing mental health in academic careers is even more urgent during the present COVID-19 pandemic. As Schroeder (2020) points out, additional workloads associated with tasks such as moving courses online have "heightened the concerns over faculty burnout. So many faculty members who already live on the edge of burnout in meeting the teaching, advising, research, and publication expectations are facing an emotional let-down or even collapse."

Finally, this volume aims to encourage and support academics who may be struggling with mental health distress and mental illness. You are not alone. I believe that research on mental health in academic careers, as well as the stories of people who experience and/or support others with mental health distress and mental illness, are absolutely needed now more than ever in today's highly uncertain global environment.

I have learned that the best response to adversity is a life well lived. Finding the courage to address the trauma that escalated my anxiety and learning to manage its symptoms has helped me return to the work where my gifts truly shine. I want any graduate students, faculty, and administrators who may be struggling with mental health challenges, and with related issues such as trauma and workplace bullying, to know that there is hope for you, too. I draw encouragement from a short poem on a wall poster that I immediately noticed when I first visited my anxiety specialist's office:

The life that was
The life that will be.

Teresa Heinz Housel

Wellington, New Zealand
January 12, 2021

REFERENCES

"What is EMDR?" EMDR Institute, 2020. https://www.emdr.com/what-is-emdr/.
Hulme, Keri. 1983. *The Bone People.* New York: Penguin Books.
Schroeder, Ray. 2020. "Online: Trending Now." *Inside Higher Ed.* October 1, 2020. https://www.insidehighered.com/digital-learning/blogs/online-trending-now/wellness-and-mental-health-2020-online-learning.

Acknowledgments

As with most large projects, this book came into being in part through support from others.

First, thank you to my loving husband, Timothy Housel, who has always supported my ambitions and offered his reasoned perspectives.

I express gratitude to Nicolette Amstutz, Senior Acquisitions Editor of Communication and Latin American Studies at Lexington Books, who championed my proposed project and guided it through the production process.

I share my sincere appreciation to this book's contributors. The COVID-19 pandemic began just as we were immersed in our chapters' research and writing. The worldwide health crisis impacted every single one of us in some way. Many contributors completed their chapters while on lockdown. Nearly all wrote their chapters while also adapting quickly to extra teaching demands as they moved their courses online, offered additional pastoral care to students, and also handled their own personal challenges around the pandemic. I am grateful for their fortitude and care as we completed this project.

Special thanks go to Diane Comer and Erinn C. Cameron, who reviewed my preface. Erinn's professional training as a psychologist helped me accurately describe my traumatic experience in my former workplace. With her gift for writing memoir, Diane advised me to write more about how I made the seemingly fearless decision to quit a tenured job and move to New Zealand in the face of sometimes nearly crippling anxiety. An American migrant herself to New Zealand who wrote about her experiences in her book, *The Braided River* (Otago University Press), Diane understands the courage and hope required to make a new country home. As I recalled difficult memories that sometimes caused emotional distress as I wrote about them, I often reflected on what Diane once told me: "Do no harm." I kept this thought close as I wrote about the human players in those memories from an explanatory motive to help readers understand my decisions.

I would like to extend appreciation to two Wellington-area people whose expertise has been instrumental to me. First, I thank Michael Burrows for giving me the tools to understand and manage anxiety and panic disorder so that I could use my gifts to help others. Second, the research on mental health and wellbeing overwhelmingly emphasizes the importance of regular physical exercise. To this end, I thank Patrick Meo, my personal trainer, whose regular sessions have strengthened my mind and body.

Toward the end of the project, Leon Salter, Whitinga Research Fellow, School of Communication, Journalism and Marketing at Massey University, took on the role of research assistant. His assistance in gathering mental health–related programming for faculty, staff, and students at different higher education institutions around the world was essential. The information will appear as an additional feature on this book's forthcoming webpage on the publisher's website. Readers can also find further resources and support on my website dedicated to mental health in academia, www.ourmindstogether.com.

I thank my astute proofreader, Nanette Norris, who helped me prepare chapters for production. Nanette also helped me untangle the Chicago Manual of Style.

When we first made the decision to migrate to New Zealand in mid-2012, little did I know how many caring people I would soon meet. They are too numerous to specifically mention here, but I am very thankful for my supportive colleagues at Massey University and other universities in New Zealand and Australia, as well as the friends I've made in the local community and elsewhere. The magic of digital communication has helped me stay in touch with others further afield. Thank you for regularly checking in and encouraging me with my mental health research.

Finally, as the book neared the production stage, I convened a research panel about mental health in academia with some of this book's contributors (Victoria McDermott, Alena Ruggerio, and Erica Knotts) and another colleague (Amy May) at the National Communication Association's annual (virtual) convention in November 2020. In our panel, "Mental Health at a Crossroads: Navigating Academia in a Time of Uncertainty," we shared our respective research projects about different aspects of mental health in academic careers. At several points during our presentations, we put our prepared notes aside as we spoke from the vulnerability of our lived experiences. In a professional career that intertwines our passions and minds, it is impossible to separate our humanness from our work's underlying goal to somehow make a positive impact on the world.

Teresa Heinz Housel
Wellington, New Zealand
January 15, 2021

Part 1

MENTAL DISTRESS AND MENTAL ILLNESS IN ACADEMIC CULTURE

Chapter 1

The Perfect Storm of Mental Health Issues in Academia and the Need for Critical Research and Policies

Teresa Heinz Housel

INTRODUCTION: INTERSECTIONS OF ACADEMIA AND MENTAL HEALTH

I have always cared deeply about mental health issues in the workplace, but I began conceptualizing this book after reading an anonymous blog, "Academics Anonymous," in *The Guardian* ("There Is" 2014). The blog described the funeral of "J.," who committed suicide and was the blogger's family friend. "J." was a British doctoral student who had long struggled with mental health issues and interrupted his studies several times to regain his health.

The blogger wondered if the stress of doctoral work had caused his friend's suicide ("There Is" 2014). "I have experienced the effects on my mental health, and I have witnessed the culture of acceptance surrounding this issue," the blogger stated. "Among the people I do know who have done PhDs, I have seen depression, sleep issues, eating disorders, alcoholism, self-harming, and suicide attempts" ("There Is" 2014). The blog received an unprecedented high response from academic readers who described the mental health impacts of their various stressors at work.

Particularly in the United States, many journalists have covered recent cases involving violent mentally ill students and faculty. On February 12, 2010, national American media outlets reported that Dr. Amy Bishop, a neuroscientist and assistant professor of biology at the University of Alabama in Huntsville, shot six colleagues at a routine department meeting that day. Three professors died while the other three were wounded (Dewan and Robbins 2010). The shootings initially appeared to result from Bishop's unsuccessful appeal of the university's decision to deny her tenure. An unpopular instructor, Bishop regularly received student complaints about her ineffective teaching and "odd, unsettling ways" (Reeves 2010).

The American news media's early focus on Bishop's tenure and appeal denial shifted as present and former colleagues described her history of erratic behavior in the workplace. Co-workers and graduate students described how Bishop rejected criticism, padded her resume to get the Alabama job, and had "cyclical 'flip-outs'" that caused students to leave her laboratory (Dewan, Saul, and Zezima 2010). In another workplace-related situation, Bishop and her husband, James Anderson, were questioned in a 1993 pipe-bomb incident against her lab supervisor, a neurology professor at Harvard University, where Bishop completed her doctorate (Ruark 2010).

Journalists soon uncovered Bishop's history of violent propensities that extended beyond the workplace. In 1986, Bishop shot and killed her eighteen-year-old brother, Seth, after a family argument at their home in Braintree, Massachusetts. The police didn't charge her after accepting the family's explanation that the shooting was accidental (Dewan, Saul, and Zezima 2010). Other violent incidents, however, suggested that Bishop "could go to great lengths to retaliate against those she felt had wronged her" (Dewan, Saul, and Zezima 2010). In 2002, Bishop was charged with punching a woman at a restaurant in Peabody, Massachusetts after accusing her of taking the last child booster seat (Dewan, Saul, and Zezima 2010).

As the Bishop case unfolded, the tragedy prompted news and academic analyses about institutional factors that may have exacerbated Bishop's possible existing mental health issues. For example, the shootings received much discussion on *The Chronicle of Higher Education*'s website about the larger, often unspoken context of stressful academic work culture ("Critical Mass" 2010; Montell 2010; "Reactions" 2010). Fox (2010) critiqued the frequent secrecy and politics around tenure processes, which are characterized by ever-increasing standards and potentially devastating professional and emotional ramifications for unsuccessful applicants.

Bishop's actions were extreme and criminal, but some critics at the time discussed the lack of mental health support for employees at many colleges and universities. For instance, Wilson (2013) pointed out that finding new work and personal direction in the terminal year of employment after tenure denial is often traumatic. Meadows (2010) stated that the "red flags" of Bishop's violent propensities "are all so obvious now," but questioned why no one at the university "connected the dots until it was too late." Most universities in the U.S. do not have formal processes for supporting professors as they deal with the loss around tenure denial (Wilson 2013, 1). Notes Kimberly Hannula, who was denied tenure in geology at Vermont's Middlebury College, that "There is so much a culture of the strong individual going off and doing brilliant things, and counseling is seen as a sign of weakness" (Wilson 2013, 1).

After pleading guilty to killing three colleagues, Bishop was sentenced to life imprisonment without parole in September 2012 (Hurley 2020; Brown 2012; Lawson 2012). Bishop has since appealed the sentence claiming that schizophrenia, allergies, and steroids caused her actions, but she was never formally diagnosed with a mental illness (Johnson 2015). Bishop's former colleague, Dr. Debra Moriarity, would have been the seventh victim, but Bishop's handgun jammed (Hurley 2020). The University of Alabama in Huntsville has counseling support available through its Employee Assistance Program, and now does background checks before hiring new faculty. However, Moriarity said she would like to see the university go further to assist faculty in the tenure process: "I really wanted the university to move forward in some type of counseling that would be automatic when letters of recommendation would be written for them and things like that. I don't see that has happened and that worries me" (Hurley 2020).

Bishop's case; a mass shooting in a bar filled with college students near a number of universities in Thousand Oaks, California in early November 2018; an undergraduate student's shootings at Virginia Tech in 2007; and the mass shooting in a movie theater in Colorado in 2012 by James Holmes, a doctoral neuroscience student at the University of Colorado, are among many recent tragic cases in the U.S. involving violence and academic employees, graduate students, or undergraduates (Price 2011). The news coverage of such high-profile cases can convey stereotypes about mentally ill people as being violent, and thus inhibit critical, informed discussions about mental health in academia and the factors that contribute to campus violence (Price 2011, 2973, 2991; Quintero Johnson and Miller 2016, 218). However, the tragedies have prompted much-needed debate in some forums about many academic institutions' inadequate mental health resources and failure to address mental health issues among their employees (Simon 2017; Cardwell 2019). Reinforcing these points, in March 2019, many colleagues and students mourned the death of Dr. Alan B. Krueger, a renowned Princeton University professor and former economics advisor to Presidents Barack Obama and Bill Clinton. Hundreds expressed shock about the "unexpectedness" of Krueger's suicide, but some colleagues spoke out about how his death was likely influenced by the isolating nature of research, "bullying culture" of economics, and the "unforgiving" competitiveness of academic culture where "no one wants to admit anything that seems like a weakness or a personal failure" (Pettit 2019; Müller 2020).

DISCOURSES ABOUT MENTAL ILLNESS IN ACADEMIC AND PUBLIC CULTURE

This volume argues that a culture of silence historically surrounds the issue of mental illness in an academic profession where not being able to cope with the rigors of research, teaching, and service is viewed as personal weakness (England 2016; Smith and Ulus 2019). The Bishop case is an extreme example of a mentally unstable faculty member's violence, but the subsequent heated discussion on *The Chronicle of Higher Education*'s website suggested how the shootings seemed to "confirm the worst of faculty workplaces" (Ruark 2010). Ruark (2010) asserts that public and academic discourses around the shootings reflect the larger and often unspoken context of stressful academic work culture. In her powerful essay about having a mental illness in academia, England (2016) describes how disclosing mental illness "is a personal and political issue" (226) in a professional culture where, despite increasing openness about mental illness and attention to undergraduates' and even graduate students' mental health, the topic is still stigmatized among faculty, administrators, and staff. This present volume seeks to help break this silence.

According to the World Health Organization (2011), mental health is the "state of well-being in which every individual realizes his or her own potential, can cope with the normal stresses of life, can work productively and fruitfully, and is able to make a contribution to her or his community." Mental distress and mental illness can interfere with one's ability to successfully manage all these areas of life. "Academic life today is a petri dish for madness," Ruark (2010) states. "The high stress of the tenure process, the pressures to be brilliant at research and teaching, the cloistered environment, the extent to which internal politics affects people's careers—it's a combination that could damage even psychologically healthy people."

Concerns about mental health among academics exist in the larger context of rapidly increasing rates of mental illness worldwide. Rates of mental illness, and particularly anxiety and depression, are increasing in the U.S. and other countries. Between 1993 and 2001, the Centers for Disease Control and Prevention (CDC) (2004) reported that incidents of frequent mental distress increased from 8.4 percent to 10.1 percent among adults in the U.S. In 2019, an estimated 20.6 percent of all American adults aged eighteen or older (or 51.5 million adults) had any mental illness (AMI). AMI is defined as a mental, behavioral, or emotional disorder, and can range from no to severe impairment (National Institute of Mental Health 2021).

The rates of mental illness are similarly increasing among the general population in comparative countries. To note some examples, nearly 4 million Canadians have a mood or anxiety disorder, the most common mental illnesses; this number is expected to increase to nearly 4.9 million people by 2041 (Mental Health Commission of Canada [MHCC] 2011, 7). A more recent MHCC (2017) report found that 7.5 million people in Canada faced a mental illness in 2017, with mood and anxiety disorders being the most common conditions. Mixed anxiety and depression is the most common mental disorder in Britain, with 7.8 percent of people meeting diagnoses criteria (Mental Health Foundation 2020a). The British charity Mind (2017) estimates that one in four people experience a mental health problem each year. Australia and New Zealand have among the world's highest suicide rates (particularly among young people), among the world's highest rates of workplace bullying, and acute mental health needs among indigenous and some immigrant populations (RANZCP 2010; Canterbury District Health Board 2020; Enoka 2017). Worldwide, mental health problems are one of the central causes of disease burden, with anxiety, depression, and drug use cited as the primary causes of disability (Mental Health Foundation 2020b).

In academic and non-academic workplaces, stress can motivate people in their work, but becomes detrimental when it exceeds a person's ability to cope (Poalses and Bezuidenhout 2018). The statistics on mental illness mirror the sharp increase in reported mental distress (depression, anxiety, and stress) in academic and other types of workplaces in the U.S. and other countries such as Canada, Britain, Australia, New Zealand, South Africa, and China ("Mental Health" 2019; Gorczynski 2018; Poalses and Bezuidenhout 2018; Collins and Mowbray 2005; Farrell et al. 2019; Raskauskas and Skrabec 2011; Marten 2009; Tytherleigh et al. 2007; Sun et al. 2011). The costs of mental ill-health to employees' personal lives and employees are high. The OECD (2015a) estimates that 30–40 percent of employees' sickness and disability caseloads in OECD countries are due to mental health problems. According to the OECD (2015b), despite increased recognition of mental health in society, and mental health's high price to employers and their families, employers, and the economy, "considerable social stigma around mental health remains."

Greater public awareness and acceptance of mental illness now leads more people to seek assistance and receive diagnoses (Benton et al. 2003). At the same time, improved medicines and counseling therapies enable students, instructors, administrators, and staff to work and attend classes, and live independently, all activities that would have been unlikely with standard treatments of mental illness in the past (Gabriel 2010; Benton et al. 2004; Rudd 2004; Sharkin 2004). In addition, academic employees' and students' frequent exposure to mental illness, either through media coverage, their own experience, or someone they know, mirrors the greater public awareness about "traumas scarcely recognized a generation ago and a willingness to seek help for those problems, including bulimia, self-cutting and childhood sexual abuse" (Gabriel 2010). Meanwhile, public discourse around mental illness is opening up as diagnoses and treatments become normalized. When public figures such as Catherine Zeta Jones, Emma Thompson, and former U.S. First Lady Michelle Obama openly discuss their mental health struggles (Payne 2013; Thorpe 2010; Rourke 2020), their willingness to share vulnerability invites audiences to reveal their struggles as well (Lee 2018). However, audiences' positive perceptions of celebrity mental health disclosures are mitigated by the type of mental illness disclosed and the audience member's perceived reputation of the celebrity, among other factors (Hoffner 2020).

Reflecting this broadening public discourse, in recent years, some faculty, administrators, and graduate students have bravely shared their mental health challenges. Margaret Price (2011), a disability studies professor at Ohio State University and Katie Rose Guest Pryal (2017), who wrote this book's Foreword, have described their experiences with mental illness and the stigma attached to disclosing one's mental illness in academia in their books and writings for mass and trade publications, such as *The Chronicle of Higher Education*. James Jones (2007), a law professor at the University of Louisville, frankly recounted his decades-long experience of bipolar disorder in a landmark academic journal essay. Elyn Saks (2009), a University of Southern California law professor, wrote about living with mental illness for *The Chronicle of Higher Education*. Like Jones, Saks (2009) expressed relief that she no longer had to hide after sharing her story.

It should be noted that many academics' disclosures of mental illness often involve advanced-career employees with likely more professional protection to reveal mental health challenges. Goodwin and Morgan (2012) point out that faculty and staff must carefully consider the impact of disclosing their conditions. "The balance of costs and benefits shifts with each level of disclosure; department chairs, colleagues, and students require different decisions" (Goodwin and Morgan 2012, 36). As Fox and Gasper (2020) note in their duoethnography about their respective decisions to disclose (or not) their mental ill-health to their universities, "Those with a mental health condition are more likely to be labeled as being untrustworthy and unstable and at best as potentially unreliable or unpredictable" (300). Even if colleagues respond well, the act of disclosing may compound the condition's symptoms. "The decision to disclose is a personal act of agency, identity and choice" (Fox and Gasper 2020, 301), but the risks, stigma, and discrimination around disclosing mental illness in the workplace are real. Britain's Equality Challenge Unit found that 38 percent of British academics with a mental health problem had not shared the information with colleagues ("Mental Illness" 2015; see also Gough 2011). The research projects across this book's chapters, which speak to important concerns about disclosure, address academics at all stages of their careers.

OVERVIEW OF MENTAL HEALTH RESEARCH IN HIGHER EDUCATION

An exhaustive compilation of the existing mental health–related research of undergraduates, graduate students, and employees in higher education is beyond this chapter's scope. The existing studies differ across methodologies, timeframe, geographical focus, type of institution, sample size, and other characteristics, and the symptom threshold that the researchers use to diagnose mental illness or distress and inclusion in their respective studies (Eleftheriades, Fiala, and Pasic 2020). However, it is important here to identify the existing research's major themes to establish this book's research context.

Mental Health Trends among Undergraduates

This chapter includes an overview of the mental health research of undergraduate students as a comparison to the studies on graduate students and academic employees. Most academic research and news coverage focus on undergraduate students' mental health at higher education institutions in America and other countries (Miles et al. 2020; Gorczynski 2018; Collins and Mowbray 2005; Roberts 2018). Recent studies about undergraduates' mental health uniformly indicate rising trends in reported mental illness in the United States (Kendler, Myers, and Dick 2015; Hunt and Eisenburg 2010; Cho et al. 2015; Gallagher 2014; Eisenberg et al. 2007) and internationally (Auerbach et al. 2016, 2018, 2019). In the U. S., the American College Health Association National College Health Assessment's (ACHA-NCHA) (2018, 2014) most recent biannual surveys report widespread and increasing depression and related mental health issues among undergraduates.

Although American undergraduate students today are more likely to seek professional psychological help for typical post-adolescent challenges such as relationship heartbreak, more now struggle with a wider range of stressors and severe mental distress (Gabriel 2010). Other research confirms that today's undergraduates face increasing stressors that manifest in mental health disorders (Kadison and DiGeronimo 2004; Lukianoff and Haidt 2015). Stressors such as financial worries, family problems, social anxiety, social isolation, assignment demands, and general health concerns can exacerbate mental illnesses (Megivern, Pellerito, and Mowbray 2003; Martin 2010; Weiner and Wiener 1997; Tinklin, Riddell, and Wilson 2005). Citing research from the American College Counseling Association, Gabriel (2010) notes that 44 percent seek counseling for depression, anxiety, suicidal thoughts, alcohol abuse, attention disorders, self-injury, and eating disorders (Gabriel 2010). Twenty-four percent take psychiatric medication, up from 16 percent in 2000, and 17 percent in 2005 (Gabriel 2010). Anxiety surpasses depression as the most common mental health diagnosis among undergraduates in the U.S. (Hoffman 2015; American College Health Association 2014). Further supporting this trend, Penn State's Center for Collegiate Mental Health's (CCMH) (2016) national survey of more than 100,000 college students found that half the students cited anxiety as a reason for visiting campus counseling services (11). Cohort subsets of the general student population, such as women (Rosenfield and Mouzon 2013), queer students (Oswalt and Wyatt 2011; Liu et al. 2019; Kerr, Santurri, and Peters 2013), international students (Koo and Nyunt 2020), and first-generation college students (FGCS) (Stephens et al. 2015; Allan, Garriott, and Keene 2016; Stebleton, Soria, and Huesman Jr. 2014; Jenkins et al. 2013) also report specific stress factors and increasing mental distress and illness. The international research collectively reflects rising rates of mental illnesses and distress in comparative countries to the U.S. (Eleftheriades, Fiala, and Pasic 2020; Adlaf, Demers, and Gliksman 2005; Collins and Mowbray 2005; Markoulakis and Kirsh 2010).

Against this background of rising rates of stress factors, mental illness, and mental distress, national American news outlets began covering campus mental health trends more frequently in the early 2000s. For example, in December 2010, the *New York Times* described the strain on student counseling centers across the country. In Gabriel's (2010) *New York Times* article, nearly half the students cited mental illness as their reason for counseling visits, double the rate in 2005. Many news media outlets in the U.S. and other countries have covered rising student mental health needs in the years since (Kenny 2019; Schackle 2019).

With more students experiencing mental illness and distress, faculty, administrators, and staff often find themselves in the position of trying to support students with mental health challenges, but without necessary professional training (Becker et al. 2002). Owen and Rodolfa (2009) point out that "college student mental health is a campus issue, not just a counseling center issue" (30). Owen and Rodolfa (2009) offer many practical suggestions for how faculty and other academic employees can assist distressed students, such as through professional development that includes a psychoeducational component or focus. This information can give employees tools, such as how to recognize warning signs of student mental health distress; understand guidelines around student confidentiality and privacy with interventions and referrals; and communicate effectively around mental health. Owen and Rodolfa (2009) also recommend that employees complete cross-cultural training that will help them understand how gender, sexuality, race, and ethnicity, as well as stigma associated with these attributes, might intersect with clinical symptoms (Owen and Rodolfa, 2009, 30–31). In this book's Foreword, Pryal discusses the resource guide, *Promoting Supportive Academic Environments for Faculty with Mental Illnesses: Resource Guide and Suggestions for Practice* (Price and Kerschbaum 2017), which is an excellent resource for institutions seeking to develop effective policies, communication, and other programming around mental illness. This book's chapters, its Appendix, and the Features tab on this book's webpage on the publisher's website (https://rowman.com/ISBN/9781793630247/Mental-Health-among-Higher-Education-Faculty-Administrators-and-Graduate-Students-A-Critical-Perspective) discuss strategies and tools that academics can use to assist students experiencing mental health challenges. In addition, this book is a companion to the website www.ourmindstogether.com. This website includes information such as a directory of campus programming in U.S. and other countries to support the mental health of academic employees and students.

Mental Health Stressors and Mental Illness among Graduate Students

Although fewer studies have examined mental illness among graduate students, a growing number of American and international studies indicate sharply rising rates in reported mental illness and contributing factors among graduate students. Researchers note that some mental health–related studies of student populations do not distinguish between undergraduate and graduate students (Pledge et al. 1998; O'Neil, Lancee, and Freeman 1984; Westefeld and Furr 1987). As another limiting factor to the research, many studies only survey graduate students who have used their institution's campus counseling services. However, Hyun et al.'s (2006) survey of the general graduate student population at the University of California, Berkeley found that half the respondents self-reported having an emotional or stress-related problem in the past year. More than half the respondents also said they knew a graduate student colleague who had experienced similar challenges in the past year (Hyun et al. 2006). In keeping with these findings, the ACHA (2018) NCHA found that 61.4 percent of graduate students self-reported greater than average stress compared to 57 percent of undergraduates.

Despite graduate students' extra pressures and work responsibilities, their overall mental health (such as incidences of anxiety and depression) tends to be better than that of undergraduates (ACHA 2018; see also Zivin 2009). Eleftheriades, Fiala, and Pasic (2020) note that graduate students must typically work to a high standard to be accepted into graduate programs, and also must manage multiple responsibilities (Eleftheriades, Fiala, and Pasic 2020, 12). Therefore, the lower rates of mental illness among graduate students may be due to selection bias because people with severe mental health issues are less likely to complete graduate studies (Eleftheriades, Fiala, and Pasic 2020, 12). Many graduate students, however, experience critical and intersecting stressors that impact their mental health.

Across studies on graduate students' mental health, researchers repeatedly cite factors ranging from social isolation to major life transitions (such as returning to school from a professional career and relationship break-up) as causes of mental distress. In Hyun et al.'s (2006) study, graduate students' self-reported data suggested that lack of a structured work schedule, financial stress, social isolation, a poor academic job market (particularly since the 2007–2009 recession and during the COVID-19 pandemic), unhealthy relationships with supervisors, relationship and childcare responsibilities, and pressure to produce innovative work contribute to anxiety and depression (248, 260; see also Johnson and Huwe 2002; Benton 2003; Nogueira-Martins et al. 2004; Toews et al. 1997; Eleftheriades, Fiala, and Pasic 2020).

As a number of this volume's chapters point out, many graduate students and faculty experience mental distress from imposture syndrome. *Imposture syndrome* is a person's self-belief that "their success was attained by fraudulence, fooling others, and luck instead of hard work and their ability" (Chakraverty 2020, 2; Clance 1985). Imposture syndrome is common across all demographics due to graduate school's competitive environment, social isolation, and low-quality mentorship for some students, or a combination of these factors (Cohen and McConnell 2019). However, women, first-generation college students (FGCS), ethnic and racial minorities, and queer graduate students particularly experience it (Housel 2019). Added to these factors, heavy workloads coupled with the often unspoken ideal of "'suffering as a badge of honour'" (Eleftheriades, Fiala, and Pasic 2020, 8) contribute to graduate students' lack of work–life balance and difficulty in recognizing their "distress as a valid mental health issue rather than just the hardship expected in higher education" (Eleftheriades, Fiala, and Pasic 2020, 9).

Social isolation, particularly, is a known trigger for mental distress during graduate studies. Unlike undergraduates, graduate students usually do not have built-in social support such as clubs and fraternal organizations. Graduate school's unstructured academic environment that heavily relies on individual motivation can lead to anxiety and depression (Peters 1997). Graduate students in certain fields, such as STEM disciplines and law, report higher rates of stress and mental health concerns such as anxiety and depression (Eleftheriades, Fiala, and Pasic 2020; Puthran et al. 2016; Tsai and Muindi 2016; Givens and Tjia 2002; Nelson et al. 2001; Clarke 2015). Certain sub-populations of graduate students, such as international students, women, racial/ethnic minorities, FGCS, and/or students with intersecting identities across any of these categories, especially experience social isolation and mental distress at greater degrees than their colleagues/peers (Perrucci and Hu 1995; Hyun et al. 2006; Straforini 2015; Potts 1992). While completing three edited volumes on FGCS (Housel 2019; Harvey and Housel 2011; Housel and Harvey 2010), I repeatedly noticed intersections between the mental health of graduate students who were also FGCS, ethnic and racial minorities, low-income, non-traditionally aged students, women, LGBTQI+, working class, or a combination of these intersecting identities (see also Eleftheriades, Fiala, and Pasic 2020; Puthran et al. 2016).

Many higher education institutions focus their campus psychological services on both undergraduates and graduate students, but fewer graduate students than undergraduates are likely to seek counseling or other mental health services. Of Hyun et al.'s (2006) graduate student sample at the University of California, Berkeley, only 30 percent of the graduate students self-reported using some form of mental health services while in graduate school (257). Additionally, cohorts of graduate students less likely to seek campus mental health services include international students, Asian students, African American students, and FGCS because of stigma against mental health services, cultural barriers, lack of commonality with the health service providers, among other factors (Zhang and Dixon 2003; Cheng, Leong, and Geist 1993; Lau and Nolan 2000; Thompson, Bazile, and Akbar 2004). When graduate students do visit campus mental health services, O'Neil, Lancee, and Freeman (1984) found that they seek counseling because they lack other social support such as extracurricular activities. Female graduate students are also more likely to report having mental health problems and seek care (Hyun et al. 2006, 255; see also Benton et al. 2003; Pledge et al. 1998).

Mental Health–Related Research of Faculty, Staff, and Administrators

Similar to the trends for undergraduate and graduate students, many higher education institutions in America and other countries report rapid increases of mental illness and mental distress among faculty, administrators, and staff (Shaw and Ward 2014). Because of the silencing stigma around mental health (including mental illness) in academia, many academics' reluctance to speak out about these matters complicates attempts to understand their experiences or develop mental health resources and institutional policies (Price et al. 2017). Similar to the studies on graduate students, research of employees at those institutions is slowly increasing, but little critical or systematic empirical research examines academics whose working conditions lead to mental ill-health (Gill 2014; Müller 2020). Although the literature in this area is expanding (Price and Kerschbaum 2017), information about faculty members with mental illnesses tends to include first-person accounts (such as autobiographical essays and autoethnographic studies) and small-scale studies (Price 2011; Price et al. 2017; Pryal 2017; Campbell 2018; Koch 2020; Lashuel 2020); posts on blogs such as *The Professor Is In* (2020)*, The Broken Academic* (Anonymous 2015), and *The Thesis Whisperer* (Resources

2020); institution- or discipline-specific studies (Shigaki et al. 2012; Horton and Tucker 2014); or studies that examine a particular phenomenon, such as academic employees' requests for accommodation (Baldridge and Veiga 2006; Baldridge and Swift 2013).

Despite the overall limited research on mental health among academic employees, the findings across countries collectively indicate how academics experience more stress than employees in other fields (Catano et al. 2010; Shaw 2014). More international comparative data is generally needed on mental health in higher education ("Being a PhD student" 2019). However, more scholars are researching this area as part of the growing public awareness of the relationship between work and well-being. To build global knowledge about mental health in academia and to respond to the increasing rates of mental distress among academics, the Cactus Foundation recently completed a multinational mental health and well-being survey of 13,000 respondents from more than 160 countries (Cactus Foundation 2020a). The survey confirmed the findings of existing research on mental health in academia, noting that long working hours, workplace bullying, pressure to perform, adequate workplace policies around work–life balance, harassment, and other areas, among other factors, negatively impact academics' mental health (Cactus Foundation 2020b). Poalses and Bezuidenhout (2018) point out that "occupational stress among university employees is a global phenomenon that does not differentiate between the socio-economic status of countries" (170; see also Shaw 2014). The *Times Higher Education*'s (2018) first global survey of university staff found that employees struggled to manage their workloads with family and personal relationships. In Britain, the University and College Union's 2014 survey on workload and stress found that two-thirds of UCU members said their job was stressful (3). Respondents cited stressors such as increased workload demands, longer hours, unpredictable working environments, and workplace bullying (UCU 2014, 5). The study also found that resources such as job support and control that traditionally protected academic employees against work-related stress had decreased in recent years (UCU 2014, 6). As academic institutions make cuts to save money, especially in the wake of the COVID-19 pandemic, their employees are expected to do more with less. Reflecting this trend, New Zealand's Tertiary Education Union's October 2020 national survey found that academics and staff reported increased levels and causes of stress, such as being expected to do more instructional, administrative, and emotional labor, in the wake of COVID-19.

The alarmingly rising rates of mental distress among academics contradict the popular perception of academic jobs as low stress with flexible hours and freedom to pursue one's intellectual interests (Vanroelen, Levecque, and Louckx 2009). The flexibility of academic work is both an important and ironic contributor to stress (Beretz 2003). Faculty can self-determine their work schedules without punching a time clock, unlike many other jobs where employees have constant supervision. Graduate students and new faculty might have idealized perceptions of faculty life, such as offering time flexibility and personal autonomy, which do not account for its realities (Bieber and Worley 2006). For example, the unstructured nature of academic work supports a "heroic stamina" culture (Beretz 2003, 53), which occurs in a hierarchical academic culture that "rewards drive and sacrifice without encouraging balance" (Djokić and Lounis 2014). Goodwin and Morgan (2012) assert that work "flexibility is what can make academic careers so challenging: because academics *can* work anytime and anywhere, we often feel we *must* work all the time and everywhere" (34). This creates an "extremely demanding work life" where "the work seems never to end" (Goodwin and Morgan 2012, 34).

Researchers cite a wide range of additional factors other than unstructured work time that contribute to mental distress and exacerbate mental illness among instructors, staff, and administrators, including perfectionism; workplace bullying; social isolation and lack of peer support in academia's competitive culture; the output-driven culture, control, and surveillance in today's neoliberal educational, political, economic, and social environments (Frank, Gowar, and Naef 2019; Gill 2010); job insecurity and dismal job markets; pressure to be always available (especially for online instructors) (Higher Education Statistics Agency 2019); and never-ending workloads that collectively increase workplace stress and mental health challenges (Poalses and Bezuidenhout 2018; O'Connor and Hagan 2016; Teelken 2015; Jackson and Rothmann 2006; Siltaloppi, Kinnunen, and Feldt 2009; Alhaseny 2014; Raskauskas and Skrabec 2011; Skinner and Machin 2017; Reevy and Deason 2014; Moulin 2020). When institutions raise tenure and annual review requirements to "superstar" levels, these high expectations present complicated challenges for employees with chronic medical conditions (Goodwin and Morgan 2012, 34). Researchers in Britain, the U.S., and other countries report that the pressure for constant and substantive research results, a long-hours culture, increasing customer-focused higher education environments, and greater job insecurity with an over-reliance on adjunct faculty are key stressors for faculty, staff, and administrators (Shaw and Ward 2014).

In worst-case scenarios, some just leave the field. Barnes, Agago, and Coombs (1998) surveyed 5,450 faculty at all levels of their careers across 306 research institutions, liberal arts colleges, and two-year colleges in the U.S. They found that high stress levels, long work hours, and lower sense of community influenced the employees' greater intent to leave academia. Nonetheless, studies indicate that even though faculty and graduate students have great stress, many do enjoy their actual work and want to stay in an academic career (Cactus Foundation 2020b; Lindfelt, Ip, and Barnett 2015; Lindfelt et al. 2018; Woolston 2017).

Certain subsets of academic employees report higher rates of mental distress and mental illness. Two cohort subsets, pre-tenured faculty and adjunct faculty, particularly experience pressure and uncertainty because of their contingent or lower academic rank with little professional leverage at their institution. In fact, the existing research repeatedly suggests that early career academics (including graduate students and non-tenured faculty) and adjuncts are especially susceptible to developing mental health challenges (Levecque et al. 2017; "Being a PhD student" 2019). Pre-tenured faculty often endure strain as they manage new work demands with personal relationships and family responsibilities (Magnuson et al. 2004; Sorcinelli 1994; Evans, Dickerson, and Carney 2015). Many first-year faculty members also relocate to new cities and institutions, and this can further increase anxiety and social isolation (Sorcinelli 1994). As institutions eliminate tenure-track positions, they increasingly rely on adjunct faculty to reduce costs. The contingency of adjunct employment, lack of benefits, and displacement across multiple campuses for many adjuncts can adversely impact mental health (MacKenna 2004, 48; Swartzlander et al. 1998).

Similar to the research on graduate students, other factors (and intersections between them) that increase mental health challenges among academics include isolation and marginalization related to gender, race, and ethnicity, being a FGCS, and LGBTQI+ identity (Hawley et al. 2016; Housel 2019; Trucks-Bordeaux 2003; Sturdivant 2015; Keim and Erickson 1998). As more women and minorities enter academic careers, they face challenges such as lack of trust from students and colleagues, workplace bullying, and racial and gender stereotypes and discrimination (Shillingford, Trice-Black, and Butler 2013; Ysseldyk 2019). Bellas (1999) examines the emotional costs of being female in academia. Female professors, especially, are frequently expected to perform emotional labor such as exhibiting friendly, caring behaviors, and offering counsel (Bellas 1999). These activities can be emotionally exhausting and are typically unpaid, and institutions usually do not value them as much as research and administration that are stereotypically coded as masculine (Bellas 1999).

The current COVID-19 pandemic is placing more stressors on academic employees and students' mental health while exacerbating existing ones (American Council on Education 2020). A year into the pandemic as of this writing, the emerging studies about COVID-19's mental health impacts heavily emphasize undergraduates' psychological and emotional needs. However, the few studies about the mental health of faculty, staff, administrators, and graduate students overwhelmingly point to significant mental health effects in this highly uncertain environment. For instructors, their institutions' demands that they place courses online at short notice while quickly learning new technologies (and often with little institutional support); expectations for faculty to provide more pastoral care and be accessible to students; anxiety around job insecurity, particularly for contract and adjunct staff; stark budget cuts and redundancy threats; expectations to manage students' mental health needs, often with little or no training; and the overall uncertainty about the general state of the world are just some stressors indicated by the early research on the pandemic's mental health impacts (Housel 2020; Sahu 2020, American Council on Education 2020; Schroeder 2020; Araújo et al. 2020). In addition to workplace-specific stressors, many academic employees (especially women) have had to manage increased home responsibilities, childcare, and homeschooling during the pandemic (Guy and Arthur 2020).

Against the context of these identified predictors of reported mental distress and mental illnesses among faculty, staff, and administrators, stigma against mental illness and other chronic illnesses often prevents them from speaking out about their conditions and/or seeking professional help. A *chronic illness* is defined as a long-term health condition that can be outwardly invisible and requires ongoing medical treatment or rest (Goodwin and Morgan 2012, 33–34). In Goodwin and Morgan's (2012) research on American academics' experiences with chronic illnesses, they discuss how academic employees often "encounter a range of negative reactions, including social avoidance, awkward social interactions, and negative stereotypes about physical, mental, or emotional competence" (35) when they reveal their condition to colleagues. Faculty with illnesses with perceived cognitive impairment, especially, say they must work twice as hard to earn their colleagues' and students' respect (Goodwin and Morgan 2012, 35; see also Brown and Leigh 2018).

Although more and more institutions now address undergraduates' wellness and mental health in student orientations and campus programming (Eva 2019), many are still slow to provide targeted programming and psychological services mental health to their academic employees (Lashuel 2020). This volume's research-based chapters offer best practices for institutions, as well as examples of existing programming around mental health and well-being.

A COMMUNICATION APPROACH TO RESEARCHING MENTAL HEALTH IN ACADEMIC CONTEXTS

This volume's chapters build on the existing studies in the under-researched area of mental health among faculty, administrators, and graduate students in higher education. Collectively, the chapters examine the complex issues around mental health in higher education. The chapters' research findings will help institutions communicate about mental health in culturally competent and person-centered ways; create work environments conducive to mental well-being; and support their academic employees who have mental health challenges. Moreover, this book argues that discussions of health and wellness, equity, workload expectations and productivity, and campus diversity must also cover chronic illness and disability, which include mental health and mental illness. To this end, institutional policies and practices must promote equity and productivity for employees with chronic illnesses, including mental illness (Goodwin and Morgan 2012, 34). "Just as academia continues to drive away talented women," Goodwin and Morgan (2012) state, "we may be driving out talented people with chronic illnesses or other disabling conditions" (38).

As this volume's chapters examine different facets of mental illness in academia, the chapters' contributors seek to remove the stigma around mental illness and create honest, person-centered communication and policies around mental illness and well-being. The chapters could be used as readings for faculty-staff workshops; new faculty training; graduate courses in organizational communication, healthcare, and interpersonal communication; pedagogy training for graduate students; staff development for campus counseling and health services personnel; and as resources for faculty and staff development centers. Campus offices or programs that assist cohorts of graduate students and employees, such as FGCS, LGBTQI+, women, and ethnic and racial minorities, would also find relevant chapters to be beneficial. In addition, the book's Appendix includes educational features such as suggested class assignments, readings, and other resources to bring mental health–related topics into the communication classroom.

Awareness and understanding are at this book's heart. In Gecker's (2007) discussion about what faculty and staff can do to assist students with mental health struggles, she points out that most mentally ill students aren't dangerous or violent. Rather, many are struggling students who fall through the cracks. Gecker (2007) states that, "The tragedy at Virginia Tech can help faculty members be a bit more alert—not just for students who might be violent, but also for any students whose behaviour reveals that they aren't able to cope with college or the world on their own" (39). This attention to mental distress should also extend to faculty, staff, and administrators.

Further reinforcing the need to support academic employees as well as students, as institutions often move quickly to assist students during the COVID-19 pandemic with flexible deadlines, hybrid or online learning, pastoral care, and changes to course structure and assessments, they must not forget that instructors, staff, and administrators must also manage constant change in a highly uncertain world. Now more than ever, academic institutions must reconsider current levels of expectations about physical and mental health, and work productivity.

Even as understanding of mental illness and mental well-being generally increases in public culture, much work is still needed to increase critical awareness. For example, Nicola Dandridge, chief executive of Universities UK, stated a few years ago that higher education institutions are "academic, not therapeutic, communities" ("Mental Illness" 2015). Such perspectives only reinforce silence and shame by creating a wall between employees who struggle with mental issues and those who do not.

In his moving narrative about his often-painful attempts over many years to hide his bipolar disorder, James Jones (2007) states that, "I want to demonstrate that those with mental illness can have full and satisfying professional and personal lives, and they need and should not endure stigma or doubt as to their ability to perform their personal or employment" (373). This book shares Jones's assertions. If academic institutions are committed to supporting the general wellness and diversity of their community, then they must also be committed to addressing mental health issues.

This commitment starts with empathic and person-centered communication that affirms the worth and talents of each person. Kreps (2020) discusses the need for people to "exhibit sensitive and caring interpersonal communication behaviors with those confronting mental health problems" (18). In their resource guide referenced earlier in this chapter, Price and Kerschbaum (2017) emphasize communication's role in creating a "culture of access" that helps create, promote, and embed policies and programming. Price and Kerschbaum (2017) state that, "'Access' means clear and effective policies *for* inclusivity, and *against* stigma and harassment; supportive structures for hiring, performance review, and promotion; a proactive, centrally located infrastructure for accommodation" (5) among other types of support that the guide covers. Institutions must build supportive cultures for faculty, administrators, and graduate students with mental distress and mental illnesses. Kreps (2020) points out that, "Effective communication can make a major contribution to addressing serious mental health challenges on an individual level and at a societal level, helping to improve mental health problems for all members of society" (19).

I choose the verb *must* when referring to institutions because academics experiencing mental health conditions are far from alone. As this chapter's overview of the existing and emerging research on mental health in academia has pointed out, mental distress and mental illness are, if anything, increasing on campuses. My hope, therefore, is that the research findings and voices of people represented in this book's chapters will help guide institutions to create effective policies, programming, and communication around mental health and well-being.

REFERENCES

Adlaf, Edward M., Andrée Demers, and Louis Gliksman. 2005. *Canadian Campus Survey 2004.* Toronto: Centre for Addiction and Mental Health.
Alhaseny, Sokaina. "Is Bullying in the Eye of the Beholder? Examining Employees' Perceptions of Workplace Bullying in the Education and Hospitality Sectors." Master's thesis, Massey University, 2014.
American College Health Association (ACHA). 2014. *National College Health Assessment: Reference Group Executive Summary Spring 2014.* Baltimore, MD: American College Health Association.
American College Health Association (ACHA). 2018. *American College Health Association: National College Health Assessment II: Canadian Reference Group Executive Summary Fall 2018.* Accessed December 1, 2020. https://www.acha.org/documents/ncha/NCHA-II_Fall_2018_Reference_Group_Executive_Summary.pdf.
American Council on Education. 2020. *Mental Health, Higher Education, and COVID-19: Strategies for Leaders to Support Campus Well-Being.* Washington, DC: American Council on Education.https://www.acenet.edu/Documents/Mental-Health-Higher-Education-Covid-19.pdf.
Anonymous. 2015. "Introducing the Toxic Academy and the Broken Academic—A Too Long Long Introduction but Much Loved." *The Broken Academic.* Accessed November 30, 2020. https://thebrokenacademic.wordpress.com/2015/10/04/introducing-the-toxic-academy-and-the-broken-academic-a-too-long-introduction-but-much-loved/.
Araújo, Francisco Jonathan de Oliveira, Ligia Samara Abrantes de Lima, Pedro Ivo Martins Cidade, Camila Bezerra Nobre, and Modesto Leite Rolin Neto. 2020. "Impact of Sars-Cov-2 and its Reverberation in Global Higher Education and Mental Health." *Psychiatry Research* 288, June 2020: 112977. doi:10.1016/j.psychres.2020.112977.
Auerbach, R. P., J. Alonso, W. G. Axinn, P. Cuijpers, D. D. Ebert, J. G. Green, I. Hwang, R. C., et al. 2016. "Mental Disorders Among College Students in the World Health Organization World Mental Health Surveys." *Psychological Medicine* 46, no. 14: 2955–2970. https://doi.org/10.1017/S0033291716001665.
Auerbach, R. P., P. Mortier, R. Bruffaerts, J. Alonso, C. Benjet, P. Cujipers, K. Demyttenaere. 2018. "The WHO World Mental Health Surveys International College Student Project: Prevalence and Distribution of Mental Disorders." *Journal of Abnormal Psychology* 127, no. 7: 623–638. https://doi.org/10.1037/abn0000362.
Auerbach, R. P., P. Mortier, R. Bruffaerts, J. Alonso, C. Benjet, P. Cuijpers, K. Demyttenaere. 2019. "Mental Disorder Comorbidity and Suicidal Thoughts and Behaviors in the World Health Organization World Mental Health Surveys International College Student Initiative." *International Journal of Methods of Psychiatric Research* 28 no. 2: 2–16. https://doi.org/10.1002/mpr.1752.
Baldridge, David C., and Michele L. Swift. 2013. "Withholding Requests for Disability Accommodation: The Role of Individual Differences and Disability

Attributes." *Journal of Management* 39, no. 3: 743–762. http://dx.doi.org//10.117 7/0149206310396375.

Barnes, Laura L. B., Menna O. Agago, and William T. Coombs. 1998. "Effects of Job-Related Stress on Faculty Intention to Leave Academia." *Research in Higher Education* 39, no. 3: 457–469. https://doi.org/10.1023/A:1018741404199.

Becker, Marion, Lee Martin, Emad Wajeeh, John Ward, and David Shern. 2002. "Students with Mental Illness in a University Setting: Faculty and Student Attitudes, Beliefs, Knowledge and Experiences." *Psychiatric Rehabilitation Journal* 25, no. 4: 359–368. https://doi.apa.org/doiLanding?doi=10.1037%2Fh0095001.

"Being a PhD Student Shouldn't Be Bad For Your Health." *Nature*, May 15, 2019. https://www.nature.com/articles/d41586-019-01492-0.

Bellas, Marcia L. 1999. "Emotional Labor in Academia: The Case of Professors." *The Annuals of the American Academy of Political and Social Science* 561, no.1: 96–110. http://dx.doi.org/10.1177/000271629956100107.

Benton, Sherry A., John M. Robertson, Wen-Chih Tseng, Fred B. Newton, and Stephen L. Benton, S. 2003. "Changes in Counseling Client Problems Across 13 Years." *Professional Psychology: Research and Practice* 34, no. 1: 68–72. https://doi.org/10.1037/0735-7028.34.1.66.

Benton, Sherry A., Stephen L. Benton, Fred B. Newton, Kathryn L. Benton, and John M. Robertson. 2004. "Changes in Client Problems: Contributions and Limitations from a 13-Year Study. *Professional Psychology: Research & Practice* 35, no. 3: 317–319. https://doi.org/10.1037/0735-7028.35.3.317.

Benton, Thomas H. 2003. "The 5 Virtues of Successful Graduate Students." *The Chronicle of Higher Education.* September 5, 2003. https://www.chronicle.com/article/the-5-virtues-of-successful-graduate-students-5060/.

Beretz, Elaine M. 2003. "Hidden Disability and an Academic Career." *Academe* 89, no. 4: 51–55. https://doi.org/10.2307/40252496.

Bieber, Jeffery P., and Worley, Linda K. 2006. "Conceptualizing the Academic Life: Graduate Students' Perspectives." *The Journal of Higher Education* 77, no. 6: 1009–1035. https://doi.org/10.1080/00221546.2006.11778954.

Brown, Robbie. "Alabama: Ex-Professor Gets Life Term in Shooting." *The New York Times*. September 12, 2012. https://www.nytimes.com/2012/09/25/us/alabama-ex-professor-gets-life-term-in-shooting.html.

Brown, Nicole, and Jennifer Leigh. 2018. "Ableism in Academia: Where are the Disabled and Ill Academics?" *Disability & Society* 33, no. 6: 985–989. https://doi.org/10.1080/09687599.2018.1455627.

Cactus Foundation 2020a. "Cactus Mental Health Survey Report 2020." Cactus Foundation. https://www.cactusglobal.com/mental-health-survey/.

Cactus Foundation. 2020b. *Joy and Stress Triggers: A Global Survey on Mental Health Among Researchers.* London: Cactus Communications.

Campbell, Elaine. 2018. "Reconstructing My Identity: An Autoethnographic Exploration of Depression and Anxiety in Academia." *Journal of Organizational Ethnography* 7, no 3: 235–246. http://doi.org/10.1108/JOE-10-2017-0045.

Canterbury District Health Board. "Mental Health and Illness." Canterbury District Health Board, 2020. https://www.cph.co.nz/your-health/mental-illness/.

Cardwell, Hamish. "Universities Say They Lack Resources to Cope with Mental Health Support." *Radio New Zealand.* October 4, 2019. https://www.rnz.co.nz/news/icymi/400319/universities-say-they-lack-resources-to-cope-with-mental-health-support.

Catano, Vic, Lori Francis, Ted Haines, Haresh Kirpalani, Harry Shannon, Bernadette Stringer, and Laura Lozanzki. 2010. "Occupational Stress in Canadian Universities: A National Survey." *International Journal of Stress Management* 17, no. 3: 232–258. doi:10.1037/a0018582.

Center for Collegiate Mental Health (CCMH). *2015 Annual Report* (Publication No. STA 15-108). State College, PA: Penn State University, January 2016.

Centers for Disease Control and Prevention (CDC). 2004. "Self-Reported Frequent Mental Distress Among Adults—United States, 1993-2001." *Morbidity and Morality Weekly Report* 53, no. 41: 963–966.

Chakraverty, Devasmita. 2020. "PhD Student Experiences with the Imposture Phenomenon in STEM." *International Journal of Doctoral Studies* 15, no. 1: 159–179. https://doi.org/10.28945/4513.

Cheng, David, Frederick T. L. Leong, and Robert Geist. 1993. "Cultural Differences in Psychological Distress between Asian and Caucasian American College Students." *Journal of Multicultural Counseling & Development-Special Multicultural Health Issues* 21, no. 3: 182–190. https://doi.org/10.1002/j.2161-1912.1993.tb00598.x.

Cho, Seung Bin, Danielle C. Llaneza, Amy E. Adkins, Megan Cooke, Kenneth S. Kendler, Shaunna L. Clark, and Danielle M. Dick. 2015. "Patterns of Substance Use Across the First Year of College and Associated Risk Factors." *Frontiers in Psychiatry* 6 (Article 152): 1–11. https://doi.org/10.3389/fpsyt.2015.00152.

Clance, Pauline Rose. 1985. *The Imposture Phenomenon: When Success Makes You Feel Like a Fake.* Atlanta: Peachtree Publishers.

Cohen, Emma D., and Will R. McConnell. 2019. "Fear of Fraudulence: Graduate School Program Environments and the Imposture Phenomenon." *Sociological Quarterly* 60, no. 3: 457–478. https://doi.org/10.1080/00380253.2019.1580552.

Collins, Mary Elizabeth, and Carol T. Mowbray. 2005. "Higher Education and Psychiatric Disabilities: National Survey of Campus Disability Services." *American Journal of Orthopsychiatry* 75, no. 2: 304–315. https://doi.org/10.1037/0002-9432.75.2.304.

Committee on the College Student, Group for the Advancement of Psychiatry, E. Silber, Chair. 1999. "Helping Students Adapt to Graduate School: Making the Grade, Chapter 1: Overview." *Journal of College Student Psychotherapy* 14, no. 2: 5–7.

"Critical Mass: What Others are Saying About the Alabama Shootings." *Chronicle of Higher Education.* February 16, 2010. https://www.chronicle.com/article/Critical-Mass-What-Others-Are/64219.

Dewan, Shaila, and Liz Robbins. "A Previous Death at the Hand of Alabama Suspect." *The New York Times.* February 13, 2010. https://www.nytimes.com/2010/02/14/us/14alabama.html.

Dewan, Shaila, Stephanie Saul, and Katie Zezima. "For Professor, Fury Just Beneath the Surface." *The New York Times.* February 20, 2010. http://www.nytimes.com/2010/02/21/us/21bishop.html.

Djokić, Denia, and Sebastien Lounis. 2014. "This is Your Mind on Grad School." *Berkeley Science Review*. April 27, 2014. http://berkeleysciencereview.com/article/mind-grad-school/.

Eisenberg, Daniel, Sarah E. Gollust, Ezra Golberstein, and Jennifer L. Hefner. 2007. "Prevalence and Correlates of Depression, Anxiety, and Suicidality Among University Students." *American Journal of Orthopsychiatry* 77, no. 4: 534–542. https://doi.org/10.1037/0002-9432.77.4.534.

Eleftheriades, Renee, Clare Fiala, and Maria D. Pasic. 2020. "The Challenges and Mental Health Issues of Academic Trainees." *F1000Research* 9, no. 104: 1–26. DOI: 10.12688/f1000research.21066.1.

England, Marcia R. 2016. "Being Open in Academia: A Personal Narrative of Mental Illness and Disclosure." *Canadian Geographer* 60, no. 2: 226–231. https://doi.org/10.1111/cag.12270.

Enoka, Mava. "When You Compare NZ's Suicide Rate to Australia's, the Stats are Shocking." *Radio New Zealand.* January 20, 2017. https://www.rnz.co.nz/news/the-wireless/374427/when-you-compare-nz-s-suicide-rate-to-australia-s-the-stats-are-shocking.

Eva, Amy L. "How Colleges Today Are Supporting Student Mental Health." January 11, 2019. https://greatergood.berkeley.edu/article/item/how_colleges_today_are_supporting_student_mental_health.

Evans, A. M., A. Dickerson, and J. Carney. 2014. "Work-Life Balance Issues: A Qualitative Analysis of Counselor Educators." *Ideas and Research You Can Use: VISTAS 2014.* Retrieved from http://www.counseling.org/docs/default-source/vistas/article_72.pdf?sfvrsn=8.

Farrell, Sarah Marie et al. 2019. "Psychological Wellbeing, Burnout and Substance Use Amongst Medical Students in New Zealand." *International Review of Psychiatry* 31, no. 7–8: 630–636. http://dx.doi.org/10.1080/09540261.2019.1681204.

Fox, James Alan. "Tenure and the Workplace Avenger." *Chronicle of Higher Education.* February 26, 2010. https://www.chronicle.com/article/Tenurethe-Workplace/64197.

Fox, Joanna, and Roz Gasper. 2020. "The Choice to Disclose (or Not) Mental Health Ill-Health in UK Higher Education Institutions: A Duoethnography by Two Female Academics." *Journal of Organizational Ethnography* 9, no. 3: 295–309. https://doi.org/10.1108/JOE-11-2019-0040.

Frank, Jefferson, Norman Gowar, and Michael Naef. 2019. *English Universities in Crisis: Markets Without Competition.* Bristol: Bristol University Press.

Gabriel, Trip. "Mental Health Needs Seen Growing at Colleges." *The New York Times.* December 19, 2010. http://www.nytimes.com/2010/12/20/health/20campus.html.

Gallagher, Robert P. *National Survey of College Counseling Centers.* The International Association of Counseling Services, 2014: http://d-scholarship.pitt.edu/28178/1/survey_2014.pdf.

Gecker, Ellen. 2007. "How Do I Know If My Student is Dangerous?" *Academe* 93, no. 6: 38–39. https://www.jstor.org/stable/40253661.

Gill, Rosalind. 2010. "Breaking the Silence: The Hidden Injuries of the Neoliberal University." In *Secrecy and Silence in the Research Process: Feminist Reflections*. Edited by Roisin Ryan-Flood and Rosalind Gill, 228–244. Abingdon: Routledge.

Gill, Rosalind. 2014. "Academics, Cultural Workers and Critical Labour Studies." *Journal of Cultural Economy* 7, no. 1: 12–30. https://doi.org/10.1080/17530350.2013.861763.

Givens, Jane, and Tjia, Jennifer. 2002. "Depressed Medical Students' Use of Mental Health Services and Barriers to Use." *Academic Medicine* 77, no. 9: 918–921. https://journals.lww.com/academicmedicine/Fulltext/2002/09000/Depressed_Medical_Students__Use_of_Mental_Health.24.aspx.

Goodwin, Stephanie A., and Susanne Morgan. 2012. "Chronic Illness and the Academic Career." *Academe* 98, no. 3: 33–38. https://www.aaup.org/article/chronic-illness-and-academic-career#.X8Q57KozaL4.

Gorczynski, Paul. "More Academics and Students Have Mental Health Problems Than Ever Before." *The Conversation*. April 18, 2018. http://theconversation.com/more-academics-and-students-have-mental-health-problems-than-ever-before-90339.

Gough, Matthew. 2011. "Looking After Your Pearls: The Dilemmas of Mental Health Self-Disclosure in Higher Education Teaching." *The Journal of Mental Health Training, Education and Practice* 6, no. 4: 203–210, doi: 10.1108/17556221111194545.

Guy, Batsheva, and Brittany Arthur. 2020. "Academic Motherhood During COVID-19: Navigating Our Dual Roles as Educators and Mothers." *Gender, Work & Organization* 27, no. 5: 887–899. https://doi.org/10.1111/gwao.12493.

Harvey, Vickie L., and Housel, Teresa Heinz. 2011. *Faculty and First-Generation College Students: Bridging the Classroom Gap Together*. San Francisco: Jossey-Bass.

Hawley, Lisa D., Michael G. MacDonald, Erica H. Wallace, Julia Smith, Brian Wummel, and Patricia A. Wren. 2016. "Baseline Assessment of Campus-Wide General Health Status and Mental Health: Opportunity for Tailored Suicide Prevention and Mental Health Awareness Programming." *Journal of American College Health* 64, no. 3: 174–183. http://dx.doi.org/10.1080/07448481.2015.1085059.

Higher Education Statistics Agency (HESA). 2019. "What Are Their Employment Conditions?" Accessed November 24, 2020. https://www.hesa.ac.uk/data-and-analysis/staff/employment-conditions.

Hoffman, Jan. "Anxious Students Strain College Mental Health Centers. *The New York Times Well* (blog). May 27, 2015. http://well.blogs.nytimes.com/2015/05/27/anxious-students-strain-college-mental-health-centers/?_r=0.

Hoffner, Cynthia A. 2020. "Responses to Celebrity Mental Health Disclosures: Parasocial Relations, Evaluations, and Perceived Media Influence." In *Communicating Mental Health: History, Contexts, and Perspectives*, 125–146. Edited by Lance R. Lippert, Robert D. Hall, Aimee E. Miller-Ott, and Daniel Coche Davis. Lanham, MD: Lexington Books.

Horton, John, and Faith Tucker. 2014. "Disabilities in Academic Workplaces: Experiences of Human and Physical Geographers." *Transactions of The Institute of British Geographers* 39, no. 1: 76–89, 1475–5661. https://doi.org/10.1111/tran.12009.

Housel, Teresa Heinz. (2020). "Connections Between Workplace Bullying and Mental Health in New Zealand's Universities." Paper presented at the National Communication Association Annual Conference, Indianapolis, Indiana, 22 November 2020.

Housel, Teresa Heinz. (Editor). (2019). *First-Generation College Student Experiences of Intersecting Marginalities.* New York: Peter Lang.

Housel, Teresa Heinz, and Harvey, Vickie L. (Editors). 2010. *The Invisibility Factor: Administrators and Faculty Reach Out to First-Generation College Students.* Boca Raton, FL: Brown Walker Press.

Hunt, Justin, and Daniel Eisenberg. 2010. "Mental Health Problems and Help-Seeking Behavior Among College Students." *Journal of Adolescent Health* 46, no. 1: 3–10. https://doi.org/10.1016/j.jadohealth.2009.08.008.

Hurley, Liz. 2020. "What's Changed 10 Years After Deadly UAH Shootings?" *WSFA12 News.* https://www.wsfa.com/2020/02/11/whats-changed-years-after-deadly-uah-shootings/.

Hyun, Jenny K., Brian C. Quinn, Temina Madon, and Steve Lustig. 2006. "Graduate Student Mental Health: Needs Assessment and Utilization of Counseling Services." *Journal of College Student Development* 47, no. 3: 247–266. doi: 10.1353/csd.2006.0030.

Jackson, Leon, and Sebastiaan Rothmann. 2006. "Occupational Stress, Organisational Commitment, and Ill-Health of Educators in the North West Province." *South African Journal of Education* 26, no. 1: 75–95.

Johnson, Alex. "After 5 Years, Alabama University Killer Apologizes For the First Time." October 19, 2015. http://www.nbcnews.com/news/us-news/after-5-years-alabama-university-killer-apologizes-first-time-n447481.

Johnson, W. Brad, and Jennifer Huwe. 2002. "Toward a Typology of Mentorship Dysfunction in Graduate School. *Psychotherapy: Theory, Research, Practice, Training* 39, no. 1: 44–55. https://doi.org/10.1037/0033-3204.39.1.44.

Jones, James T. R. (2007). "Walking the Tightrope of Bipolar Disorder: The Secret Life of a Law Professor." *Journal of Legal Education* 57, no. 2: 349–374. https://www.jstor.org/stable/42894032.

Kadison, Rirchard, and Theresa Foy DiGeronimo. 2004. *College of the Overwhelmed: The Campus Mental Health Crisis and What to Do About It.* San Francisco: Jossey-Bass.

Keim, Jeanmarie S., and Chris D. Erickson. 1998. "Women in Academia: Work-Related Stressors." *Equity & Excellence in Education* 31, no. 2: 61–67.

Kendler, Kenneth S., John Myers, Danielle Dick. 2015. "The Stability and Predictors of Peer Group Deviance in University Students." *Social Psychiatry and Psychiatric Epidemiology* 50, no. 9: 1463–1470. https://doi.org/10.1007/s00127-015-1031-4.

Kenny, Lee. "Universities Seeing 'Sustained' Rise in Mental Distress." Stuff.co.nz, September 28, 2019. https://www.stuff.co.nz/national/116152181/universities-seeing-sustained-rise-in-mental-distress.

Kerr, Dianne Lynne, Laura E. Santurri, and Patricia Peters. 2013. "A Comparison of Lesbian, Bisexual, and Heterosexual College Undergraduate Women on Selected Mental Health Issues." *Journal of American College Health* 61, no. 4: 185–194. https://doi.org/10.1080/07448481.2013.787619.

Koch, Lynn C. 2020. "Disclosure in the Classroom and Beyond: The Perspectives of a Professor with Mental Illness." *Psychological Services*: 1541–1559. https://doi.org/10.1037/ser0000514.

Koo, Katie, and Gudrun Nyunt. 2020. "Culturally Sensitive Assessment of Mental Health for International Students. Special Issue: Voices from the Margins: Conducting Inclusive Assessment for Minoritized Students in Higher Education." *New Directions for Student Services* 169: 43–52. http://dx.doi.org/10.1002/ss.20343.

Kreps, Gary L. 2020. "The Chilling Influences of Social Stigma on Mental Health Communication: Implications for Promotion Health Equity." In *Communicating Mental Health: History, Contexts, and Perspectives,* 11–24. Edited by Lance R. Lippert, Robert D. Hall, Aimee E. Miller-Ott, and Daniel Coche Davis, Lanham, MD: Lexington Books.

Lashuel, Hilal A. 2020. "Mental Health in Academia: What About Faculty?" *eLife.* January 8, 2020. https://elifesciences.org/articles/54551.

Lau, Anna, and Nolan Zane. 2000. "Examining the Effects of Ethnic-Specific Services: An Analysis of Cost-Utilization and Treatment Outcome for Asian American Clients." *Journal of Community Psychology* 28, no. 1: 63–77. https://doi.org/10.1002/(SICI)1520-6629(200001)28:1<63::AID-JCOP7>3.0.CO;2-Z.

Lawson, Brian. "Amy Bishop Will Be in Prison for Life, Victims Did Not Want Her to Get Death Penalty." Alabama.com (blog). 24 September, 2012. https://www.al.com/breaking/2012/09/amy_bishop_will_be_in_prison_f.html.

Levecque, Katia, Frederik Anseel, Alain De Beuckelaer, Johan Van der Heyden, and Lydia Gisle. 2017. "Work Organization and Mental Health Problems in PhD Students." *Research Policy* 46 (no. 4): 868–879. https://doi.org/10.1016/j.respol.2017.02.008.

Lindfelt, Tristan, Eric J. Ip, Alejandra Gomez, and Mitchell J. Barnett. 2018. "The Impact of Work-Life Balance on Intention to Stay in Academia: Results from a National Survey of Pharmacy Faculty." *Research in Social and Administrative Pharmacy* 14, no. 4: 387–390. https://doi.org/10.1016/j.sapharm.2017.04.008.

Lindfelt, Tristan. A, Eric J. Ip, and Mitchell J. Barnett. 2015. "Survey of Career Satisfaction, Lifestyle, and Stress Levels Among Pharmacy School Faculty." *American Journal of Health-System Pharmacy* 72, no. 18: 1573–1578. https://doi.org/10.2146/ajhp140654.

Liu, Cindy H., Courtney Stevens, Sylvia H. M. Wong, Miwa Yasui, and Justin A. Chen. 2019. "The Prevalence and Predictors of Mental Health Diagnoses and Suicide Among U.S. College Students: Implications for Addressing Disparities in Service Use." *Depression and Anxiety* 36, no. 1: 8–17. doi: 10.1002/da.22830.

Lukianoff, Greg, and Jonathan Haidt. "The Coddling of the American Mind: How Trigger Warnings are Hurting Mental Health on Campus." *The Atlantic,* September 2015. https://www.theatlantic.com/magazine/archive/2015/09/the-coddling-of-the-american-mind/399356/.

MacKenna, Erin. 2004. "Contingent Performances: Between the Acts of Adjunct Faculty." *The Journal of the Midwest Modern Language Association* 37, no. 2: 45–48. https://www.jstor.org/stable/4144698.

Magnuson, Sandy, Holly Shaw, Bosmat Tubin, and Ken Norem. 2004. "Assistant Professors of Counselor Education: First and Second Year Experiences. *Journal of Professional Counseling: Practice, Theory, & Research* 32, no. 1: 3–18. http://dx.doi.org/10.1080/15566382.2004.12033797.

Markoulakis, Roula, and Bonnie Kirsh. 2010. "Difficulties for University Students with Mental Health Problems: A Critical Interpretive Analysis." *The Review of Higher Education* 37, no. 1: 77–100. https://doi.org/10.1353/rhe.2013.0073.

Marten, Sarah. "The Challenges Facing Academic Staff in UK Universities." 2009. https://career-advice.jobs.ac.uk/academic/the-challenges-facing-academic-staff-in-uk-universities/.

Martin, Jennifer Marie. 2010. "Stigma and Student Mental Health in Higher Education." *Higher Education Research & Development* 29, no. 3: 259–274. ttps://doi.org/10.1080/07294360903470969.

Meadows, Bob. "Murder on Campus: A Professor's Rage." *People*. March 8, 2010. https://people.com/archive/murder-on-campus-a-professors-rage-vol-73-no-9/.

Megivern, Deborah, Sue Pellerito, and Carol Mowbray. 2003. "Barriers to Higher Education for Individuals with Psychiatric Disabilities." *Psychiatric Rehabilitation Journal* 26, no. 3: 217–231. https://doi.org/10.2975/26.2003.217.231.

"The Mental Health of PhD Researchers Demands Urgent Attention." *Nature*. November 13, 2019. https://www.nature.com/articles/d41586-019-03489-1?fbclid=IwAR0OOYIJmDxuWOKXv-r-MPjn6eO0ijKuiylnPagwwQ_WNWQ9P6zvm4HTKZs.

Mental Health Commission of Canada [MHCC]. 2011. *Making the Case for Investing in Mental Health in Canada*. Accessed November 30, 2020. https://www.mentalhealthcommission.ca/sites/default/files/2016-06/Investing_in_Mental_Health_FINAL_Version_ENG.pdf.

Mental Health Commission of Canada [MHCC]. 2017. *Case Study Research Project Findings*. Accessed January 16, 2020. https://www.mentalhealthcommission.ca/sites/default/files/2017-03/case_study_research_project_findings_2017_eng.pdf.

Mental Health Foundation. 2020a. "Mental Health Statistics: The Most Common Mental Health Problems." Mental Health Foundation. Accessed November 30, 2020. https://www.mentalhealth.org.uk/statistics/mental-health-statistics-most-common-mental-health-problems.

Mental Health Foundation. 2020b. "Mental Health Statistics: UK and Worldwide." *Mental Health Foundation*. Accessed November 30, 2010. https://www.mentalhealth.org.uk/statistics/mental-health-statistics-uk-and-worldwide.

"Mental Illness: I Keep Mine Hidden." 2015. *Times Higher Education*. April 16. https://www.timeshighereducation.com/comment/opinion/mental-illness-i-keep-mine-hidden/2019639.article.

Miles, Rona, Laura Rabin, Anjali Krishnan, Evan Grandoit, and Kamil Kloskowski. 2020. "Mental Health Literacy in a Diverse Sample of Undergraduate Students:

Demographic, Psychological, and Academic Correlates." *BMC Public Health* 20, no. 1: 1–13. doi: 10.1186/s12889-020-09696-0.

Mind. 2017. "Mental Health Facts and Statistics." *Mind.* Accessed November 30, 2020. https://www.mind.org.uk/information-support/types-of-mental-health-problems/statistics-and-facts-about-mental-health/how-common-are-mental-health-problems/.

Montell, Gabriela. "Do the Faculty Shootings in Alabama Say Something About Academic Culture?" *Chronicle of Higher Education.* February 15, 2010. https://www.chronicle.com/article/Do-the-Faculty-Shootings-in/64195.

Moulin, Thiago C. 2020. "Mental Health in Academia: The Role of Workplace Relationships." *Frontiers in Pyschology* 11 (September): https://doi.org/10.3389/fpsyg.2020.562457.

Müller, Astrid. 2020. "Mental Health Disorders: Prevalent but Widely Ignored in Academia?" *The Journal of Physiology* 598, no. 7: 1279–1281.

National Institute of Mental Health (NIH). 2021. "Mental Illness." https://www.nimh.nih.gov/health/statistics/mental-illness.shtml.

Nelson, Nancy G., Carol Dell'Oliver, Chris Koch, and Robert Buckler. 2001. "Stress, Coping, and Success Among Graduate Students in Clinical Psychology." *Psychological Reports* 88, no. 3: 759–767. http://dx.doi.org/10.2466/pr0.2001.88.3.759.

Nogueira-Martins, L., R. Fagnani Neto, P. Macedo, V. Citero, and J. Mari. 2004. "The Mental Health of Graduate Students at the Federal University of Sao Paulo: A Preliminary Report." *Brazilian Journal of Medical and Biological Research* 37, no. 10: 1519–1524. https://doi.org/10.1590/S0100-879X2004001000011.

O'Connor, Pat, and Clare O'Hagan. 2016. "Excellence in University Academic Staff Evaluation: A Problematic Reality?" *Studies in Higher Education* 41, no. 11: 1943–1957. https://doi.org/10.1080/03075079.2014.1000292.

OECD. 2015a. *Fit Mind, Fit Job: From Evidence to Practice in Mental Health and Work.* Paris: OECD Publishing. https://dx.doi.org/10.1787/9789264228283-en.

OECD. 2015b. "New Approach Needed to Tackle Mental Ill-Health at Work." April 3, 2015. https://www.oecd.org/newsroom/new-approach-needed-to-tackle-mental-ill-health-at-work.htm.

O'Neil, Mary Kay, Lancee, William J., and Stanley J. J. Freeman. 1984. "Help-Seeking Behaviour of Depressed Students." *Social Science & Medicine* 18, no. 6: 511–514. doi: 10.1016/0277-9536(84)90009-1.

Oswalt, Sara B., and Tammy J. Wyatt. 2011. "Sexual Orientation and Differences in Mental Health, Stress, and Academic Performance in a National Sample of US College Students." *Journal of Homosexuality* 58, no. 9: 1255–1280. https://doi.org/10.1080/00918369.2011.605738.

Owen, Jesse, and Rodolfa, Emil. 2009. "Prevention Through Connection: Creating a Campus Climate of Care. *Planning for Higher Education Journal* 37, no. 2: 26–33.

Perrucci, Robert, and Hu, Hong 1995. "Satisfaction with Social and Educational Experiences Among International Graduate Students." *Research in Higher Education* 36, no. 4: 491–508. http://dx.doi.org/10.1007/BF02207908.

Peters, Robert L. 1997. *Getting What You Came For: The Smart Student's Guide to Earning a Master's or Ph.D.* New York: Farrar, Straus, and Grioux.
Pettit, Emma. "A Prominent Economist's Death Prompts Talk of Mental Health in the Professoriate." *Chronicle of Higher Education.* March 19, 2019. https://www.chronicle.com/article/a-prominent-economists-death-prompts-talk-of-mental-health-in-the-professoriate/.
Pledge, Deanna S., Richard T. Lapan, P. Paul Heppner, Dennis Kivlighan, and Helen J. Roehlke. 1998. "Stability and Severity of Presenting Problems at a University Counseling Center: A 6-Year Analysis." *Professional Psychology: Research & Practice* 29, no. 4: 386–389. https://doi.org/10.1037/0735-7028.29.4.386.
Poalses, Jacolize, and Bezuidenhout, Adéle. 2018. "Mental Health in Higher Education: A Comparitive Stress Risk Assessment at an Open. Distance Learning University in South Africa." *International Review of Research in Open and Distributed Learning* 19, no. 2: 169–190. https://doi.org/10.19173/irrodl.v19i2.3391.
Potts, Marilyn K. 1992. "Adjustment of Graduate Students to the Educational Process: Effects of Part-Time Enrolment and Extracurricular Roles." *Journal of Social Work Education* 28, no. 1: 61–76. http://dx.doi.org/10.1080/10437797.1992.10778758.
Price, Margaret. 2011. *Mad at School: Rhetorics of Mental Disability and Academic Life.* Ann Arbor: University of Michigan Press.
Price, Margaret, and Stephanie L. Kerschbaum. 2017. *Promoting Supportive Academic Environments for Faculty with Mental Illnesses: Resource Guide and Suggestions for Practice.* Philadelphia, PA: Temple University Collaborative.
Price, Margaret, Mark S. Salzer, Amber O'Shea, and Stephanie L. Kerschbaum. 2017. "Disclosure of Mental Disability by College and University Faculty: The Negotiation of Accommodations, Supports, and Barriers." *Disability Studies Quarterly* 37, no. 2. http://dx.doi.org/10.18061/dsq.v37i2.5487.
The Professor Is In. 2020. Accessed November 30, 2020. https://theprofessorisin.com/category/mental-illness-and-academia/.
Pryal, Katie R. Guest. 2017. *Life of the Mind Interrupted: Essays on Mental Health and Disability in Higher Education.* Chapel Hill, NC: Snowraven Books.
Puthran Rohan, Melvyn W. B. Zhang, Wilson W. Tam, and Roger C. Ho. 2016. "Prevalence of Depression Amongst Medical Students: A Meta-Analysis." *Medical Education* 50, no. 4: 456–468. doi: 10.1111/medu.12962.
Quintero Johnson, Jessie M., and Bonnie Miller. 2016. "When Women 'Snap': The Use of Mental Illness to Contextualize Women's Acts of Violence in Contemporary Popular Media." *Women's Studies in Communication* 39, no. 2: 211–227. https://doi.org/10.1080/07491409.2016.1172530.
Raskauskas, Juliana, and Chris Skrabec. 2011. "Bullying and Occupational Stress in Academia: Experiences of Workplace Bullying in New Zealand Universities." *Journal of Intergroup Relations* 35, no. 1: 18–36.
"Reactions: Is Tenure a Matter of Life or Death?" *Chronicle of Higher Education.* March 5, 2010. https://www.chronicle.com/article/Reactions-Is-Tenure-a-Matter/64321.

Reeves, Jay. "Students Complained About Prof Charged in Rampage." *The Monitor.* February 17, 2010. https://archive.vn/20150313063142/http://www.themonitor.com/students-complained-about-prof-charged-in-rampage/article_3e2e4d5f-c6a8-5ad0-98ef-5d72a778604a.html.

Reevy, Gretchen M., and Grace Deason. 2014. "Predictors of Depression, Stress, and Anxiety Among Non-Tenure Faculty." *Frontiers in Psychology,* 5 (July): 701. https://doi.org/10.3389/fpsyg.2014.00701.

Resources. 2020. *The Thesis Whisperer.* Accessed November 30, 2020. https://thesiswhisperer.com/useful-resources-for-students-and-supervisors/.

Roberts, Laura Weiss (Editor). 2018. *Student Mental Health: A Guide for Psychiatrists, Psychologists, and Leaders Serving in Higher Education.* Washington, DC: American Psychiatric Association Publishing.

Rosenfield, Sarah, and Mouzon, Dawne. 2013. "Gender and Mental Health." In *Handbook of the Sociology of Mental Health.* Edited by Carol S. Aneshensel, Jo C. Phelan, and Alex Bierman, 277–296. Dordrecht, Netherlands: Springer Netherlands. https://doi.org/10.1007/978-94-007-4276-5_14.

The Royal Australian and New Zealand College of Psychiatrists (RANZCP). *Improving Mental Health in Australia and New Zealand.* Melbourne: RANZCP, 2010, October). Accessed November 30, 2020. https://www.ranzcp.org/files/resources/reports/improving-mental-health-in-australia-and-new-zeala.aspx.

Ruark, Jennifer. "In Academic Culture, Mental-Health Problems are Hard to Recognize and Hard to Treat. *The Chronicle of Higher Education.* February 16, 2010. http://www.chronicle.com/article/In-Academe-Mental-Health/64246/.

Rudd, M. David. 2004. "University Counseling Centers: Looking More and More Like Community Clinics." *Professional Psychology: Research & Practice* 35, no. 3: 316–317. https://doi.org/10.1037/0735-7028.35.3.316.

Sahu, Pradeep. 2020. "Closure of Universities Due to Coronavirus Disease 2019 (COVID-19): Impact on Education and Mental Health of Students and Academic Staff." *Cureus* 12, no. 4: e7541. http://dx.doi.org/10.7759/cureus.7541.

Saks, Elyn R. "Mental Illness in Academe." *Chronicle of Higher Education.* November 25, 2009. https://www.chronicle.com/article/Mental-Illness-in-Academe/49233.

Schroeder, Ray. 2020. "Online: Trending Now." *Inside Higher Ed.* October 1, 2020. https://www.insidehighered.com/digital-learning/blogs/online-trending-now/wellness-and-mental-health-2020-online-learning.

Shackle, Samira. 'The Way Universities are Run is Making Us Ill': Inside the Student Mental Health Crisis." *The Guardian.* September 27, 2019. https://www.theguardian.com/society/2019/sep/27/anxiety-mental-breakdowns-depression-uk-students.

Sharkin, Bruce S. 2004. "Assessing Changes in Categories But Not Severity of Counseling Center Clients' Problems Across 13 Years: Comment on Benton, Robertson, Tseng, Newton, and Benton (2003)." *Professional Psychology: Research & Practice* 35, no. 3: 313–315. https://doi.org/10.1037/0735-7028.35.3.313.

Shaw, Claire. "Overworked and Isolated–Work Pressure Fuels Mental Illness in Academia." *The Guardian,* May 8, 2014. https://www.theguardian.com/hi

gher-education-network/blog/2014/may/08/work-pressure-fuels-academic-mental-illness-guardian-study-health.

Shaw, Claire, and Lucy Ward. "Dark Thoughts: Why Mental Illness is on the Rise in Academia." *The Guardian*. March 6, 2014. https://www.theguardian.com/higher-education-network/2014/mar/06/mental-health-academics-growing-problem-pressure-university.

Shigaki, Cheryl L., Kim M. Anderson, Carol Howald, Lee Henson, and Bonnie E. Gregg. 2012. "Disability on Campus: A Perspective from Faculty and Staff." *Work* 42, no. 4: 559–571. http://dx.doi.org/10.3233/WOR-2012-1409.

Shillingford, M. Ann, Trice-Black, Shannon, and Butler, S. Kent. 2013. "Wellness of Minority Female Counselor Educators." *Counselor Education and Supervision* 52, no. 4: 255–269. http://dx.doi.org/10.1002/j.1556-6978.2013.00041.x.

Siltaloppi, Marjo, Ulla Kinnunen, and Taru Feldt. 2009. "Recovery Experiences as Moderators Between Psychosocial Work Characteristics and Occupational Well-Being." *Work & Stress* 23, no. 4: 330–348. http://dx.doi.org/10.1080/02678370903415572.

Simon, Caroline. "More and More Students Need Mental Health Services. But Colleges Struggle to Keep Up." *USA Today*. May 4, 2017. https://www.usatoday.com/story/college/2017/05/04/more-and-more-students-need-mental-health-services-but-colleges-struggle-to-keep-up/37431099/.

Skinner, Natalie, and M. Anthony Machin. 2017. "Work Intensification, Work–Life Interference, Stress, and Well-Being in Australian Workers." *International Studies of Management & Organization* 47, no. 4: 360–371. http://dx.doi.org/10.1080/00208825.2017.1382271.

Smith, Charlie, and Eda Ulus. 2019. "Who Cares for Academics? We Need to Talk About Emotional Well-Being Including What We Avoid and Intellectualize Through Macro-Discourses." *Organization* 27, no. 6: 840–857. https://doi.org/10.1177/1350508419867201.

Sorcinelli, Mary Deane. 1994. "Effective Approaches to New Faculty Development." *Journal of Counseling and Development* 72, no. 5: 474–479. http://dx.doi.org/10.1002/j.1556-6676.1994.tb00976.x.

Sun, Wei, Wu, Hui, and Wang, Lie. 2011. "Occupational Stress and its Related Factors Among University Teachers in China." *Journal of Occupational Health* 53, no. 4: 280–286. https://doi.org/10.1539/joh.10-0058-OA.

Straforini, Carol Morrison. 2015. "Dissertation as Life Chapter: Managing Emotions, Relationships, and Time." *Journal of College Student Psychotherapy* 29, no 4: 296–313. https://doi.org/10.1080/87568225.2015.1074021.

Sturdivant, C. 2015. "Silencing the Stigma." *Diverse: Issues in Higher Education* 32, no. 1: 8.

Swartzlander, LuAnn, Raymond Garcia, Marilyn Sweeney, Barbara Dayton, Anne L. Hunter, Patricia Stoll, Silvija Meija, Tammie Bob, Lauren Hahn, and Helen Hoffman. 1998. "That Adjunct Situation: Exploitation, Dilettantism, and the Downsizing of Academia." *The Journal of the Midwest Modern Language Association* 31, no. 3: 65–113. https://www.jstor.org/stable/1315358.

Teelken, Christine. 2015. "Hybridity, Coping Mechanisms, and Academic Performance Management: Comparing Three Countries." *Public Administration* 93, no. 2: 307–323. https://doi.org/10.1111/padm.12138.

Tertiary Education Union. 2020. *Tertiary Lives: COVID-19*. Wellington, New Zealand: Tertiary Education Union.

"There is a Culture of Acceptance Around Mental Health Issues in Academia." March 1, 2014. *The Guardian*. https://www.theguardian.com/higher-education-network/blog/2014/mar/01/mental-health-issue-phd-research-university.

Thompson, Vetta L. Sanders, Anita Bazile, and Maysa Akbar. 2004. "African Americans' Perceptions of Psychotherapy and Psychotherapists." *Professional Psychology: Research & Practice* 35, no. 1: 19–26. http://dx.doi.org/10.1037/0735-7028.35.1.19.

Times Higher Education. 2018. "Work-Life Balance Survey 2018: Long Hours Take Their Toll on Academics." Accessed Nov. 24, 2020. https://www.timeshighereducation.com/features/work-life-balance-survey-2018-long-hours-take-their-toll-academics.

Tinklin, Teresa, Riddell, Sheila, and Wilson, Alastair. 2005. "Support for Students with Mental Health Difficulties in Higher Education: The Students' Perspective." *British Journal of Guidance and Counselling* 33, no. 4: 495–512. https://doi.org/10.1080/03069880500327496.

Toews, J. A., J. M. Lockyer, D. J. Dobson, E. Simpson, A. K. Brownell, F. Brenneis, and K. M. MacPherson. 1997. "Analysis of Stress Levels Among Medical Students, Residents, and Graduate Students at Four Canadian Schools of Medicine." *Academic Medicine* 72, no. 11: 997–1002. doi: 10.1097/00001888-199711000-00019.

Trucks-Bordeaux, Tammy. 2003. "Academic Massacres: The Story of Two American Indian Women and Their Struggle to Survive Academia." *American Indian Quarterly* 27, no. 1/2: 416–419. https://doi.org/10.1353/aiq.2004.0057.

Tsai, Jessica W., and Fanuel Muindi. 2016. "Towards Sustaining a Culture of Mental Health and Wellness for Trainees in the Biosciences." *Nature Biotechnology* 34: 353–355. http://dx.doi.org/10.1038/nbt.3490.

Tytherleigh, Michelle, C. Webb, C. L. Cooper, and C. Ricketts. 2007. "Occupational Stress in UK Higher Education Institutions: A Comparative Study of All Staff Categories." *Higher Education Research and Development* 24, no. 1: 41–61. https://doi.org/10.1080/07294360520003185 69.

University and College Union (UCU). 2014. *Taking Its Toll: Rising Stress Levels in Further Education*. Accessed January 13, 2021. https://www.ucu.org.uk/media/7264/UCU-stress-survey-2014/pdf/ucu_festressreport14.pdf.

Vanroelen, Christophe, Katia Levecque, and Fred Louckx. 2009. "Psychosocial Working Conditions and Self-Reported Health in a Representative Sample of Wage-Earners: A Test of the Different Hypotheses of the Demand-Control-Support-Model." *International Archives of Occupational and Environmental Health* 82, no. 3: 329–342. https://doi.org/10.1007/s00420-008-0340-2.

Weiner, Enid, and Judith Wiener. 1997. "University Students with Psychiatric Illness: Factors Involved in the Decision to Withdraw from Their Studies." *Psychiatric Rehabilitation Journal* 20, no. 4: 88–91.

Westefeld, John S., and Susan R Furr. 1987. "Suicide and Depression Among College Students." *Professional Psychology: Research & Practice* 18, no. 2: 119–123. https://doi.org/10.1037/0735-7028.18.2.119.

Wilson, Robin. "'Terminal Year' for Professors Denied Tenure Can Be Difficult, If Not Risky." August 13, 2013. *Chronicle of Higher Education.* https://www.chronicle.com/article/Terminal-Year-Granted-to/141145

Woolston, Chris. 2017. "Graduate Survey: A Love-Hurt Relationship." *Nature* 550: 549–552. https://doi.org/10.1038/nj7677-549a.

World Health Organization. "Mental Health Evidence and Research (MER)." 2011. http://www.who.int/mental_health/evidence/en/.

Ysseldyk, Renate, Katherine H. Greenaway, Elena Hassinger, Sarah Zutrauen, Jana Lintz, Maya P. Bhatia, Margaret Frye, Else Starkenburg, and Vera Tai. 2019. "A Leak in the Academic Pipeline: Identity and Health Among Postdoctoral Women." *Frontiers in Psychology* 10: 1297. https://doi.org/10.3389/fpsyg.2019.01297.

Zhang, Naijian, and David N. Dixon. 2003. "Acculturation and Attitudes of Asian International Students Toward Seeking Psychological Help." *Multicultural Counseling and Development* 31, no. 3: 205–222. https://doi.org/10.1002/j.2161-1912.2003.tb00544.x.

Zivin, Kara, Daniel Eisenberg, and Sarah E. Gollust, and Ezra Golberstein. 2009. "Prevalence of Mental Health Problems and Needs in a College Population." *Journal of Affective Disorders* 117, no. 3: 180–185. https://doi.org/10.1016/j.jad.2009.01.001.

Chapter 2

Anxiety in Academia

An Autoethnographic Account

Andrea L. Meluch

There are few things that cause me more anxiety than writing about my anxiety. I realize the ironic nature of this statement and that the obvious answer to this conundrum may be to just not write about my struggles with anxiety. However, I feel that it is incumbent upon me as a health communication researcher to consider how my personal experiences intersect with my research and pedagogy.

I am not alone in living and struggling with mental health. One in five adults in the United States lives with some form of mental illness (National Institute of Mental Health 2019). However, the prevalence of mental health issues in the United States does little to explain the stigma around these issues. Culturally, mental health issues such as anxiety and depression are often framed negatively by public culture, the popular media, and in professions such as academia (Bauer 2011, 193; Kreps 2020, 14). When someone is struggling with mental health issues, they are stigmatized and often perceived as incompetent, weak, and even dangerous (Smith and Applegate 2018, 383). This is especially the case in demanding professions such as academia, where not being able to cope with the job's daily rigors and seemingly never-ending workload are often viewed as personal weakness.

The day-to-day experience of living with a mental health issue as a faculty member is quite different from the cultural portrayals of mental illness. Popular culture often portrays people with mental illness as unable to fit into regular society and even dangerous (Heath 2019, 4; Stout, Villegas, and Jennings 2004, 543; Wahl 2003, 3). Few examples of faculty struggling with mental illness exist in popular culture, with the exception of *A Beautiful Mind*, which also is problematic in framing a faculty member as brilliant but aloof, eccentric, and unable to live a normal life due to mental illness. Portrayals of mental illness in the media, which are often framed by stereotypes and blame the person for their situation, are usually untrue because individual experiences often vary widely (Heath 2019, 4). In my own experience, I have found that my anxiety is something that is constantly present in my life. I do my best to dismiss and ignore it when I am able to do so, but I also realize that my anxiety is a continuous struggle that I have just come to accept.

In many ways, I am a typical tenure-track academic at a large public university. I teach, conduct research, and complete service for my institution. I have managed to accomplish many, but not all, of my academic goals while managing an ongoing anxiety disorder. Unfortunately, struggles with mental health issues like mine are on the rise across academia (Gorczynski 2018). I use my personal story in this autoethnographic chapter to highlight the lived experience of being an academic who is living with anxiety. I believe that, although my story may be different from others, it does have the potential to shed light on the experience of working in academia while managing a mental health issue. Drawing from my experiences and the existing research on mental health in academia, the chapter will also conclude with some recommendations for managing mental health issues in academia.

CHOOSING AUTOETHNOGRAPHY TO EXPLORE PERSONAL EXPERIENCES

Autoethnography is an approach to qualitative research in which one's personal story is connected to concepts and theories in order to explore and interrogate a specific lived experience (Denzin 1997, 227). As a method of inquiry, autoethnography has been deemed to be a rigorous method of analysis (Duncan 2004, 31). However, autoethnography is not without its criticisms. For example, because autoethnography relies on the author's memory of events (some of which occurred long ago), it can be questioned whether autoethnography has the same legitimacy as other qualitative methods of inquiry such as grounded theory or phenomenology (Altheide and Johnson 2011, 581). Furthermore, autoethnographies vary in form and function and, thus, can be difficult to apply (Wall 2008, 39). As such, I believe it is critical to delineate the scope of this autoethnographic work for clarity and precision.

Autoethnography has been used to explore a variety of health issues (Doshi 2014, 840; Small 2019, 515), including mental health (Burnard 2007, 808). However, few scholars use autoethnography to deeply explore mental health from a personal perspective, marking a significant gap in the literature. Although there are many reasons why individuals may not choose to use autoethnography to explore mental health issues, I believe one of the most pressing reasons for this lack of literature is the stigmatizing nature of mental health: many individuals are unwilling to "out" themselves in publications.

As many academics are aware, they face professional and personal risk by coming forward to discuss mental health issues publicly (Flaherty 2017). At this particular juncture, my personal experiences have guided me toward using autoethnography in my research despite (potentially in spite of) the risks because I believe personal accounts are one of the most powerful ways to share difficult and painful experiences.

As a research method, autoethnography is particularly challenging because it requires me to be vulnerable as I share my deeply personal and painful experiences of living with anxiety as an academic. I would much rather be writing up the findings of a study where my own experiences and feelings are not the focus of the analysis. However, I also realize that sharing stories can powerfully bring attention to important issues. Even my story has this potential. That is, storytelling has the ability to shape and define one's reality (Lawler 2002, 242). Specifically, storytelling can be used to speak out against harmful stigmas and legitimize stigmatized and marginalized experiences (Kellett 2019, ix).

This chapter explores my memories and experiences living and working as an academic with anxiety. Although there have been individuals who I have known both personally and professionally throughout my academic career who have shaped my experiences in both positive and negative ways, I will not examine any specific interpersonal relationship in great detail. Our interpersonal relationships have the power to shape our lived experiences, but the focus of this particular piece is on my cumulative experiences navigating academia as an individual living with an anxiety disorder. As such, I will provide examples of when I chose to discuss and when I chose to conceal my anxiety disorder throughout my academic career to date, and the results of these decisions. The communicative aspects and outcomes of my decisions to reveal or conceal my anxiety disorder will also be addressed from a health communication perspective. Throughout this narrative, I also draw upon literature on stigma and imposter syndrome in higher education, to further delineate how my own experience fits within the broader understandings of mental health experiences in academia.

MENTAL HEALTH AND ACADEMIA: WHAT WE KNOW

Increasingly, mental health issues among academics are the center of scholarly and mainstream media attention (Fowler 2015, 157; Gonçalves 2017; Price and Kerschbaum 2017, 5; Szetela 2018). The discussion around mental health in higher education contexts may lead some to believe that there is a great deal of work being done on the subject. However, few analyses consider how institutional and societal norms contribute to the problem. In addition, few studies use a narrative or autoethnographic approach to consider how individuals experience mental health issues across roles in higher education (e.g., undergraduate, graduate, faculty) (Pryal 2017, 5; Saks 2007, 1). The following section summarizes the state of the current literature on mental health in higher education and highlights where these gaps exist.

In 2018, Adam Szetela wrote in *The Chronicle of Higher Education* that the culture of academia is to constantly experience an "uneasy feeling that there is always something left to do." Although academics may have a passion for research and teaching, this constant pressure to perform is a ripe environment for mental health issues like anxiety to flourish. Academia as a profession is generally one that is chosen out of a passion for knowledge. Like many who have come before me, I chose academia as a career path because I had a burning desire to create new knowledge and impart that knowledge to eager students. However, my path through academia has not been without its roadblocks. Academia can give you the freedom to pursue a deep interest while simultaneously putting the work you produce under intense scrutiny. Academics work fairly autonomously, which provides great freedom over our time and how we wish to spend it. However, that same freedom can be accompanied by guilt if time is spent on non-academic pursuits. These dichotomies are the reality of life as an academic today.

The advent of the neoliberal university and the associated economic pressures that such universities face have increased the pressure on faculty to perform with greater scrutiny if they do not meet high expectations for publications, teaching, service, and unpaid emotional labor (Seal 2018). Specifically, the decreasing number of tenure-track job openings and the increasing reliance on contingent faculty send the message to faculty who are on tenure-track that they should just be grateful for what they have and not question the status quo (Childress 2019, 101). For someone living with anxiety, this lifestyle of non-stop work and pressure from within can produce a cycle of uncertainty and stress that only amplifies the everyday anxiety that one is living with and can create a situation ripe for burnout.

Today, academics are more interested in mental health issues than ever before. The main focus of much of the mental health–related research in higher education examines undergraduate student experiences (Aloia and McTigue 2019, 128; American College Health Association 2018, 14; Hartley 2011, 596; Hunt and Eisenberg 2010, 3). Researchers have noted the stigmatized nature of mental illness on college campuses (Smith and Applegate 2018, 384), and the importance of constructing narratives in higher education classrooms that reduce students' feelings of shame (Goldman 2018, 400). However, undergraduates are not alone in their mental health struggles and, often, graduate students (Barry et al. 2018, 469; Russell-Pinson and Harris 2019, 64; Waight and Giordano 2018, 392) and faculty (Fowler 2015, 157;

Gonçalves 2017; Price and Kerschbaum 2017, 5; Szetela 2018) experience these same issues. For example, Fowler (2015) discusses how students and faculty experience intense stress and subsequent burnout in their academic roles (157). Fowler explains that the norms within academia, such as expectations for high productivity and for the emotional labor of providing pastoral care to students, create stress for faculty that may result in increased depression and burnout (162).

Mental health issues are steadily increasing in the U.S., as noted earlier in this chapter (National Institute of Mental Health [NIMH] 2019). Mental health issues in academia mirror these trends. The American College Health Association (2018) reports that 41.9 percent of college students are so depressed that they find it difficult to function and 63.4 percent feel overwhelming anxiety (14). Furthermore, graduate students are reporting similarly high levels of mental health problems, with one study finding 41 percent of graduate students struggling with anxiety and 39 percent struggling with depression (Evans et al. 2018, 283).

Less is known about the prevalence of mental health issues among faculty members. The pervasiveness of mental health issues in academia presents a unique context for examining how people with mental health conditions like anxiety handle obstacles, such as the stigmatized nature of mental health. In the following sections, I will explain my own experiences navigating these obstacles and how my anxiety has interfered and even inhibited my ability to be a productive and confident academic.

Anxiety from the Onset

I vividly remember the late afternoon in March 2012 when I opened the envelope that contained my acceptance letter into my doctoral program. My family was thrilled when I read the acceptance letter. I, on the other hand, immediately felt anxiety and dread. After the initial excitement abated, I had to quickly make the decision about whether or not I would actually pursue the PhD. As much as I wanted to be an academic, I also knew that doctoral programs were intense, and I seriously wondered whether I could handle the demands. I had already struggled with anxiety throughout my adolescence, and I knew that a doctoral program would likely amplify my anxiety. What I did not realize at the time was the full extent to which academia could often be an isolating, grueling, and uncertain career path.

I mostly decided to pursue being an academic because I love higher education. I love the classroom discussions, conferences, and research. While pursuing my master's program, I fell in love with teaching and with having the freedom to pursue my research passions. However, I also decided to pursue academia to prove something to all of the people throughout my life who had made me feel like I was not smart enough. It was as if, in many ways, none of my academic accomplishments had ever stacked up high enough for me, and obtaining a PhD was the only way that I could actually prove, maybe more to myself than to others, that I was smart enough. My insecurities about my abilities were only heightened by the fact that I struggled with anxiety. I have often felt that I needed to prove my worth through my academic work, and that any struggles with mental health need to be hidden so that they can never be used against me.

Like many academics and non-academics, I struggle with *imposter syndrome*, which is when someone who may be competent and high achieving actually feels as if he or she is a fraud or imposter (Clance and Imes 1978, 243). Feeling like an imposter is a very real obstacle for many individuals in academia (Ramsey and Spencer 2019, 504). Particularly, research points out how certain groups such as women, first-generation college students, and people of color experience imposter syndrome in higher education (Gardner and Holley 2011, 87; Peetet, Montgomery, and Weekes 2015, 175). My feelings of imposter syndrome intensified when I attended my doctoral program, and these feelings still exist in many ways today. I have often wondered when everyone will figure me out and realize that I am not, in fact, as capable and intelligent as I should be. These thoughts of being a fraud invade my mind at the most inopportune times. For example, after a major presentation, or if I have made a comment in a meeting, my mind will start the constant stream of questioning:

Did you really just say that?!
Wow, now everyone knows how little you really know.
What were you thinking?

These negative, self-defeating thoughts are intrusive; they often begin to take on a life of their own until I find myself no longer focusing on the task at hand. They can become a barrier to any real progress in my work. I know deep down that these internalized feelings are not true and are just my anxiety about my abilities getting the best of me. However, pushing aside my anxiety and feelings of being an imposter can be a monumental feat. Further, feeling like an imposter can make it even harder to want to open up to peers and colleagues since I already feel like I do not belong. Thus, the default becomes to conceal one's feelings of inadequacy and one's struggles with anxiety.

Working through Graduate School with Anxiety

I do not believe that it is possible to talk about living with anxiety as a tenure-track academic without first talking about living with anxiety as a graduate student. Graduate students often live with worse mental health than any other sub-group of individuals in higher education (Evans et al. 2018, 283; Russell-Pinson and Harris 2019, 64). Not only is graduate school demanding for even the most competent students, but it is also infused with unceasing uncertainty about the future ahead. The current academic job market for tenure-track positions, especially in the humanities, is dismal, to say the least. In today's neoliberal educational system, institutions seek to cut costs, extract the most work for the least amount of money, quantify intellectual labor, and remove job security in favor of insecure contract work (Kelsky 2015, 7; Kramnick 2018). As a result, most graduate students are left in the vulnerable position of meeting arduous demands for low stipends with an exceedingly ambiguous future ahead of them. As such, anxiety and depression are rampant among graduate students (Evans et al. 2018, 283).

Although I had lived with anxiety for the majority of my life when I started graduate school, I do not think anything could have prepared me for the struggles ahead. Throughout my coursework, comprehensive exams, job search, and dissertation writing process, I lived in a state of panic. I was always either working on my studies or feeling guilty that I was not working on my studies. Having been raised as a Catholic, I was somewhat used to the guilt that can accompany an individual in daily life. However, I believe that academic guilt puts Catholic guilt to shame. Academic guilt is feeling like there should be no life outside of academia and it is instilled in many graduate students pretty early in our careers. I was point-blank told by a professor that I should not spend time with family because they are a distraction from my research. Another faculty member told me that my marriage would probably fail because I was pursuing a PhD. These messages are hurtful and damaging. In particular, I found these messages took on lives of their own and provided me with all the more reason to be anxious when I was spending time with my family and friends or not spending time with my partner.

Graduate school is also difficult for someone who is struggling with anxiety because of how isolating the experience can be. Although today I love the autonomous nature of my job, there have been moments in which working autonomously is actually the opposite of a healthy work environment. Throughout my dissertation writing process, I spent most days completely alone in my home office, working at a card table I had set up, with only my dogs as company. Being isolated with only my anxious thoughts for company was not healthy. I would sit and write and edit and allow anxious feelings to take control of my mind. Sometimes I was very productive. Sometimes I would work on a sentence for what felt like eternity, and still find that I was not making progress because my anxiety kept me from being able to move forward.

I rarely speak about my anxiety to other people. *I do not like to talk about it.* It is often something I do not even mention to my husband unless it is really getting in the way of my daily activities. I usually try to brush off my anxiety as best as I can. If it is really bad, I will tell my husband, "My anxiety is really bad today." If I feel that I need to explain why I am being quiet or pacing the house I might say, "I've really been struggling." I am lucky that my partner accepts me for who I am. However, I am embarrassed by my anxiety and would prefer to just ignore it instead of talking about it.

Throughout graduate school, I did my best to not talk about my anxiety. I would put on my armor for the day—planned talking points in classes, social situations, and other interactions with colleagues—and do my best. However, there were a few times when my anxiety could not be contained. After a conversation with other graduate students, I found myself running to the restroom to stand in a stall and breathe deeply. I felt like the world was crashing in and I did not want them to see me get upset. On another occasion, after a meeting with my advisor, I felt myself unable to breathe or even start my car to drive home, so I sat in my parked car and replayed that conversation in my mind over and over. I was ashamed of my anxiety and afraid that, if I sought out any help, it would just make things worse.

Although I have used counseling at certain points in my life, I avoided counseling services for the duration of my PhD program. Many undergraduate and graduate students avoid seeking out help to deal with their mental health issues for fear of being stigmatized (Smith and Applegate 2018, 384). Further, studies in health communication similarly find that, on college campuses, students are particularly careful with whom they discuss their mental health (Venetis, Chemichky-Karcher, and Gettings 2018, 661; White and LaBelle 2019, 141). I avoided seeking help throughout my PhD program because, at the time, going to counseling felt like admitting defeat. For the longest time, I avoided counseling and medical help because I believed, incorrectly, that if I needed help to deal with my anxiety, I was not capable of being a successful academic.

It is odd even to me that I avoided help so ardently. I had gone to counseling during my undergraduate career and had experienced success with it. However, something in me felt that exposing myself to a counselor in graduate school was a paramount failure. If I could go back in time, I would force myself to seek help during those struggles. I believe that I probably would have managed my anxiety much better had I spoken to a professional about it.

Toward the end of my graduate career, my anxiety worsened and I did end up sharing my experience with some other graduate students. In my conversations, I found that I was not alone. Some of them experienced mental health issues much more severe than my own. Many were also struggling in silence.

Today, it makes me frustrated that graduate students live with this pain and often suffer alone. When I was in graduate school, conversations about mental health were very "hush hush" among students and almost never discussed between students and faculty. I have made it a point in recent years to talk to my classes about mental health services on campus and, on occasion, when a student shares their struggles with me, to open up, if only briefly, about my own struggles, as well. These small, even imperceptible steps are perhaps the best way to change the culture of silence and suffering alone that many undergraduate and graduate students experience.

The period of my life when I was in graduate school was when my anxiety was at its highest levels. In the years since graduating, I have tried to manage my anxiety and keep myself from being beholden to it in the ways I was throughout the four years of my doctoral program. However, finishing my PhD did not cure my anxiety. Completing my PhD provided me with greater security in my work and life, which has helped me to not get bogged down by the career-related "what ifs" that used to plague me. However, moving to the next stage of my career created new obstacles that I am still learning to manage.

Anxiety in Day-to-Day Academia

My anxiety feels like I have a critic constantly following me around and telling me how I am failing or could potentially fail. My mind incessantly catastrophizes even the most mundane tasks. Sometimes these thoughts are warranted and even helpful. When I am preparing for a major trip or a difficult task, it can be helpful to think of all of the ways something could go wrong and try to prepare to prevent those things from happening. However, more often than not, these thoughts and feelings get in the way of being a productive individual and feeling confident in my abilities.

When I was hired in my first tenure-track job the critic—my anxiety— was especially present. I am an individual who does not handle stress well. In fact, I have never managed stress well in my entire life. When I am in a new situation these feelings of anxiety can be particularly immobilizing. After the challenges of my job search and finishing my dissertation, my nerves were completely fried. I existed in almost a constant state of complete anxiety. Starting a new job is hard in the best of circumstances. However, starting a new job as an academic coming off of a year of constant pressure and stress can feel like trying to pour more tea into an already full cup.

In the weeks leading up to my first semester in the new job, my panic attacks began intensifying. Not only was I starting a new position, but I had also moved to a new city by myself for the first time in my life. I would sit in my apartment and feel tingling in my chest. My brain would simultaneously feel foggy and like it was racing. I would liken this experience to standing in the middle of a highway. Thoughts were zooming in and out of my mind so quickly that I would not be able to stop one long enough to actually think about it. In these moments, I tried to focus on my breathing or distract myself with the absolute worst reality television on the planet. I would be able to calm down eventually and put myself to work on whatever I needed to do, but these panic attacks were immobilizing. They made me question whether I was even capable of anything in my life, let alone being a scholar.

Throughout my years on the tenure-track, I have found myself working in bursts and busts. Sometimes I am extremely productive and amaze even myself with how much I can get done. At other times, I turn to bad reality television and amaze myself with how little I get done. One of the many peculiar elements of anxiety is how it seeps into all aspects of my life. When I am busy working on my courses, a new research project, or committee work, my anxiety can feel like it is in the passenger's seat; it is still present, but not necessarily driving my actions. When I am feeling lethargic and unmotivated, my anxiety usually takes those opportunities to get into the driver's seat and steer me even further off course. In moments of rest and respite, my anxiety often fills the moment with a long list of tasks that I am not currently accomplishing.

Anxiety Informing Pedagogy: An Unlikely Pairing

Over the course of my academic career, I have had many students talk to me about their struggles with depression and anxiety. As a college professor and health communication researcher, I find that it is necessary to incorporate my personal experiences with anxiety and my research into my pedagogy. Faculty can take on an empathetic listening role by providing a safe context for students to share their experiences of mental illness and how it has affected their lives. This sharing can be done without guilt or shame. Further, through opening up and supporting students, instructors may find that they make students who are struggling with mental health more comfortable and less stigmatized (Meluch and Starcher 2020, 157).

Not too long ago, I taught a class for a new college program designed to help contingent-admitted students on my campus. On the first day of class, I went over where to find campus resources: the tutoring center, advising, disability services, and counseling. I told my class that the student counseling center is available to all students free of charge. I made sure to also tell them that many students struggle with mental health issues and that they should not be embarrassed.

At the end of class some students came up to me to ask questions. I answered them and saw one student keeping back. The other students finished asking their questions and left. The student toward the back of the group then walked up to the front of the room and said she had something to tell me. She told me that she has severe anxiety. I could see her starting to tear up as she explained how nervous she was about this class. I looked at her and told her that she could be successful in my class. She started to relax a little and told me how her anxiety had affected her in high school and how she wanted to have a better experience in college. I gave her the space to tell her story to me and I listened closely. At the end of the conversation, I told her to consider using the counseling center and to check in with disability services about any accommodations she may need for all of her classes.

Over the course of the semester, I worked directly with this student and provided her with the opportunity to share with me her struggles related to mental health and academic goals. On more than one occasion, it was readily apparent to me that the student needed some flexible deadlines to be successful in the class. In these instances, having already established a dialogue related to the issue with the student was useful because I was able to encourage her to reach out early on and provide the appropriate documentation so that I could make accommodations. If this dialogue had not been established previously, it may have been harder for both the student to feel comfortable reaching out for help and for me, as an instructor, to provide support.

As an instructor, I have found that being able to assist students who are struggling with mental health issues can have a transformative impact on the student's academic pursuits and their persistence toward their degree. I believe it is critical for instructors to be open to accommodating students who are struggling with mental illness. Further, in my own teaching I have found that encouraging students to share their struggles related to mental health has provided greater opportunities for me to be supportive and help students be successful in my classes. However, I am unsure whether I would have the understanding to encourage students to seek help for mental illness if I had not experienced similar struggles.

In addition, I find that my interactions and relationships with students are more likely to evolve when I incorporate openness to understanding their experiences into my pedagogy. Through developing these relationships and providing a safe outlet for difficult conversations about mental health, I have seen my students excel academically. Instructors in higher education face a variety of challenges, and helping students to manage mental health issues is one of the most pressing today. Allowing my experiences with anxiety to shape my interactions with students as well as elements of my pedagogy has made me a more thoughtful instructor.

RECOMMENDATIONS

As my own experiences and extant research indicate, it is important for students and faculty struggling with mental health issues to seek out support services, such as counseling (Price and Kerschbaum 2017, 5; Waight and Giordano 2018, 392). Beyond individual-level interventions, such as referrals to counseling, it is also important to consider how academic culture can make mental health a greater priority and services more accessible. Individual institutions must also consider how they can remove barriers to mental health support and create greater access for undergraduate students, graduate students, and faculty. Price and Kerschbaum (2017) recommend developing campus-wide policies, such as confidentiality and accommodation policies, that encourage faculty to seek out support (9).

As a health communication scholar, I have noted particular ways in which faculty can contribute to meaningful campus-wide initiatives focusing on mental health. First, in the classroom, instructors can destigmatize mental health issues by discussing the prevalence of mental health problems that undergraduate and graduate students face (Goldman 2018, 400). These types of conversations early on can change the classroom conversation to be more inclusive toward those who are struggling with mental health. Next, faculty and institutions should use quality training programs aimed at intervening when students are struggling and opening a dialogue (QPR, 2019). Finally, faculty can take the first steps with each other to address imposter syndrome by creating inclusive spaces on campus for those who are marginalized (e.g., people of color, those diagnosed with mental health conditions, LGBTQ+ community members). Many faculty members are disenfranchised by the current cultural, institutional, and social norms that pervade the neoliberal university (Rodriguez, Dutta, and Desnoyers-Colas 2019, 3). Discussing these barriers and challenges openly, even if they are controversial, is one of the major steps that faculty can take to dismantle structures that marginalize individuals by reinforcing a culture of silence around stigmatized identities, such as mental illness.

From my own experience, I contend that being open about mental health issues on college campuses is the first step we can take to change the culture for both students and faculty. I believe telling our stories is an important step in removing the stigma attached to mental illness. As faculty, we should also consider how we can provide students a safe space to discuss their own struggles. By incorporating the discussion of mental health into our courses and encouraging help-seeking behaviors, we may be able to make changes that have far-reaching effects.

CONCLUDING THOUGHTS

Recently, I attended a concert. It was a beautiful summer night—cool and pleasant. I sat listening to the music and trying to enjoy the night air, but I found my mind returning to my to-do list. At one point, I pulled out my phone and started writing the list:

1) *Mental health autoethnography*
2) *Order business cards*
3) *Set up learning management system*
4) *Finish syllabi*

The list went on and into even greater detail. I felt relieved when I looked at the list, but extremely frustrated with myself. My anxiety kept me from enjoying something that I had decided to do for pure entertainment value. This is the academic guilt that I live with. This is the anxiety that keeps me constantly coming back to all of the tasks I need to do and prevents me from living in the moment or even accomplishing the tasks at hand. It is immobilizing, and frustrating, and makes me feel incredibly exhausted.

I know from firsthand experience that my students are probably struggling with similar issues. I do my best to listen to their experiences, send them to the appropriate resources, and enact compassion in any way that I can. My work as a researcher has provided me with the tools I need to investigate the social world and provide recommendations for how we can improve understanding. Much of what I have learned through my research is that, when individuals are struggling with their health, whether physical, mental, or emotional, it is by showing each other compassion that healing has the best chance of taking place.

I hate feeling vulnerable, and my mental health issues make me feel extremely vulnerable. Writing about myself is not a natural process for me. I am a private person and I only want to share certain parts of myself with certain individuals who I have carefully selected. Writing about something as painful and shameful as my mental health issues is not something that I do lightly. I know that I am "putting it out there" into the world and allowing others to draw their own conclusions about my experiences. This is difficult for me to do.

This autoethnography was a piece that I avoided writing for as long as I could. I waited until the deadline for this chapter was looming and, even then, I told myself that I could wait a little longer. The process of digging deep and telling my story has been more stressful than cathartic. Still, I think that my experience is worth sharing. I have spoken to many students and colleagues who are afraid to talk about their anxiety or depression, and who, instead, keep these feelings hidden away from view. As mental illness continues to increase in the United States and other countries and, especially, in higher education environments, we do a disservice to everyone affected to choose to avoid talking about it. Most individuals who struggle with mental health keep their experiences hidden to ensure they are not stigmatized by others. However, the cycle of silence only perpetuates the stigma surrounding mental illness.

REFERENCES

Aloia, Lindsey Susan, and Megan Mctigue. 2019. "Buffering Against Sources of Academic Stress: The Influence of Supportive Informational and Emotional Communication on Psychological Well-Being." *Communication Research Reports* 36, no. 2: 126–135. https://doi.org/10.1080/08824096.2019.1590191.

Altheide, David L., and John M. Johnson. 2011. "Reflections on Interpretive Adequacy in Qualitative Research." In *The SAGE Handbook of Qualitative Research,* edited by Norman K. Denzin and Yvonna S. Lincoln, 581–594. Thousand Oaks, CA: Sage.

"American College Health Association—National College Health Assessment II: Reference Group Executive Summary Spring 2018." American College Health Association. Hanover, MD: American College Health Association.

Bauer, Erica. 2011. "Mental Illness, Stigma, and Disclosure." In *Family Communication, Connections, and Health Transitions: Going Through this Together,* edited by Michelle Miller-Day, 193–225. New York: Peter Lang.

Barry, K. M., M. Woods, E. Warnecke, C. Stirling, and A. Martin. 2018. "Psychological Health of Doctoral Candidates, Study-Related Challenges and Perceived Performance." *Higher Education Research & Development* 37, no.3: 468–483. https://doi.org/10.1080/07294360.2018.1425979.

Burnard, P. 2007. "Seeing the Psychiatrist: An Autoethnographic Account." *Journal of Psychiatric and Mental Health Nursing* 14: 808–813. https://doi.org/10.1111/j.1365-2850.2007.01186.x.

Childress, Herb. 2019. *The Adjunct Underclass: How America's Colleges Betrayed Their Faculty, Their Students, and Their Mission.* Chicago, IL: University of Chicago Press.

Clance, Pauline Rose, and Suzanne Ament Imes. 1978. "The Imposter Phenomenon in High Achieving Women: Dynamics and Therapeutic Intervention." *Psychotherapy: Theory, Research, and Practice* 15, no. 3: 241–247. https://doi.org/10.1037/h0086006.

Denzin, Norman K. 1997. *Interpretive Ethnography: Ethnographic Practices for the 21st Century.* Thousand Oaks, CA: Sage.
Doshi, Marissa Joanna. 2014. "Help(less): An Autoethnography About Caring for My Mother with Terminal Cancer." *Health Communication* 29, no. 8: 840–842. https://doi.org/10.1080/10410236.2013.809502.
Duncan, Margot. 2004. "Autoethnography: Critical Appreciation of an Emerging Art." *International Journal of Qualitative Methods* 3, no. 4: 1–14. https://journals.library.ualberta.ca/ijqm/index.php/IJQM/index.
Evans, Teresa M., Lindsay Bira, Jazmin Beltran Gastelum, L. Todd Weiss, and Nathan L. Vanderford. 2018. "Evidence for a Mental Health Crisis in Graduate Education." *Nature Biotechnology* 36, no. 3: 282–284. https://doi.org/10.1038/nbt.4089.
Flaherty, Colleen. 2017. "Portrait of Faculty Mental Health." *Inside Higher Ed.* June 8, 2017. https://www.insidehighered.com/news/2017/06/08/study-faculty-members-mental-health-issues-finds-mix-attitudes-disclosing-and.
Fowler, Sean. 2015. "Burnout and Depression in Academia: A Look at the Discourse of the University." *Empedocles: European Journal for the Philosophy of Communication* 6, no. 2: 155–167. https://doi.org/10.1386/ejpc.6.2.155_1.ws.
Gardner, Susan K., and Karri A. Holley. 2011. "Those Invisible Barriers are Real: The Progression of First-Generation Students through Doctoral Education." *Equity & Excellence in Education* 4, no. 1: 77–92. https://doi.org/10.1080/10665684.2011.529791.
Goldman, Zachary W. 2018. "Responding to Mental Health Issues in the College Classroom." *Communication Education* 67, no. 3: 399–404. https://doi.org/10.1080/10665684.2011.529791.
Gonçalves, Francisco Valente. 2017. "Mental Health in Academia: What's Happening and What Can We Do to Address It." *Psychreg.* August 5, 2017. https://www.psychreg.org/mental-health-academia/.
Gorczynski, Paul. 2018. "More Academics and Students have Mental Health Problems than Ever Before." *The Conversation.* April 18, 2018. http://theconversation.com/more-academics-and-students-have-mental-health-problems-than-ever-before-90339.
Hartley, Michael T. 2011. "Examining the Relationships between Resilience, Mental Health, and Academic Persistence in Undergraduate College Students." *Journal of American College Health* 59, no. 7: 596–604. https://doi.org/10.1080/07448481.2010.515632.
Heath, Erin. 2019. "Introduction." In *Mental Disorders in Popular Film: How Hollywood Uses, Shames, and Obscures Mental Diversity*, edited by Erin Heath, 1–10. Lanham, MD: Lexington Books.
Hunt, Justin, and Daniel Eisenberg. 2010. "Mental Health Problems and Help-Seeking Behaviors among College Students." *Journal of Adolescent Health* 46, no.1: 3–10. https://doi.org/ 10.1016/j.jadohealth.2009.08.008.
Kellett, Peter M. 2019. "Introduction." In *Narrating Patienthood: Engaging Diverse Voices on Health, Communication, and the Patient Experience*, edited by Peter M. Kellett, ix–xii. Lanham, MD: Lexington Books.

Kelsky, Karen. 2015. *The Professor is In: The Essential Guide to Turning Your Ph.D. into a Job.* New York: Three Rivers Press.

Kramnick, Jonathan. 2018. "How the Jobs Crisis has Transformed Faculty Hiring." *The Chronicle of Higher Education.* August 26, 2018. www.chronicle.com/article/How-the-Jobs-Crisis-Has/244324.

Kreps, Gary L. 2020. "The Chilling Influences of Social Stigma on Mental Health Communication: Implications for Promoting Health Equity." In *Communicating Mental Health: History, Contexts, and Perspectives*, edited by Lance R. Lippert, Robbie D. Hall, Aimee Miller-Ott, and Daniel Cochece Davis, 11–26. Lanham, MD: Lexington Books.

Lawler, Steph. 2002. "Narrative in Social Research." In *Qualitative Research in Action*, edited by Tim May, 242–258. London: Sage.

Meluch, Andrea Lauren, and Shawn Starcher. 2020. "The Stigmatization of Mental Health Disclosure in the College Classroom: Student Perceptions of Instructor Credibility and the Benefits of Disclosure." In *Communicating Mental Health: History, Contexts, and Perspectives*, edited by Lance R. Lippert, Robbie D. Hall, Aimee Miller-Ott, and Daniel Cochece Davis, 147–166. Lanham, MD: Lexington Books.

"Mental illness." 2019. *National Institute of Mental Health.* April 27, 2020.https://www.nimh.nih.gov/health/statistics/mental-illness.shtml.

Peetet, Bridgette J., LaTrice Montgomery, and Jerren C. Weekes. 2015. "Predictors of Imposter Phenomenon Among Talented Ethnic Minority Undergraduate Students." *The Journal of Negro Education* 84, no. 2: 175–186. https://doi.org/10.7709/jnegroeducation.84.2.0175.

Price, Margaret, and Stephanie L. Kerschbaum. 2017. "Promoting Supportive Academic Environments for Faculty with Mental Illnesses: Resource Guide and Suggestions for Practice." *Temple University Collaborative on Community Inclusion.* http://tucollaborative.org.

Pryal, Katie R. Guest. 2017. *Life of the Mind Interrupted: Essays on Mental Health and Disability in Higher Education.* Chapel Hill, NC: Blue Crow Books.

Ramsey, Jennifer L., and Abby L. Spencer. 2019. "Interns and Imposter Syndrome: Proactively Addressing Resilience." *Medical Education* 53, no. 5: 504–505. https://dx.doi.org/10.1111/medu.13852.

Rodriguez, Amardo, Mohan J. Dutta, and Elizabeth F. Desnoyers-Colas. 2019. "Introduction to Special issue on Merit, Whiteness, and Privilege." *Departures in Critical Qualitative Research* 8, no. 4: 3–9. https://doi.org/10.1525/dcqr.2019.8.4.3.

Russell-Pinson, Lisa, and M. Lynne Harris. 2019. "Anguish and Anxiety, Stress and Strain: Attending to Writers' Stress in the Dissertation Process." *Journal of Second Language Writing* 43: 63–71. https://doi.org/10.1016/j.jslw.2017.11.005.

Saks, Elyn. 2007. *The Center Cannot Hold: My Journey through Madness.* New York: Hachette Books.

Seal, Andrew. 2018. "How the University Became Neoliberal." *The Chronicle of Higher Education.* June 8, 2018. https://www.chronicle.com/article/How-the-University-Became/243622.

Small, Dan. 2019. "Defining Moments and Healing Emplotment: 'I Have Cancer; It Doesn't Have Me." *Health Communication* 34, no. 4: 515–517. https://doi.org/ 10.1080/10410236.2017.1418190.
Smith, Rachel A., and Amanda Applegate. 2018. "Mental Health Stigma and Communication and Their Intersections with Education." *Communication Education* 67, no. 3: 382–393. https://doi.org/10.1080/03634523.2018.1465988.
Stout, Patricia A., Jorge Villegas, and Nancy A. Jennings. "Images of Mental Illness in the Media: Identifying Gaps in the Research." 2004. *Schizophrenia Bulletin* 30, no. 3: 543–561. https://doi.org/10.1093/oxfordjournals.schbul.a007099.
Szetela, Adam. 2018. "Feeling Anxious? You're Not the Only One." *The Chronicle of Higher Education*. April 13, 2018. https://www.chronicle.com/article/feeling-anx ious-youre-not-the-only-one/.
Venetis, Maria K, Skye Chernichky-Karcher, and Patricia E. Gettings. 2018. "Disclosing Mental Illness Information to a Friend: Exploring How the Disclosure Decision-Making Model Informs Strategy Selection." *Health Communication* 33, no. 6: 653–663. https://doi.org/10.1080/10410236.2017.1294231.
Waight, Emma, and Aline Giordano. 2018. "Doctoral Students' Access to Non-academic Support for Mental Health." *Journal of Higher Education Policy and Management* 40, no. 4: 390–412. https://doi.org/10.1080/1360080X.2018.1478613.
Wahl, Otto F. 2003. *Media Madness: Public Images of Mental Illness*. New Brunswick, NJ: Rutgers University Press.
Wall, Sarah. 2008. "Easier Said than Done: Writing an Autoethnography." *International Journal of Qualitative Methods* 7: 38–53. https://doi.org/10.1177/1 60940690800700103.
White, Allie, and Sara LaBelle. 2019. "A Qualitative Investigation of Instructors' Perceived Communicative Roles in Students' Mental Health Management." *Communication Education* 68, no. 2: 133–155. https://doi.org/10.1080/03634523 .2019.1571620.

Chapter 3

Structuration of U.S. Communication Graduate Students' Stress

Rahul Mitra, Nubia Brewster, Patrice M. Buzzanell, Julia Grzywinski, Elizabeth-Ann Pandzich

Recent academic studies document the epidemic of stress faced by graduate students when they encounter an uncertain job market and unsupportive institutional environments (Arnold 2014). However, the existing studies on this topic include either anecdotal accounts or macro-level data, and rarely consider the underlying disciplinary or geographical contexts. In contrast, this present study is a situated analysis of graduate students' experiences of stress and burnout in the communication discipline. Communication is regarded as both a social science and humanities field, depending on the expertise in the department and subfield. We emphasize graduate school's role as a professional space, where career norms and professional expectations are formed (primarily for academic jobs), even as graduate students are employed as institutional workers in teaching, research, administrative, and miscellaneous jobs (Gardner 2008). Our inductive analysis, based on in-depth interviews with fifty graduate students from universities across the United States, uses structuration theory (Giddens 1984) to examine the dialectical interplay of structure and action across micro-, meso-, and macro-levels. Using this theoretical approach, we address how graduate students' experiences of stress are shaped by broader institutional ideologies (macro), departmental rules and resources (meso), and interpersonal dynamics with faculty and cohort members (micro) (Stones 2005). Our findings will strengthen the understanding of stressors that graduate students face so that institutions can create meaningful solutions to mental health issues on their campuses.

LITERATURE REVIEW

Increasingly, education researchers and policymakers recognize that academia's professional demands and institutional norms produce significant stress, anxiety, and other mental health challenges. Graduate students particularly have a stressful work environment where they must manage not only their program's intellectual rigor, but also the changing and precarious academic job market (Golde 1998; Hyun, Quinn, Madon, and Lustig 2006; Mazzola, Walker, Shockley, and Spector 2011). Using a sample in Belgium, Levecque et al. (2017) found that PhD students were far more likely to experience mental health problems such as depression compared to other highly educated individuals or undergraduates. Levecque et al. (2017) also found that work–family conflicts, job demands, and control over the job situation/role best predicted these mental conditions.

However, graduate school stressors are not restricted to finding a tenure-track job. Graduate school is also where students are socialized into norms of what it means to be a *successful* academic: having multiple peer-reviewed papers, defending a dissertation, doing interdisciplinary collaborations, and/or having good teaching evaluations (Gardner 2008). This urgency of professional development adds to schoolwork and job market pressures, creating a mixture of stress, anxiety, depression, fear, and frustration with the status quo.

Previous researchers have demonstrated that social support networks can buffer stress and help professionals cope (Singh and Singhi 2015). However, in some cases, peer social support might have negative consequences; for example, when graduate students find solace in commiserating with classmates, this activity could lead to co-rumination, which can lead to internalizing problems and increased emotional exhaustion among students (Boren 2013; Spendelow, Simonds and Avery 2017). Rumination and co-rumination can impair problem-solving skills and cause or exacerbate anxiety, depression, and embitterment (Dunn and Sensky 2018). Co-rumination is frequently part of peer commiseration. In these situations, commiseration can build on itself and deter students' abilities to develop creative solutions and take empowered actions on behalf of oneself and peers (Dunn and Sensky 2018). This destructiveness is exacerbated when graduate students are in a larger, unsupportive or hostile work environment, where the institutional apparatus seems designed to thwart their prospects, leading to a vicious cycle of stress and toxic relationships.

This chapter uses structuration theory to trace the intersection of micro-, meso-, and macro-levels of stress formation and experience in graduate school. Structuration theory also emphasizes the duality of structure, such that social structures and social actors' actions are inherently reinforced and challenged through each other (Giddens 1984; Stones 2005). Thus, our study traces the many discourses that flow across macro- through micro- contexts, shaping graduate students' experiences of stress, as well as the networks that perpetuate connection and marginalization in such instances. Our guiding research question is: How do graduate school structures and processes contribute to communication graduate students' stress?

METHOD

After obtaining permission from the first and third authors' Institutional Review Board, we collected interview data between 2012 and 2013 using Skype and telephone calls with fifty graduate students enrolled in communication programs at American universities. The data was collected as part of a larger project examining resilience and meaningful work among graduate students. Interviews ranged from forty-five to sixty minutes each. The sample included thirty-six female and seventeen male participants. Of the participants, twenty-two were enrolled in a master's program, while twenty-eight were doctoral students. The semi-structured interviews included questions about participants' daily and usual work routines; the kinds of social support they enjoyed; memorable incidents and messages encountered at graduate school; stressful experiences (and their consequences); and key turning points that caused them to rethink their perceptions of graduate school. The interviews were transcribed, with all identifying information masked to preserve participants' anonymity through pseudonyms and deleting the names of their graduate schools and institutions. Our research yielded approximately twenty-four hours of data and 608 single-spaced transcribed pages.

Three trained coders analyzed the data using the constructivist constant comparative approach that enables researchers to incorporate their own knowledge to assist interpretations of findings and contributions (Charmaz 2006). Repeated interactions among the coders and the two authors who originally designed this project resulted in consensus of meaning during open coding and mutual agreement when authors and coders did not agree on code labels. Selective coding yielded families of open codes along categories such as destructive relationships, hostile work environments, and lack of support. This structurational perspective allowed us to further refine these categories by deconstructing them to tell a more complex story connecting macro-, meso-, and micro-levels.

FINDINGS

Our intention is to explain continuities across macro-, meso-, and micro-levels, rather than imply distinct boundaries between each of them, or even unidirectional causality.

Macro Themes

Graduate students, and even those at non-research-intensive institutions, frequently cited macro-level discourses of *publish or perish*. This imperative to continually publish stems from institutional prestige and changing academic job market expectations. The graduate student participants linked *publish or perish* to harsh (bordering on abusive) criticism they faced about their work from faculty and mentors and to toxic hyper-competition among peers. Harry, a graduate student with a pre-existing anxiety diagnosis, discussed his program's hostile environment. He described the difference between his undergraduate and graduate experiences:

> I won't say that it's been harder to handle that mental health issue since starting graduate school. Largely because I think it's an environment calculated to create a sort of insecurity that at least my undergraduate experience was not.

Harry's statement about the environment led to his further comments about competitiveness and jealousy. For example, he described how his program's structure pitted him against a classmate. The two students were up against one another to have a book review published. Harry said that he and this classmate often competed for publications. When the other student's review was selected for publication over Harry's, Harry was unsatisfied with the outcome.

> It was widely thought that he and I were the most likely to be published. He ended up being the one that was. I got jealous, so I immediately went and wrote a different book review, and I did get it published in a different publication. There is that.

Meanwhile, Dottie, a doctoral student with a health communication emphasis, recounted her experiences with unsupportive advisors and faculty. Dottie hoped to take a qualitative research approach to her academic work, but her administration did not support her methodological objective. Dottie stated:

> The problem isn't so much that they're doing quantitative work. I think the problem is that they don't have too much sympathy towards qualitative work or an understanding of it. There's no way to have them on my committee and have a supportive committee. I'd just have a committee that was squabbling.

Participants cited other institutional influences such as ongoing debates about the *incommensurability* among different sub-fields and epistemologies that characterize the communication discipline (Corman 2000). To this end, some participants shared how perceived incommensurability led to tensions among department faculty and harsh criticism of graduate work that did not satisfy partisan notions of communication theory. This situation led these students to experience professional insecurity and departmental marginalization. For example, one graduate student, Penelope, said she initially thought her institution would be culturally inclusive, but she became incredibly frustrated and upset about its exclusivity. Penelope stated, "I just thought it was gonna be this idealistic place, where there were so many brown, critical people. I got here, and it was all white. It was very pretentious. It was very upsetting." For Penelope, it was not simply diversity in terms of racial and ethnic representation, but it was also the lack of "critical people" or those who would challenge the status quo and embody difference in critical inquiry.

Finally, participants described how societal discourses that valorized diversity and multiculturalism compelled universities to recruit students from multiethnic backgrounds, but without adequately investing in them or understanding their lived experiences. Consequently, interviewees criticized their programs' tokenism and rampant stereotyping. For instance, Penelope described her experiences in being the only gay student, as well as one of very few students of color in her department. Penelope said that students were not subtle in their thoughts about her:

> I had folks tell me. I had people in my cohort tell me that they thought that I was a minority admission. They said, that therefore, I didn't really belong in the same ways that they did. I got in on some kind of social advantage, that they got it on the merit of their work. It's not just once that I heard that. I wish the program had more of a recognition of that, and addressed it, instead of pretending that it doesn't exist.

Meso Contexts

At the meso-level, participants highlighted departmental politics, unclear policies, inadequate resources, and lack of mentorship as key reasons for their stress. Participants cited examples of departmental politics such as arguments about field incommensurability and interpersonal conflict. Grace identified politics as leading to her unconstructive relationship in the department and disheartening graduate school experience:

> I was so disappointed by the politics, so disappointed. I didn't see it in my master's program because I think sometimes master's students are kind of sheltered from that, but the PhD program—and I don't know if this is unique to my program or not, but you get more responsibilities and you work more intimately with faculty members. You take part on committees and what not out there, and

the politics is so disappointing because you realize quickly that people aren't doing things because they love learning. That was really disappointing for me.

Unclear rules and policies at the department level also intensified these situations because graduate students had little recourse and were consequently marginalized. One student, Helen, described her interactions with a professor who refused to allow her to attend an international trip that explored her interest area. Helen had done the trip the previous year. Helen felt that she and the particular professor developed a positive working relationship as she learned more about her specialty area through their collaboration. When the trip was announced again the next year, the professor did not allow her to attend for reasons not disclosed to her.

> I didn't just get passed over. I was actively passed over, and that my advisor went to him and said, "Don't forget, here's this student. She's really—this is really, strongly her research area, and this is exactly what she wants to do," and he said, "No, she can't go." She said, "Well, I don't understand," and then he said, "Well, she can't go." She said, "Well, are there any reasons, and the answer was no. I'm not telling you why. She can't go," and I just was so bitterly disappointed, because I mean, this is my career.

Helen felt betrayed by her professor. She was discouraged and confused about the actions in light of their previous positive relationship. When another professor went to the same location for a different trip, Helen was offered a spot. However, the initial professor who actively denied Helen the first trip presumably spoke with the professor now offering her a position. After the conversation, the new professor suddenly refused to allow Helen to attend the trip.

> So, it was just like at every turn he kind of went out of his way to actively work against me, but nobody understands why. Nobody understands what—what did I do? What did I do—three of his classes I got "A's," and so, I was producing decent work, but it just was so baffling. That whole experience was really frustrating, and if—everyone kind of just agreed, it's clearly a personality conflict.

Although Helen explained that she and the professor could have had a personality conflict, the professor's inconsistent and unexplained behavior contributed to graduate school's competitive environment.

Helen's example also reflects departmental politics, the remaining source for unhealthy competition. Interviewees said that crucial professional development resources were either missing or denied to graduating students when faculty and administrators considered the students' actions to be inconsistent with departmental (or college and institutional) priorities and power hierarchies (Pelletier, Kottke, and Sirotnik 2019). Students lacked adequate graduate student funding, prestigious teaching or research opportunities, and pedagogical training. One doctoral interviewee, Jewel, was given useless resources during her graduate program. She said, "There's a lot of resources at the university, but then coming here, realizing, okay, there are a lot of resources, but not necessarily the ones that I had wanted so much."

Finally, several participants described the lack of useful and compassionate mentors among department faculty, either because they were too busy in their own lives and careers to adequately guide graduate students, or they were disinterested in graduate students' work because of field incommensurability issues. When Dottie found an advisor to confide in, she still felt unsupported and that there was truly no way for her to do the work that she wanted to pursue:

> He said something like, "You need to follow your passion. If you're passionate about health, then you need to stick with health." I was like, "Well, then that's bullshit because there's no support for it. How the hell am I going to stick with health if none of the people have any sympathy?"

Another student, Tara, explained that her attempts to find supportive faculty were seemingly unsuccessful, so she turned elsewhere for support: "Well, finally after giving up on trying to work with professors and make a connection because that's impossible [laughter] unfortunately, I pretty much just turned to other grad students."

These themes were all nested in participants' accounts. For instance, despite institutional directives to value diversity, inadequate funding and other resources such as mentoring often accompanied other departmental practices such as unclear policies and racial stereotyping. One example of stereotyping occurred when international students were asked to teach intercultural communication classes, despite no subject training, simply because of their non-U.S. country of origin. For instance, Shar felt that stereotyping played a role in her perception of the discrimination that she experienced. Shar said that her department routinely asked international students to teach cross-cultural and intercultural communication, while her American-born counterparts did not have the same request:

> There are a couple of other international students in our department. So, we were kind of slated to teach intercultural classes just because we were international students, even though we did not have any kind of background in . . . scholarly background in the cultural communication. So, people who did have a background who were not international students were passed over, and people who were international students were given those kinds of classes to teach. So, that was an interesting thing that happened.

Shar explained that she attempted to speak with faculty about her lack of experience in intercultural theory, but faculty subtly told her that she was eligible to teach the course simply because she was an international student.

> Basically, went and talked to people who were supposed to be giving these kinds of things out... the positions to me... made the positions... and I basically said that I did not have any experience in teaching this kind of stuff. So, they basically talked about—they did not refer to my international status, but they basically said that depending on the needs of the department, we thought you were the best person to teach.

In this section on meso-level contexts, participants described a number of departmental procedures, policies, and norms that they perceived as contributing to their stress in graduate school. Participants expressed their frustrations, anger, and sometimes simply resignation that there seemed to be little that they could do to find out answers or change the system.

Micro Interactions

Regarding everyday micro-level interactions, participants described several manifestations of graduate school stress. *Toxic hyper-competition* among peers was attributed to a confluence of macro- and meso-factors (e.g., publish or perish imperative, lack of funding, departmental politics), so that participants reported being pitted against their peers by faculty or the larger cohort. Although hyper-competition sometimes motivated students to perform better, it usually created fragmentation and envy among peers. Some students felt socially disconnected, while others felt socially shunned by their classmates. Grace explained her disappointment about her academic work, and passion for learning, and her peers' receptiveness to herself:

> You realize that even though there are these people who should be like minded and just love to learn and love to make new discoveries, that there's still a whole lot of ego involved, that you're still going to deal with people who treat others poorly. They don't respect opinions or ideas. They don't listen well. They're arrogant, just random things like that.

The participants said that resentment among the cohort grew when successful graduate students were rewarded with scarce resources such as funding and research opportunities, while others were not. This situation created what many viewed as division between the haves and have-nots, and perpetuated the vicious hyper-competitive cycle. One student, Hallie, described this environment:

The master's program that I was in, it was only 20 percent of the students were fully-funded, and it created really radical divides, because the school never released who was funded, but you obviously figure it out pretty quickly, and as one of the students who was receiving funding, there was two kinds of backlashes. There was the one where students were almost angry because they felt as though their tuition money was supporting your education, which, I mean, it probably was, given how expensive the tuition was and the stipends we were getting, but the other problem that occurred was we were able to get so much more work done than the students that were paying for their degrees that, first, when they graded on a curve, we would always come out ahead.

Participants also reported deep *professional insecurity*, resulting from inadequate funding, training, resources, or mentorship, or because they felt the department devalued their work and expertise. Another doctoral student, Carrie, explained her frustration about how not having adequate resources inhibited her teaching assistant role at her institution:

Well, my school for example, doesn't give you any—or doesn't require any pedagogy courses or [silence] experience . . . . No pedagogy courses, no certification. They drop you into a classroom and then they never really follow up to see if I'm actually teaching what the kids should be learning.

One student, Renee, recalled being told that her work would not lead to future success: "I was told very early on by some people in my department that being an applied scholar would land me homeless and that I would never find a job as an applied scholar and that I needed to pick a methodology and that I couldn't do interdisciplinary work."

Such insecurities often led graduate students to abandon their original research trajectories for something more aligned with faculty imperatives. In other cases, the students simply stopped asking faculty and departmental staff for help. For example, Dottie changed her project's focus after determining that she would probably not earn faculty or peer support. "It was a hard decision. It really was. It made me rethink a lot of things, to the point where it was almost like, should I drop out of (university) and go to another place, like transfer to another place or what? I felt like I had to. I felt pressured, in that sense."

Dottie's story reflects the negative relationship that can form when students don't have a proper support system in graduate school. They may feel pressured to change their paths to find support. In the latter case, participants either eventually disengaged from the graduate program altogether, or fell back on a small group of trusted peers for social support, but probably missed out on valuable professional development. As quoted earlier, Tara also explained how she turned elsewhere for encouragement following unsuccessful, even *impossible* attempts to connect with faculty.

Lack of institutional or department support commonly stemmed from irrelevant or inadequate resources for students. Jewel explained that, "There's a lot of resources at the university, but then coming here, realizing, okay, there are a lot of resources, but not necessarily the ones that I had wanted so much." Jewel and Tara described how their institutions did not meet their expectations and inhibited their success. We observed that students felt as if their peers or organizations' lack of support led them to experience negative relationships.

Disconnection also occurred for reasons other than lack of trust. Some participants isolated themselves because they found the tokenism, stereotyping, and even racism in their departments—sometimes from their peers—too stressful. International students frequently discussed discrimination and racism during their interviews. They described subtle to more obvious displays of marginalization. Greg, an international student, explained that coming to America allowed him to learn what racism truly was: "Well, at the interpersonal level here, I have been—well, the experience here taught me about what racism is, so this is at the interpersonal level."

Greg went on to further explore his encounter with racism. As a student, he experienced obvious intense discrimination from one of his cohort members. He recalled a female student who constantly talked with him and asked to spend time with him. Greg asked the student to accompany him to his hometown in China during their break. Although Greg believed that his classmate enjoyed the trip, the other student told false stories about her experience to others after the new semester began:

> She keeps telling the department what bad person I was, I'm behaving and telling a story I'm mistreating her and I give her food poisoning. There's so many stories. She just walk around the department telling people her bad experience with me and with my family back home. I say, "This is not true. I mean, you really enjoyed it, and then with our trip, you only bought your ticket. You said they were happy, and how come you tell the whole department that I'm mistreating you?"

Furthering the harassment, the student began to publicly embarrass Greg during class. Aggressively asking Greg questions, the student would then complain to the department head (who Greg also identified as his boss) that Greg did not respond to her requests. The harassment was unwarranted and inexplicable. Greg could not recall a time where the university willingly stepped in. He said:

> This goes worse and worse. Sometimes in class, she will try to falsely talk. She will ask me, like five minutes' questions, and then I don't know how to answer. I just look at her like I don't know. Then, my boss once called me to talk with

him. He said, "How come you don't answer your cohort's question? What's wrong with you?" I was like, I said, "I'm not able to. I just don't know how to respond in appropriate way, and you were pushing me."

The ongoing destructive relationship greatly marred how Greg felt about school and his experiences there. He said, "Here in grad school . . . . I particularly feel isolated because some way, because of my skin color." His poor experience with the classmate further isolated him from his cohort. No faculty members addressed the harassment, even after Greg made several inquiries. He began to feel like his department did not value him: "I'm just an invisible person in a department."

Other interviewees desired meaningful peer connections, but they could not obtain it. This led them to lack a support network for managing graduate school anxieties. One doctoral student, Fergie, identified how the absence of social connection contributed to her anxiety toward school. Lacking interpersonal connection made it difficult for her to navigate school and build positive peer relationships.

> That social, I don't know, bonding and getting together just didn't happen. It was really frustrating. Everyone always talks about when you first get to grad school you always have to plan for the meltdown because there will be one whether you want it to happen or not. I think for the most part my meltdown happened not because of classes and stress of adjusting to the level of work that it takes to be a grad student, but the fact that I didn't have anyone to share my frustrations with. Even the good days, there was just nobody there.

In sum, some participants reported being marginalized by their peers (often in departments divided by incommensurability concerns and hyper-competitiveness or resource disparities; e.g., Renee and Dottie), or by peers and faculty members who no longer wanted to work with them (and persuaded others to shun them as well and/or treat them in discriminatory ways, e.g., Greg).

DISCUSSION

Our findings from the interview data demonstrate a multilevel structurational account of communication graduate students' experiences of stress at American institutions. This perspective traces the intersections between institutional ideologies (macro-level), departmental policies (meso-level), and interpersonal dynamics (micro-level) that shape stress, providing a situated understanding of the problems at stake.

Moreover, our inductive and situated study demonstrates how discipline-specific concerns about field incommensurability, diversity, and the academic job market crucially shape experiences of graduate school stress. We acknowledge that concerns expressed by graduate students in our study are not endemic to the entire discipline, nor are concerns always manifest in the same ways as our participants noted. In other words, although the existing research in this area indicates general stressors related to graduate school (Hyun et al. 2006; Levecque et al. 2017; Mazzola et al. 2011), our study demonstrates how interpersonal-, departmental-, field- and institutional-specific stressors can form a culture of stress and toxicity in communication departments (Pelletier, Kottke, and Sirotnik 2019). Communication graduate students struggle to figure out how to change the toxic environment on their own, or to find others with whom they can develop alliances for meso- and macro-level change. Our findings suggest that a locale- and field-specific approach to graduate student stress and mental health is needed to develop targeted institutional policies to support graduate students.

First, our study demonstrates that *toxic hyper-competition* stems from both macro- and meso-levels. Therefore, rather than complain about the *publish or perish* ideology, and otherwise plead helplessness, administrators and faculty can take concrete steps to address the issue. These steps might range from providing more support forums and messages to overstressed graduate students, to instituting policies on disbursing key resources, to adopting a zero-toleration stance on department politics that harm graduate students' prospects. As one example of resources, more than 230 institutions of higher education in the United States subscribe to the National Center for Faculty Development and Diversity (NCFDD 2020), which has been dedicated to "independent professional development, training, and mentoring community for faculty members, postdocs, and graduate students" since 2010. In addition, communication departments could sync their in-house trainings on professionalism and best practices with the Council of Graduate Schools' Preparing Future Faculty (PFF) program so that graduate students can learn about the support that they can expect or request during their graduate, postdoc, and faculty experiences (Council of Graduate Schools 1993). Departments could also encourage members to participate in the National Communication Association's (NCA) and International Communication Association's (ICA) regularly sponsored pre-conferences, conference sessions, and career-developmental and support networks, particularly those listed under NCA's "Convention & Events" and "Academic & Professional Resources" such as the annual NCA Doctoral Honors Seminar and NCA Institute for Faculty Development's annual summer conference. The monthly ICA Newsletter (under "Publications") has columns on graduate student life and career opportunities, among other resources. ICA's online "Resources" has a section called "Career Center."

Second, our participants highlighted *hidden discrimination* that stems from race, ethnicity, gender, national origin, research area, methodology, and faculty mentor identity, to mention a few biases. Administrators can address the issue by streamlining policies on reporting discriminatory instances. These policies can prevent tokenism and stereotyping in teaching assignments, ensure transparency in dispersal of key professional resources, and support superlative mentoring for students of color. For their part, graduate students can organize workshops on tokenism and stereotyping, as well as social gatherings to downplay toxic competition and marginalization of diverse students. They do so at NCA, ICA, and regional conferences. In the Communication Department at University of South Florida, graduate students work with their department leadership and communication graduate associations to develop sessions and standing committees on equity, inclusiveness, social justice, and accountability. This department also has a graduate student mission statement and Student Bill of Rights and Responsibilities.

Finally, administrators and graduate student organizations can build *meaningful support networks* to help students deal with stress, anxiety, and professional insecurities. For instance, our research raises questions whether faculty receive proper training to create a supportive and compassionate communication environment for their mentées and other students. Likewise, targeted training could help graduate students create productive advising mentorships. For example, training could help students understand reasonable expectations for mentor–mentée contributions to the relationship. This training could also enable students to identify when mentorships are dysfunctional, and what to do about it (Eddington and Buzzanell 2018; Johnson and Huwe 2002).

In addition, graduate student organizations could survey their members to map the diverse landscape of newcomers and current graduate students—age, first-generation graduate student, race and ethnicity, cultural heritage, military veteran status, visa status, and proximity of family members, among other potential areas of commonality and difference—to display and work with the composition of each communication graduate student cohort and the larger program. In theory, departmental programming and social gatherings could better welcome diverse experiences to decrease stress, and especially during difficult disruptions such as COVID-19.

Our recommendations for interventions affirm graduate students' agency and the responsibilities that communication departments and educational institutions have to support these students. We present our multilevel structurational analysis of communication graduate students' reported stressors to describe where students feel as though their peers, professors, departmental administrators, institutions, and communication associations could assist them more fully during their moments of uncertainty and of socialization into the discipline. We encourage graduate students and members of the professoriate to consider how changes in what they do regularly, and how they enact their departmental and institutional cultures can promote graduate students' well-being and connections to others.

REFERENCES

Arnold, Carrie. 2014. "Paying Graduate School's Mental Toll." *Science Careers*, Feb. 4, 2014. https://www.sciencemag.org/careers/2014/02/paying-graduate-schools-mental-toll.

Boren, Justin. 2013. "Co-Rumination Partially Mediates the Relationship between Social Support and Emotional Exhaustion among Graduate Students." *Communication Quarterly* 61, no. 3 (June): 253–267. https://doi.org/10.1080/01463373.2012.751436.

Charmaz, Kathy. 2006. *Constructing Grounded Theory: A Practical Guide through Qualitative Analysis*. Thousand Oaks, CA: Sage.

Corman, Steven. 2000. "The Need for Common Ground." In *Perspectives on Organizational Communication: Finding Common Ground*, edited by Steven Corman and M. Scott Poole, 3–13. New York: Guilford.

Council of Graduate Schools. 1993. "Preparing Future Faculty." https://preparing-faculty.org/.

Dunn, Joanne, and Tom Sensk. 2018. "Psychological Processes in Chronic Embitterment: The Potential Contribution of Rumination." *Psychological Trauma: Theory, Research, Practice, and Policy* 10, no. 1: 7–13. https://doi.org/10.1037/tra0000291.

Eddington, Sean, and Patrice M. Buzzanell. 2018. "Tensions within Bullying and Career Resilience in Higher Education." In *The Routledge Handbook of Communication and Bullying*, edited by Richard West and Christina Beck, 164–172. New York: Routledge.

Gardner, Susan. 2008. "Fitting the Mold of Graduate School: A Qualitative Study of Socialization in Doctoral Education." *Innovative Higher Education* 33, no. 2: 125–138. https://doi.org/10.1007/s10755-008-9068-x.

Giddens, Anthony. 1984. *The Constitution of Society: Outline of the theory of Structuration*. Berkeley, CA: University of California Press.

Golde, Chris. 1998. "Beginning Graduate School: Explaining First-year Doctoral Attrition." *New Directions for Higher Education* 1998, no. 101: 55–64. https://doi.org/10.1002/he.10105.

Hyun, Jenny, Brian C. Quinn, Temina Madon, and Steve Lustig. 2006. "Graduate Student Mental Health: Needs Assessment and Utilization of Counseling Services." *Journal of College Student Development* 47, no. 3: 247–266. http://dx.doi.org/10.1353/csd.2006.0030.

International Communication Association (ICA). n.d. https://www.icahdq.org/.

Johnson, W. Brad, and Jennifer M. Huwe. 2002. "Toward a Typology of Mentorship Dysfunction in Graduate School." *Psychotherapy: Theory, Research, Practice, Training* 39, no. 1: 44–55. https://doi.org/10.1037/0033-3204.39.1.44.

Levecque, Katia, Frederik Anseel, Alain De Beuckelaer, Johan Van der Heyden, and Lydia Gisle. 2017. "Work Organization and Mental Health Problems in PhD Students." *Research Policy* 46, no. 4: 868–879. https://doi.org/10.1016/j.respol.20 17.02.008.

Mazzola, Joseph, Erin J. Walker, Kristen M. Shockley, and Paul E. Spector. 2011. "Examining Stress in Graduate Assistants: Combining Qualitative and Quantitative Survey Methods." *Journal of Mixed Methods Research* 5, no. 3: 198–211. https://doi.org/10.1177/1558689811402086.

National Center for Faculty Development and Diversity (NCFDD). 2020. "Changing the Face of Power in the Academy." https://www.facultydiversity.org/ncfddmission.

National Communication Association (NCA). n.d. https://www.natcom.org.

Singh, Ashak, and Nitu Singhi. 2015. "Organizational Role Stress and Social Support as Predictors of Job Satisfaction among Managerial Personnel." *Journal of Psychosocial Research* 10, no. 1: 1–10.

Pelletier, Kathie, Janet L. Kottke, and Barbara W. Sirotnik. 2019. "The Toxic Triangle in Academia: A Case Analysis of the Emergence and Manifestation of Toxicity in a Public University." *Leadership* 15, no. 4: 405–432. https://doi.org/10.1177/1742715018773828.

Spendelow, Jason, Laura M. Simonds, and Rachel E. Avery. 2017. "The Relationship between Co-rumination and Internalizing Problems: A Systematic Review and Meta-analysis." *Clinical Psychology & Psychotherapy* 24, no. 2 (March/April): 512–527. https://doi.org/10.1002/cpp.2023.

Stones, Rob. 2005. *Structuration Theory*. London: Macmillan International Higher Education.

Chapter 4

"Burn It Down"

The Graduate Student Burnout Experience

Victoria McDermott and Nike Bahr

Although education research extensively validates predicting factors and long-term impacts of burnout on people employed in academic careers (Bilge 2006, 1725; Stoeber, Childs, Hayward, and Feast 2011, 523–524; Watts and Robertson 2011, 33), research has yet to examine the impact of stigmatized career paths on people's perceptions of burnout. Stigma, with its potential to influence people's sensemaking process and worldview, may negatively characterize people's perceptions of careers such as public service and medical fields that are widely known to cause burnout. As such, this chapter explores how the stigma of academic culture impacts the graduate student experience. Through evaluating the survey responses of 139 eligible graduate students using thematic coding (Lindlof and Taylor 2017, 320; Owen 1984, 275), our findings suggest that graduate students in the United States face extensive and continual stress in their personal and professional lives due to academic expectations and procedures. Our survey responses also suggest that although students expected stress in graduate school, the lack of support from mentors, as well as their experiences in observing mentors and advisors' experiences with burnout, leads graduate students to expect and often romanticize burnout. Based on our study's findings, we recommend that institutions increase support for graduate students, change the portrayal of mental health, and reform academic culture to improve graduate students' experience and reduce burnout in higher education.

BURNOUT

Burnout is defined as a syndrome of emotional exhaustion and depersonalization that leads to decreased effectiveness at work (Maslach, Jackson, and Leiter

1996, 192). Burnout can manifest in a variety of ways that range from an inability to perform professionally to suicide in extreme cases (Maslach, Jackson, and Leiter 1996, 192). According to the World Health Organization (WHO), burnout has become a more severe and pervasive health issue because of Western workplace culture's emphasis on overwork as productivity. This situation has led the WHO to recognize burnout as a factor that influences health status (Cassella 2019, para. 1–2; World Health Organization 2019, para. 3–6).

Over time, burnout can potentially negatively impact people's physical and mental health. For example, in a 2012 study of 9,000 employed adults, workers scoring in the top 20 percent on the workplace burnout scale had a 79 percent increased risk of being diagnosed with coronary heart disease (Toker et al. 2012, 843–844). These employees were also at an increased risk for high cholesterol, type 2 diabetes, hospitalization due to a cardiovascular disorder, musculoskeletal pain, prolonged fatigue, headaches, gastrointestinal issues, respiratory problems, severe injuries, and even mortality before age forty-five (Salvagioni et al. 2017, 5–16; Cassella 2019, para. 16). Burnout's psychological effects include insomnia, depression, use of psychotropic and antidepressant medications, hospitalization for mental disorders, and psychological ill-health symptoms (para. 16). Previous research indicates that the profound emotional exhaustion and negativity caused by burnout can alter a person's brain, making it more challenging to deal with stress in the future (Golkar et al. 2014, 8–9). The longer a person experiences burnout, the more difficult it becomes to recover physically and mentally (Cassella 2019, para. 12).

STIGMA OF BURNOUT IN WESTERN CULTURE

Since becoming an "occupational syndrome" (Cassella 2019, para. 2), the term *burnout* has also become a label-related stigma. In the United States, burnout is viewed as shameful and a sign of personal and professional weakness (Bianchi et al. 2016, 92; Cresswell and Eklund 2006, 219; Dyrbye et al. 2015, 964–967). Schaufeli (2017) suggests that sociocultural development in the United States, such as increasing social fragmentation and the rise of individualistic *me culture*, further fuel the heavy stigmatization of burnout (121–124). Workplace culture in the United States values assertiveness, efficiency, and emphasizes the individual over the group while celebrating relentless productivity, aka, "Hustle Culture" (Griffith 2019, para. 3). Coined by Erin Griffith in a *New York Times* article (2019), the term *Hustle Culture* describes an obsession with avid productivity and striving to accomplish more with little rest (para. 3). Griffith (2019) concludes that the "logical endpoint of excessively avid work, of course, is burnout" (para. 22). "Hustle

Culture," coupled with the overall globalization, privatization, and liberalization of the Western workplace, causes rapid changes in a person's working life that require agile adaptation to navigate successfully (Schaufeli 2017, 119). Additionally, the individualistic "Hustle Culture" demonizes taking time off from "the grind" (Griffith 2019, para. 4), and stigmatizes self-care, chastising those who prioritize mental health over productivity. This general workplace acceleration, increased workload, fast-paced adaptation, and heightened temporal pressure with little rest or time off may be optimal for breeding burnout (Schaufeli 2017, 120).

Furthermore, stigma can have far-reaching implications for those who have a stigmatized condition such as a mental illness (Goffman 1986). Stigmatized labels, such as being *burned out* or having depression, can prevent people from seeking help. Researchers indicate that stigma can negatively impact people's willingness to seek out resources such as counseling when experiencing burnout (Andrew and Brenner 2018, under "Problems with Treating Physician Depression"). For example, many medical professionals have reported that they are reluctant to seek mental health treatment because of the fear of stigma, shame, or losing their employment (Farmer 2018, para. 24). In August 2018, it was estimated that around 300–400 physicians commit suicide each year because of burnout (Andrew and Brenner 2018, under "Depression in Physicians"). For those who do seek help, the fear of the burnout stigma is so severe that physicians have been known to take measures such as using false names when using support services and searching for therapy miles outside their local communities (Farmer 2018, para. 25). Moreover, a 2016 study of burnout found that people with higher levels of burnout more frequently perpetuated the negative stigma around seeking help to improve one's mental health (Endriulaitiene et al. 2016, 255). Previous research even suggests that stigma itself might serve as a potential workplace stressor that can eventually create or increase a person's burnout (Corrigan et al. 2014, 4–5; Endriulaitiene et al. 2016, 259–260; Mårtensson et al. 2014, 785–787; Schulze 2007, 137).

CULTURE OF ACADEMIA

Both academic researchers and journalists acknowledge that academia is a difficult place to be employed: Academic careers have a highly competitive atmosphere that requires one to commit to long, irregular hours and limited leisure time for a healthy work–life balance to be successful (Bell, Rajendran, and Teiler 2012, 26–27). For example, the perceived freedom of flexible work hours and research topics gives academics "the freedom to work all the time" (Tierney 1997, 11). Often described as a "prestige economy" (Fyfe et al. 2017, 3), academia operates on the symbolic wealth system driven by publishing as a critical motivator for career progression (Fyfe et al. 2017, 10–13). "Publish or perish" (coined by Coolidge 1932, 308) is now the harsh reality for most academics (Rawat and Meena 2014, 87). To be considered a success in academia and get a tenured position, graduate students, faculty, and professors must work tirelessly to build their academic resumes with teaching opportunities, research publications, service to their discipline, and in many cases, involvement in their local communities.

Additionally, in 2016, Yu, Chae, and Chang (2016) found that academia was rife with socially prescribed perfectionism, which is the idea that others have unrealistic expectations for behavior and that people cannot meet these standards (53–54). Many studies examine the impact of the *perfectionism* required in academia for career success (Abouserie 1996, 49; Cazan and Nastsa 2015, 1577–1578; Chang, Seong, and Lee 2020, 8–10; Hill and Curran 2015, 23–26; Karimi et al. 2014, 61; Zhang, Gan, and Cham 2007, 1529). Professors believe there is external pressure to be perfect and that others will evaluate them critically if perfection is not maintained. To this end, many academics are unofficially expected to work seven days a week while the academic year is in session, including late nights, weekends, and even dedicating personal time to their department or university to maintain this perfectionist facade (Moore and Amey 1993, 29–32). In the summer months, a time many might consider an extended vacation, academics are expected to conduct research, teach, or make extra money to financially prepare for the upcoming academic year. For many past, current, and future members of academia, this career path becomes a lifestyle requiring an unquestioned drive for achievement and dedication, rather than merely a career (Tierney 1997, 12). Over time, the long workdays paired with the need to attain a socially prescribed level of perfection can lead to negative long-term impacts on mental health and academic self-efficacy.

HISTORY OF THE GRADUATE STUDENT EXPERIENCE

Graduate school has had a tenuous history with regard to graduate student mental health. Previous research suggests that the graduate student experience can be difficult, stressful, and occasionally mentally and physically detrimental (Berezow 2018, para. 1; Braxton et al. 2011; Evans et al. 2018, 282–283; Goodboy, Martin, and Johnson 2015, 277–278). The American Council on Science and Health reported in 2018 that students in subjects such as the hard sciences, law, and medicine will devote as many as fifty, sixty, and even eighty hours a week to reading, studying, and completing school work (Berezow 2018, para. 2). These strenuous work hours can lead to feelings of isolation and exhaustion (Tierney 1997, 11–12). Some contributing factors to this exhaustion include managing multiple academic assignments and the pressure to complete ongoing tasks such as teaching classes, or conducting and publishing research (Rahmati 2015, 54). Other triggering factors for negative mental and physical health impacts include the perceived lack of work–life balance, the financial burdens of graduate school, and mentor relationships that can be fraught with tension (Evans et al. 2018, 282). Because many graduate students must fulfill teaching obligations, on top of schoolwork and publishing, they have little time left for sleep, personal care, and social engagements.

According to a University of California, Berkeley study (2014), 43–46 percent of graduate students in the university's biosciences program reported having experienced depression (7). In a subsequent study at the University of Arizona (Smith and Brooks 2015), a majority of doctoral students reported rates of "more than average" or "tremendous" levels of stress provoked by school and education-related issues (1–2). Most recently, in 2018, a study of 2,279 PhD candidates in the biological/physical science, engineering, and humanities/social sciences found that 41 percent of respondents expressed suffering from moderate to severe anxiety, and 39 percent reported moderate to severe depression (Evans et al. 2018, 282–283). When compared to the general population, anxiety, and depression were found to be six times more common among PhD students than their non-academic counterparts (Evans et al. 2018, 282).

These increased rates of mental health issues among graduate students reflect generally rising rates of psychological distress in adolescents and young adults, many of whom are undergraduate students (Auerbach et al. 2018, 623–624; Mojtabai, Olfson, and Han 2016, 4–8; Twenge et al. 2018, 3). According to a study by Twenge et al. (2019), which draws on the results of the National Survey of Drug Use and Health, "serious psychological distress in the last month and suicide-related outcomes (suicidal ideation, plans, attempts, and deaths by suicide) in the last year [have] also increased among young adults 18–25 from 2008–2017" (185). With rising rates of mental distress in adolescents and young adults, the already mentally demanding task of completing graduate school can become exacerbated.

Over time, long-term mental distress and perceived unrelenting stress can lead to graduate student burnout. Research indicates that students in PhD programs report higher levels of stress than those in Master's degrees or certification programs, with ultimately 43.4 percent of doctoral students leaving their program without completing their degree (Cassuto 2013, para. 3; Sowell et al. 2008, 6). In 2017, Bullock and colleagues (2017) found a high prevalence of burnout in graduate healthcare programs (94). These findings suggest that graduate-level healthcare students have higher levels of burnout than their age-matched peers (Bullock et al. 2017, 94). Upon entering their graduate programs, the students did not differ from their peers; however, as students progressed through their graduate degree, their mental health deteriorated, and they experienced higher levels of dissatisfaction (Dyrbye et al. 2008, 339–340; Kjeldstadli et al. 2006, 5–7). Although burnout spans across disciplines, research suggests that those who pursue graduate degrees in public service, such as the medical and education fields, report higher rates of burnout (Watts and Robertson 2011, 33). While there is no research directly comparing the rates of burnout among different disciplines, the current literature focuses heavily on those in medical fields such as nurses, residents, and surgeons, as well as teachers ranging from pre-K to higher education (Campbell et al. 2010, 1630; Bauer et al. 2006, 202–203; Dyrbye et al. 2014, 443; Fore, Martin, and Bender 2002, 36; Suzuki et al. 2006, 101–102).

In academia, the pressure to produce work and achieve specific goals while entertaining superiors' high expectations begins with graduate students who have a unique position within the academic hierarchy as both student and faculty members. Their dual role requires graduate students to juggle multiple role identities in a system that requires perfectionism and results above all else. Ultimately, the pressures of graduate school coupled with academic culture create the optimal scenario for cultivating burnout (Yu, Chae, and Chang 2016, 53–54). Academia can, therefore, become a greedy institution to one's physical and mental well-being.

WEICK'S SENSEMAKING

The present study uses Weick's sensemaking process to understand the stigmatization of academia on graduate students' perceptions and their experiences with burnout. *Sensemaking* is the process by which people give meaning to their collective experiences (Weick, Sutcliffe, and Obstfeld 2005, 409–413). It is defined as "the ongoing retrospective development of plausible images that rationalize what people are doing" (Weick, Sutcliffe, and Obstfeld 2005, 409). The sensemaking process is explained through seven properties: identity, retrospection, enact, social activity, ongoing, extract cues, and plausibility over accuracy (Abolafia 2010, 363–364; Currie and Brown, 2003, 25–32; Kumar and Singhal 2012, 138; Weick, 1995, ch. 2). Sensemaking encompasses "presumption and entails actively connecting the abstract and concrete in a way that draws on experience" (Rhodes et al. 2016, 281).

Researchers can apply sensemaking's retrospective nature and shared narratives to understand common meanings of a situation (Currie and Brown

2003, 25–32). Previously, Weick's sensemaking has been used in a variety of studies to understand burnout and workplace factors that may lead to burnout. Rom and Eyal (2019, 26–30) analyzed how educators construct meaning within policy-dense work environments. Rom and Eyal (2019) suggest that the policy implementation process impacts educators' identity, and ultimately determines educators' positive or negative attitudes toward an institutional policy (26–30). Through this sensemaking lens, administrators may better understand the factors that impact the success of policy implementation in their institution (Rom and Eyal 2019, 26–30). Lehmann-Willenbrock, Allen, and Belyeu (2016) explored meeting exhaustion through the lens of sensemaking (1304–1307). Their findings suggest meetings that were considered counterproductive were linked to increased emotional exhaustion (Lehmann-Willenbrock et al. 2016, 1304–1307). As such, managers may be able to predict their employees' responses to and energy levels after a meeting (Lehmann-Willenbrock et al. 2016, 1308). Knowing this information, managers can plan meetings according to these potential dips in emotional energy (i.e., a meeting before lunch or at the end of the day as opposed to the beginning of the day) (Lehmann-Willenbrock et al. 2016, 1308). When faculty and staff experience burnout, their mental and emotional symptoms become part of the narrative for academic employees. Thus, the present study uses the sensemaking model to understand the factors and shared sensemaking that lead to graduate students' understanding and attitudes of burnout.

CURRENT ISSUE

Ultimately, graduate students who take on dual positions as students and faculty often experience many negative aspects of academia, such as a lack of funding, the pressure to frequently publish, intolerant administration, and negative-minded faculty. Currently, little research addresses the stigmatization of career fields such as academia that have high burnout rates. Much research addresses the stigmatization of burnout within medical professions and service industries. For example, Mitake et al. (2019) found that occupational mental health staff with a higher perceived stigma against mental distress experienced more severe burnout (3–4). Wallace (2012) discusses the stress of medical training and points out the acute need to destigmatize mental distress in medical professions (13). Bove and Pervan (2013) discuss how service workers have poor mental health when they experience stigmatization, despite their work's societal value (259). The emotional labor of dealing with this stigma and a lack of available mental health resources can ultimately lead to burnout (Bove and Pervan 2013, 259).

Some researchers have investigated burnout and its consequences on university faculty (Armour et al. 1987, 3; Bell, Rajendran, and Theiler 2012, 26–27;

Fowler 2015, 824.e5–824.e8; Lackritz 2004, 13–15; Watts and Robertson 2011, 33), but none has examined how the stigmatization of burnout in academia impacts the graduate student experience. Thus, we explore graduate students' sensemaking process of burnout and the associated stigma of academia that generates burnout. The fact that faculty (including tenured professors) experience high-stress levels that lead to burnout raises the question of how graduate students mitigate their current stress while being aware that their chosen career path likely poses future tenure burnout. As we consider the portrayal and communication of mental health in academia, the question becomes: Why do graduate students continue to pursue an academic career?

METHODS

Population and Sampling

To be eligible for the survey, participants had to be over age eighteen. Participants were required to be current or past graduate students at a university in the United States and had to be planning on pursuing a career in academia. We did not provide a limit on time passed since graduation, as we felt it was essential to allow graduate students from different generations to provide their burnout experiences. To obtain a diverse sample of respondents, we used a variety of recruitment strategies, including posting survey links on flyers around campus, emailing flyers to professors to share with their graduate students, and using a variety of social media platforms such as personal Facebook pages and Reddit to gain a diverse sample population. We also used a variety of listservs, such as the graduate student listserv at our university and the Communication Research and Theory Network listserv (now COMMNotes). No incentives were offered for participation.

Instrument

We developed an anonymous online survey to collect participant responses. The online survey contained a mix of open-ended, Likert scale, and close-ended survey questions (see Appendix A). The survey questions aimed to assess the specific variables of sensemaking burnout, the culture of academia, the stigma of mental health, the stigma of burnout, the impact of mentor-communicated perceptions, and coping with stress. To define these variables, we used previous literature to create the survey. To measure burnout, the survey used research from Maslach's Burnout Inventory to define *burnout* and assess factors that may cultivate burnout (Maslach and Jackson 1981, 100; Maslach, Jackson, and Leiter 1996, 193). Using the properties of Weick's sensemaking process such as retrospection, identity, and extracting cues, the survey sought to facilitate narrative development from each respondent (Weick 1995, ch. 2; Weick, Sutcliffe, and Obstfeld, 2005, 409). At the end of the survey, we used three close-ended survey questions to gather demographic data on participants' gender identity, ethnicity/race, and age.

Qualitative Analysis

Once the survey responses were collected, we analyzed the data to determine thematic patterns. We read through the responses three times. The first time we read through the responses individually without taking notes to get a foundational understanding of the data. The second time, we took notes and highlighted keywords and similar conceptualizations based on recurrence, forcefulness, and repetition (Owen 1984, 275; Lindlof and Taylor 2017, 320). As patterns emerged, they were organized into categories (Owen 1984, 275). During the third review of responses, we came together to discuss similarities and differences in the categories we identified separately. We then reorganized the categories into overarching themes to answer the research question (Lindlof and Taylor 2017, 320). Representative quotes were identified and used to exemplify each theme.

RESULTS

The online survey yielded 139 responses. In total, 109 participants—the majority—were between the ages eighteen and thirty-four; twenty-eight participants identified with the thirty-four to fifty-three age range; and three between the ages fifty-four and sixty-nine. Of the respondent sample, 62.6 percent of participants identified as women while 33.1 percent identified as men. One participant identified as a trans male/transman and four identified as genderqueer/gender non-conforming. Of all the participants, 111 identified as white, 11 reported being of Hispanic or Latino origin, and 6 identified as Asian. Two participants identified as black or African American, three identified as American Indian or Alaska Native, and six identified as other.

RQ: How does the characterization of the academy impact graduate students' perception of burnout and academia?

Students Expect Stress and Burnout

Collectively, this study's participants stated that they expected burnout in graduate school. The participants said they were aware that, once in graduate school, they would be constantly stressed, overwhelmed, and overworked.

Many mentioned they had friends or family who had shared their graduate school horror stories; however, respondents still believed they were prepared for the constant pressure.

Nevertheless, graduate school is more stressful than expected. When asked if their degree program matched their stress expectations, respondents stated that graduate school was more stressful than they anticipated. One participant stated, "I felt I was the victim of a bait and switch with my assistantship. I experienced more stress than I ever would have expected." When provided with the definition of *burnout*, 56.68 percent of respondents stated that the definition was very applicable to themselves, and 31.55 percent responded that the definition was somewhat applicable. When asked later in the survey if they had ever experienced burnout, 89 percent of participants responded "Yes.".

Participants explained that the stress in graduate school could be easier to overcome if it were not as frequent. They stated that the triggers that caused stress or stressful interactions occurred too often, leaving them with little time to recover from the last stressful event. One participant stated, "On a scale of one to 10, I'd say I existed at a constant stress level of 12." Respondents who completed the survey said they felt like they were always putting out a fire or running to jump on the next big project. The continued stress of overcoming each problematic situation led to an overall base level of fatigue and animosity toward their degree program.

Looking with Rose-Colored Glasses

While many of the participants cast academia in a harsh light, some respondents romanticized the idea that academia has the potential to become *something different*. In this hypothetical utopia, academia would be an inspiring and innovative place. One respondent explained that:

> I want it to be a place of innovation; a place where ideas are exchanged and we all work to better our fields/society, etc. I want it to be a place where good teaching is recognized and those who are willing to go above and beyond are recognized and rewarded (not taken advantage of). I want it to be a place for learning and the love of learning.

One graduate student stated that they wanted academia to be "focused on expanding knowledge and on educating new generations of intellectuals." Overall, participants stated that they wanted to pursue an academic career because of its potential to become an intellectual paradise. Another participant explained:

> I love the existence of a space to constantly pursue knowledge and have resources available to help me pursue it, and I love that it allows me to teach,

do research, and also serve in ways which help people, which to me seems like a dream job.

In its best possible outcome, academia provides the space for fostering learning and understanding to support its members. Ultimately, however, respondents indicated that their idea of the expected graduate experience did not equate to their actual experiences.

Its Own Insular World

When removing the rose-colored glasses, some participants evaluated academia much more cynically. Due to the exclusivity that is cultivated within academia, participants characterized academia as an elitist establishment. Some survey responses included terms such as "toxic" and "all-consuming." Other respondents used words such as "classist," "elitist," "abusive," and "dog-eat-dog world" to describe academic careers. One participant personified academia, saying:

> If it were a person, it would definitely be a toxic person and that I have toxic ties to it. It asks for more and more while hardly giving back. It is thankless. It is persistent. It demands time and attention and makes you feel guilty for giving time and attention elsewhere.

The negative characterization of academia continued when students compared the gap between the imagined purpose of academia and their actual academic experience. Although most participants pursuing a career in academia focused on the goal of global improvement, academia's exclusive nature, impregnable structure, and dated ideologies made them feel like it was impossible to accomplish their goals. Participants described it as "freedom, but only for the privileged few," and as "rigorous yet out of touch with the business world." Many participants stated that the field's hyper-focus on small, detailed things made academia challenging to translate to the outside world. One participant elaborated:

> Academia has a rigid culture which is very resistant to change. Norms of dress, speaking, writing, and interaction are based around White (mostly male) traditions and values, and it is difficult to create change. It's difficult to discern if most research is making an impact on real lives, so there is an overall sense of hopelessness for those who want to promote social justice with their work. Imposter syndrome is everywhere and academics feel guilt whenever they are not working, because the job never ends and there is always more that needs to be done.

The lack of flexibility within academia presents its members with continual resistance to change and, ultimately, with hopelessness. Participants also described academia as "an industry full of egos," "demanding," "inaccessible," "esoteric," "indentured servitude," and "cult-like." One participant stated, "It's a club. Which is great if you're on the inside of the club, but it can be catty and political as well." For those who are not members of the club, academia can be an exhausting and isolating experience that further perpetuates its negative impact on mental health.

Mental Health in Academia

Academia was noted to have a culture of "praising burnout." If you are not burned out, you are not doing *it* right. Participants frequently acknowledged that they had no possibility for work–life balance while earning a graduate degree and that being burned out was admired. One participant explained, "Academics are obsessed with being stressed out, looking 'busy' all the time, and overworked even though every job is stressful." Students felt that burnout was "publicly accepted, expected ('mad scientist'), yet culturally invisible."

In this same vein, students mentioned that burnout could also become a competition. They would compare themselves to their peers' level of productivity and burnout to gauge how successfully they believed they were doing in their graduate program. For example, one respondent stated, "I see publishing and conference awards as very flawed ways of measuring academic impact.... [however] my identity and sense of self-worth are becoming so increasingly tied to publishing, attending conferences, and getting awards." Moreover, students saw burnout being used as a badge of honor: "Your mental health is supposed to suffer through graduate school, and you're supposed to be able to work through it if you're actually worthy of being in academia," stated one respondent. The present findings suggest that mental health is not a priority in academia, graduate programs, or for graduate students. This lack of focus on mental well-being is exacerbated by romanticizing burnout.

A small minority of participants did note that their schools highlighted the importance of mental health. Even in this minority, participants were aware of how lucky they were to have that support from their university and department, knowing many other institutions did not focus as heavily on mental health. One respondent pointed out, "I'm very lucky to have [profs] who care about me."

Overall, participants reported that their universities did not see mental health as a priority. For many students, departments and universities were focused solely on productivity, such as class evaluations, publications, and grants. This extreme pressure meant that participants did not feel comfortable taking a "day off." Even on the weekends, students felt guilty if they were not writing or researching. Participants also stated that they felt uncomfortable asking for mental health days off. The lack of available resources for maintaining a healthy mental state impacted students' perspective of burnout and their future with encountering burnout.

Participants responded that burnout significantly impacted their sense of self. Graduate students lost self-confidence after becoming burned out. They also mentioned that the effects of burnout left them wanting to quit academia. When asked if they had ever considered another career path, 87.5 percent of respondents answered that they had considered paths other than academia because of burnout and the fear of failure if they stayed in academia. Many participants were left questioning the worth of academia. Additionally, these negative hits to their self-efficacy led to the fear of a self-fulfilling prophecy that they could never succeed in academia.

Mentors Make the Most Significant Impact

Advisors and mentors have the biggest impact on the graduate student experience. Respondents frequently mentioned that the nature of their graduate experience was closely tied to one's subject and advisor. The mentor experience was a predicting factor in whether a graduate student would continue in academia or not. Thus, watching a mentor burnout had a tremendous impact on students' confidence in continuing in academia. One student explained, "I've heard a lot of narratives about it being tough, it not being fair, it requiring thick skin." This characterization made it difficult for respondents to feel hopeful for their future careers. Participants mentioned that they "came to expect a similar life for [themselves]" after watching mentors and other close faculty burnout. Other people stated that watching mentors suffer through burnout was "worrisome" and "disheartening."

Furthermore, students learned about the cultural norms and expectations of academia through their mentors. For many, their understanding of a future in academia was characterized by their mentors. When mentors characterized academia in a negative light, students came to interpret the culture similarly. For example, one respondent described hearing a mentor complain often about "why-can't-you-just-let-me-do-what-I-was-trained-to-do?" regarding their academic work and research, which left the survey participant feeling skeptical about their long-term happiness if they stayed in academia. Hearing bits and pieces of their mentors' experiences and perceptions of academia impacted the sensemaking process for graduate students. A respondent noted that she heard an advisor describe "a clear hierarchy with good old boy professors and administrators that cover for abusive professors that supervise graduate students." Ultimately, the negative experiences shared by mentors who had already gone through the same graduate school process led to the graduate students' fear of the future and failure in academia.

DISCUSSION

Historically, academia has been rife with the condition of chronic stress, also known as burnout (Armour et al. 1987, 3; Parker 2018, 30–31). Burnout does not discriminate based on hierarchical level, and impacts even the newest members of academia—graduate students. The present study reinforces previous research that the main stressors among graduate students are work–life balance or lack of leisure time, academic cultural requirements such as research or curriculum work, and insecurity of professional future (Shetty et al. 2015, 34–35). Our study finds that while graduate students expected stress throughout their graduate experience, the reality far exceeded the previously expected levels of mental distress. Moreover, the frequency at which stressful interactions or incidents occurred left little time for students to recover. Over time, continual stress without breaks potentially leads to graduate student burnout (Maslach, Jackson, and Leiter 1996, 295) and, in extreme cases, causes affected individuals to leave academia.

Furthermore, participant responses revealed a great difference between what students expected academia to be and their actual experiences. This difference between expectation and reality became a silent stressor for many participants. Participants first imagined academia to be a place for intellectual exploration, innovation, and inspiration. In reality, students found the workload overwhelming (Bell, Rajendran, and Teiler 2012, 26–27; Moore and Amey 1993, 29–32) and the process for promotion and recognition impregnable and elitist, accessible only for the "privileged few."

Our study's findings contribute to the existing literature by suggesting that graduate students sensemake (Weick, Sutcliffe, and Obstfeld 2005, 409–413) their understanding of academic culture through mentors' experiences and shared narratives. Watching advisors and mentors struggle with work–life balance and burnout painted a bleak picture for the participants' futures. How mentors characterize their academic experiences and journey significantly impacts graduate students' expectations and understanding of academic career paths. Our findings suggest that the negative characterization of academia can highly discourage graduate students from thinking about a career in academia or even finishing their degree program. While the rate of doctoral students quitting programs without completing a degree is already 43.4 percent (Cassuto 2013, para. 3; Sowell, Zhange, Redd, and King 2008, 6), the findings in the present study indicate that these numbers could be on the rise. When we consider the increasing rates of mental distress among young adults (Twenge et al. 2019, 185) alongside our findings that 87.5 percent of participants said they had considered leaving academia due to burnout and the fear of failure, the number of graduate students who quit academia could be impacted if the workplace culture remains the same.

The presentation of burnout and mental health in academia through advisors and cultural norms can leave graduate students with unfavorable perceptions of academic career paths. Watching the struggle for a healthy work–life balance and an almost inevitable path to burnout causes students to worry about preserving their mental health if they were to continue in an academic career. When mentors negatively stigmatize burnout, this ultimately presents graduate students with a discouraging narrative and future expectations of burnout and job dissatisfaction.

RECOMMENDATIONS

Although the survey responses indicate a negative picture of academic work and burnout, the respondents' experiences form invaluable recommendations for improving the graduate students' experience. These recommendations come directly from participants, as well as from the literature in response to many themes highlighted in this chapter's results section. The recommendations have three overarching themes: support for graduate students, portrayal of mental health, and a cultural shift.

Support for Graduate Students

To support graduate students more effectively, institutions must focus more substantially on quality mentorship from faculty. This study identified that mentorship makes or breaks the graduate student experience and profoundly influences a student's desire to continue in academia. Previous research shows that professors spend between 2 and 6 percent of their working time one-on-one with students (Olwell 2017, para. 5). This is drastically less time than they spend on meetings, teaching, or research (Olwell 2017, para. 9). Due to academia's competitive nature, students need positive guidance and assistance to feel prepared for entering the academic job market. Mentoring has been recognized as one of the keys to long-term student success (Olwell 2017, para. 6). For many, a dedicated mentor reduces the stress of having to navigate academia on their own and provides support in areas where graduate students' knowledge is still developing. Understanding the grave implications of mentorship and providing avenues for developing positive mentoring skills are vital for reducing graduate student burnout.

Due to the significant role mentorship plays in graduate students' sensemaking process, universities should implement more training for faculty mentors. Mentors should be trained on best practices for advising students, providing support, setting students up for success, managing interpersonal relationships, and characterizing academia in a positive light. To develop stronger mentors, more universities must invest in developing mentorship programs and networks. For example, Rackham Graduate School of the University of Michigan, West Texas A&M University, and the University of Illinois provide literature on their website specifically for mentoring graduate students. Because graduate students require different resources, access, and knowledge than undergraduate students, this literature provides tips for serving the niche graduate student community. The information on these web pages ranges from the definition and value of mentoring to the steps in the mentorship process and setting boundaries with mentées (University of Illinois n.d.; The Regents 2020, 8–12; West Texas n.d.).

Additionally, beginning training and development opportunities to cultivate these skills in master's and PhD programs will help to ingrain these skills in academics as they rise through the ranks. Universities such as Princeton provide teaching and mentorship programs, events, fellowships, and webinars to provide graduate students with mentorship training (Princeton University n.d.). Additionally, highly qualified faculty mentors should be acknowledged and rewarded for their commitment to developing future academics. Portraying mentorship as a vital aspect of a faculty's job role and career development, as well as providing compensation for, or recognition of, faculty who take on more mentorship roles will help to solidify the importance of mentorship within academic culture. It will also allow faculty to spend more time with graduate students, without negatively impacting their perceived *productivity* among administrators.

Finally, mentors need to model positive behaviors for succeeding in academia. Graduate students see more than faculty think. Graduate students sensemake their expectations from the experiences shared by close mentors. Therefore, how faculty behave and speak about academia becomes even more crucial for developing a positive work climate and habits. Because professors and mentors play a significant role in graduate students' sensemaking of academia and how to perform academic roles efficiently, they must model and validate the importance of mental health to overcome or even potentially avoid burnout. Wearing stress and burnout as a *badge of honor* does not provide students with realistic expectations for a life-long academic career. These unhealthy behaviors can also reinforce the idea that maintaining healthy mental well-being is insignificant if workaholic behaviors are being modeled. Setting goals and work–life boundaries will show students that there are ways to avoid burnout and maintain a healthy career in academia.

Portrayal of Mental Health

Graduate students need more support when it comes to maintaining their mental health.

In addition to emphasizing seeking help and taking care of students' mental health, there needs to be a wider cultural change in the current stigma of mental health. Burnout should not be glorified and expected from academics. Our research participants noted that burnout is "publicly accepted, expected," and it is a "standard thing that many experience." While members of academia are aware that burnout is an issue in their field, research participants also understand burnout as taboo: "It's a stigma. It's put up and shut up" and "Something to be dealt with and gotten over." If institutions and academics perpetuate the idea that burnout equals success, this will only continue to negatively impact the sustainability of working in academia. One participant described this situation:

> At my institution, mental health issues are very stigmatized. In academia, more generally, amongst younger people, mental health issues are openly discussed to the point of becoming a desirable identity. Both at my institution and in academia, more widely, chronic burnout, anxiety, depression, and substance abuse are almost expected. Being exhausted makes you look productive, and there is a constant competition to be the most productive.

When poor mental health is viewed as normal and as a trait that one should possess to show productivity and success, stigmatization thrives, and affected individuals feel as if they cannot seek the help they need. Universities need to recognize this and provide graduate students with resources to address mental distress and promote self-care for a better work–life balance. For example, the Jed Foundation (2019), "a nonprofit that protects emotional health and prevents suicide for our nation's teens and young adults," partners with universities to assist them in establishing prevention and intervention strategies to protect students' mental health. Across the country, academic institutions now have programs that give their students access to free resources to support personal well-being. For example, Duke University's DuWell project (2020a) uses a holistic approach to help students manage stress, reduce anxiety, and focus on overall well-being. This includes teaching students about healthy practices in their private, social, and religious lives, offering classes such as knitting, Thai Chi or meditation, drug and alcohol education, as well as offering professional care providers (Duke 2020b). Other resources may include the CampusWell program (Duke 2020c), an interdepartmental platform for student affairs at universities that connects departments that are involved in student wellness. The health communication program provides "high quality, research-based content, and proven marketing strategies" (Duke 2020c); that is, it disseminates mental health and well-being research and information to students through mobile, social media, print, and digital channels and platforms.

Additionally, universities should make mental health and well-being a part of their discourse with students to normalize the concept and support the student population (including graduate students) struggling with mental health. For example, getting help and taking *mental health* days should be met with positive reactions instead of being reprimanded. Through the lens of health communication, addressing mental health issues in a more positive and open format will help destigmatize burnout and make graduate students feel more comfortable seeking mental health support. Different programs in the United States, such as Kognito, Active Minds, and 24-hour texting hotlines, help students with mental and emotional distress. Currently, at least 350 colleges use an online simulation program called Kognito to help students learn how to talk to friends who may be suffering emotionally and direct them to appropriate resources (Kognito 2017). Active Minds is a nationwide organization dedicated to mental health advocacy (Active Minds 2020). A 2018 study of Active Minds that surveyed 1,129 students across 12 universities found that even students with low engagement in Active Minds at the start of the school year reported an increase in mental health awareness and a decrease in negative stigmatizing attitudes about mental illness by the end of the year (Sontag-Padilla et al. 2018, 500). Similarly, the University of Sioux Falls created a free texting hotline for students to talk with trained professionals 24/7 (Eva 2019, para. 21). The university also provides encouraging notes, stories, and quotes on their Instagram feed to promote community and decrease the stigma of reaching out for help for mental illness or distress (Eva 2019, para. 21).

Overall, institutions need to increase mental health training for mentors and graduate students. This training must identify warning signs and symptoms of common mental health issues such as depression and burnout. Many mentors and graduate students may be unaware of the small signs leading up to a graduate student breakdown or a faculty member's inevitable spiral into burnout. Furthermore, mental health training can be used as a platform to help destigmatize mental health issues such as burnout and provide students with actionable steps for seeking treatment.

As well as providing more mental health resources and addressing the stigma of mental distress, research participants mentioned needing more avenues to air grievances about faculty or advisors without repercussions in their professional lives. Much of the stress from graduate school was ascribed to mismanagement or abuse from advisors. Due to the advisors' essential role in graduate student success, with everything from passing a dissertation to future job references, students do not believe they can adequately self-advocate in toxic situations. Many students were afraid of advisors slandering their reputation, failing their dissertations, or even kicking them out of a lab, if they were to report toxic workplace behavior. Institutions should develop systems for anonymous reporting of toxic behaviors such as abuse and harassment. Many respondents reported there was no way for them to report harmful behavior from faculty without risking their future career success.

We want to note that, while many universities may have mental health resources for their undergraduate students, there is little information regarding mental health programs and resources for graduate students. Due to their unique position as being part of the student body while also working as faculty, doing research, and teaching classes, undergraduate mental health programs and resources may not be helpful or applicable for graduate students. Thus, taking into account the nuances of the graduate school experience while developing mental health resources, programs, and training is vital for improving the portrayal of mental health among graduate students.

Shift in Academic Culture

Overall, academic culture must change to allow its members opportunities to work in environments that do not foster excess levels of burnout. Decades of previous research have documented the current academic culture's negative impact on job satisfaction and sustainability, which ultimately leads to extreme stress and often burnout (Bell, Rajendran, and Teiler 2012, 26–27; Maslach, Jackson, and Leiter 1996, 205; Moore and Amey 1993, 29–31; Rawat and Meena 2014, 87; Tierney 1997, 8–12; Yu, Chae, and Chang 2016, 53–54). For academia to effectively address burnout, the culture must change to encourage administrations to develop new measures of productivity and promote more career paths for people with PhDs.

Conflict between administration and faculty is well documented (Campbell and Newell 1973, 3; Coltrin and Glueck 1977, 101; Haseeb and Sattar 2018, 31–32; Holton and Philips 1995, 43–50). As higher education shifts to a more prestige economy, it is progressively apparent that faculty and administration have different goals within the same institution. For example, administrators feel the pressure to *sell* the idea of higher education to current and potential stakeholders through evidence of accountability, efficiency, and effectiveness. In 2010, the Texas A&M system developed an index to determine whether faculty were generating more revenue than their payroll costs, for calculating employee efficiency (Mangan 2010, para. 1). The university calculated the total value of tuition generated by the classes taught by a faculty member and then subtracted that faculty member's salary and benefits from the amount (Mangan 2010, para. 3), promoting a neoliberal environment in which faculty have to continuously prove their worth.

While this may seem like a useful measurement scale, these accountability initiatives failed to measure the entirety of faculty members' work (Bess and Dee 2014, ch. 1). Professors are required to be proficient in three distinct areas: teaching, research, and service. However, if only one of the three is evaluated by administrators, it invalidates many expected job tasks that faculty must complete for job promotion and success. Developing new ways to calculate staff and faculty accountability and efficiency will help change academia's toxic and competitive culture. For example, the New York University (NYU) Langone Medical Center developed a dashboard system for tracking academic and clinical performance. The dashboard measures four work areas that include grants, publications, innovations (such as patents), and efficiency, in conjunction with open dialogue among faculty and administrators (Tachibana 2017). This system provides a more complete view of a faculty member's job performance and productivity. Moreover, dashboard results have been used to evaluate the university's strengths and weaknesses, as well as to provide data to monitor and support the career trajectory of faculty through the identification of needed resources (Tachibana 2017, para. 10).

The pressure to research and publish comprised one of the most significant collective stressors for this study's respondents. Publishing eventually equated to students' sense of self-worth, leading to a heightened focus on quantity over quality when publishing. The idea of "publish or perish" (Coolidge 1932, 308) may adversely affect mental health, job satisfaction, and work-flow sustainability over time. Many respondents felt that they had turned in work they were not proud of or spent their entire free time writing for the sake of increasing their number of publications. Developing other forms of performance metrics could help quell the publication-based promotion system. For example, at the University of Washington, Associate Professor Trevor Branch created a database of the most cited papers in his field. This database includes a metric for estimating individual contributions to studies with multiple authors (Tachibana 2017, para. 18). Instead of counting published papers, this system accounts for the overall impact and importance a published work has in its field (Tachibana 2017, para. 18). Since academia's prestige economy (Fyfe et al. 2017, 3) contributes to eventual burnout, shifting the culture to focus on quality publications instead of high numbers of curriculum vitae line items may help boost morale and career sustainability.

Presently, there is a stigma associated with PhDs that they limit and/or narrow potential career paths, leaving doctoral candidates feeling as though they have little to no choice but to stay in academia. This anxiety has crept into the graduate student experience, and as students are completing their degrees, they fear for their future. Providing alternative career paths for people with

PhDs will help lessen the pre-graduation dread for many graduate students. Additionally, lack of support from administration and mentors makes graduate students second-guess their academic career choice. One participant states the following:

> My time in this graduate program has made me want to leave academia. Like so many of us that go into teaching, I was inspired to continue my education and become a professor because of my undergraduate advising relationships. I was extremely well-supported by a handful of incredible faculty at my undergrad and again at my Master's program. I expected to have the same situation in my doctoral program but seeing how little faculty seem to care about both their undergrad and grad students, in combination with working in a student services office and thus being privy to structural, administrative problems, has made me question whether academia is a worthwhile locus of change—whether social change or change in individual students' lives.

Knowing the problematic nature of their possible career choice, many research participants confirmed they have second-guessed their choice to continue in academia and have considered abandoning their ultimate goal of tenure track in favor of their mental health. One participant stated that, "Sometimes I don't think the process is worth the outcome, I don't know if the detriments to my mental health are worth it . . . and I don't know if I can survive through this much stress for that long." Students fear that if they leave academia they will not be viewed as competitive in the job market outside higher education. Students should be able to follow their chosen career path without the expectation of poor mental health, as well as have the ability to change career paths without fear of being unemployable. Promoting career paths other than tenure-track positions at highly regarded research universities is a way to better support graduate students and lessen their fear of failure post-graduation.

LIMITATIONS AND FUTURE RESEARCH

Although this research is just a starting point for understanding the graduate student burnout experience, there were some limitations to this study. Overall, the sample size was limited to 139 participants and only represents a small sample of graduate students from across the U.S. The majority of participants were white, which possibly limited insight into how ethnicity/race might impact graduate student burnout. The researchers did not inquire about socioeconomic status, which has been known to impact stress levels and burnout (Adams, Meyers, and Beidas 2016, 362; Lou, Wang, Zhang, and Chen 2016, 2111; Mompremier 2009, para. 1–2). Future studies should further address the burnout experience of graduate students of different ethnicities and socioeconomic status.

This study about graduate student burnout was also posted at the end of a semester; therefore, there could have been biased responses from participants ending a stressful semester. In addition, this study was conducted by two recent graduate students who may have been biased toward the graduate student burnout experience. Finally, as two female researchers completed this analysis, our lived experiences as women in academia could have impacted the data analysis' results.

Based on this study's findings, future research must focus on strategies to implement preventative burnout strategies to improve the graduate student experience. More in-depth stories should be collected from graduate students so that their experiences can help institutions, faculty, and administrators better understand the unique dynamics and stressors that may occur during a graduate degree program. Additionally, future research should explore the sensemaking experience of advisor burnout and the subsequent impact on mentor-mentée communication. Overall, this vital research area should be explored in more depth, given the dearth of research on the subject.

CONCLUSION

The romanticization of burnout in the academy can have detrimental effects on people's physical and mental well-being, as well as on their decision to stay in academia. The portrayals of burnout such as "needing to be burned out to be considered successful" and "not seeking out mental health help to combat burnout" compound the already difficult journey of completing a graduate degree. In order to improve the graduate student experience and increase degree completion rates, universities are challenged to change their organizational culture from that of *publish or perish* to focus more on long-term community impacts and promote the importance of mental health among their faculty members. Maintaining the ideals of the *hustle culture* will only negatively impact the retention of valuable scholars and continue to stigmatize higher education as a toxic career path. Ultimately, promoting and supporting a sustainable work–life balance, as well as destigmatizing mental health help and resources, will benefit students, faculty, administrators, and universities in the long term.

REFERENCES

AAUP. 2018. "Data Snapshot: Contingent Faculty in US Higher Ed." https://www.aaup.org/sites/default/files/10112018%20Data%20Snapshot%20Tenure.pdf.

Abolafia, Mitchell Y. 2010. "Narrative Construction as Sensemaking: How a Central Bank Thinks." *Organization Studies* 31, no. 3 (April): 349–367. https://doi.org/10.1177/0170840609357380.

Abouserie, Reda. 1996. "Stress Coping Strategies and Job Satisfaction in University Academic Staff." *Educational Psychology: An International Journal of Experimental Educational Psychology* 16, no. 1 (September): 49–56. https://doi.org/10.1080/0144341960160104.

Active Minds. 2020. "Mission and Impact." Accessed March 26, 2020. https://www.activeminds.org/about-us/mission-and-impact/.

Adams, Danielle R., Steven A. Meyers, and Rinad S. Beidas. 2016. "The Relationship Between Financial Strain, Perceived Stress, Psychological Symptoms, and Academic and Social Integration in Undergraduate Students." *Journal of American College Health* 64, no. 5 (April): 362–370. https://doi.org/10.1080/07448481.2016.1154559.

Andrew, Louise B., and B. E. Brenner. 2018. "Physician Suicide." Medscape. Last updated August 1, 2018. https://emedicine.medscape.com/article/806779-overview#a1.

Armour, Robert A., Rosemary S. Caffarella, Barbara S. Fuhrmann, and Jon F. Wergin. 1987. "Academic Burnout: Faculty Responsibility and Institutional Climate." *New Directions for Teaching and Learning* 1987, no. 29 (March): 3–11. https://doi.org/10.1002/tl.37219872903.

Auerbach, Randy P., Philippe Mortier, Ronny Bruffaerts, Jordi Alonso, Corina Benjet, Pim Cuijpers, Koen Demyttenaere et al. 2018. "WHO World Mental Health Surveys International College Student Project: Prevalence and Distribution of Mental Disorders." *Journal of Abnormal Psychology* 127, no. 7 (October): 623–638. https://doi.org/10.1037/abn0000362.

Bauer, Joachim, Axel Stamm, Katharina Virnich, Karen Wissing, Udo Müller, Michael Wirsching, and Uwe Schaarschmidt. 2006. "Correlation Between Burnout Syndrome and Psychological and Psychosomatic Symptoms Among Teachers." *International Archives of Occupational and Environmental Health* 79, no. 3 (October), 199–204. https://doi.org/10.1007/s00420-005-0050-y.

Bell, Amanda S., Diana Rajendran, and Stephen Theiler. 2012. "Job Stress, Wellbeing, Work-Life Balance and Work-Life Conflict Among Australian Academics." *E-Journal of Applied Psychology* 8, no. 1: 25–37. https://doi.org/10.7790/ejap.v8i1.320.

Berezow, Alex. 2018. "Is There a Mental Health Crisis Among Graduate School Students?" *American Council on Science and Health*. Last updated March 7, 2018. https://www.acsh.org/news/2018/03/07/there-mental-health-crisis-among-graduate-school-students-12672.

Bess, James L., and Jay R. Dee. 2014. *Bridging the Divide Between Faculty and Administration: A Guide to Understanding Conflict in the Academy*. New York: Routledge.

Bianchi, Renzo, Jay Verkuilen, Romain Brisson, Irvin Sam Schonfeld, and Eric Laurent. 2016. "Burnout and Depression: Label-Related Stigma, Help-Seeking, and Syndrome Overlap." *Psychiatry Research* 254, no. 1 (November): 91–98. https://doi.org/10.1016/j.psychres.2016.08.025.

Bilge, Filiz. 2006. "Examining the Burnout of Academics in Relation to Job Satisfaction and Other Factors." *Social Behavior and Personality* 34, no. 9 (November): 1151–1160. https://doi.org/10.2224/sbp.2006.34.9.1151.

Bove, Liliana L., and Simon J. Pervan. 2013. "Stigmatized Labour: An Overlooked Service Worker's Stress." *Australasian Marketing Journal (AMJ)* 21, no. 4 (November): 259–263. https://doi.org/10.1016/j.ausmj.2013.08.006.

Braxton, John M., Eve M. Proper, and Alan E. Bayer. 2011. *Professors Behaving Badly: Faculty Misconduct in Graduate Education*. Baltimore: John Hopkins University Press.

Bullock, Garrett, Lynnea Kraft, Katherine Amsden, Whitney Gore, Bobby Prengle, Jeffrey Wimsatt, Leila Ledbetter, Kyle Covington, and Adam Goode. 2017. "The Prevalence and Effect of Burnout on Graduate Healthcare Students." *Canadian Medical Education Journal* 8, no. 3 (June): e90–e108. https://doi.org/10.36834/cmej.36890.

Campbell, Jessica, Allan V. Prochazka, Traci Yamashita, and Ravi Gopal. 2010. "Predictors of Persistent Burnout in Internal Medicine Residents: A Prospective Cohort Study." *Academic Medicine* 85, no. 10 (October): 1630–1634. https://doi.org/10.1097/ACM.0b013e3181f0c4e7.

Campbell, Roald F., and L. Jackson Newell. 1973. "A Study of Professors of Education Administration: A Summary." *Educational Administration Quarterly* 9, no. 3 (October): 3–27. https://doi.org/10.1177/0013161X7300900302.

Cassella, Carly. 2019. "'Burn-Out' is Now a Legitimate Syndrome According to the WHO. Here Are the Symptoms." *Science Alert*. May 29, 2019. https://www.sciencealert.com/burn-out-is-now-officially-recognised-as-a-legitimatesyndrome-by-the-world-health-organisation.

Cassuto, Leonard. 2013. "Ph.D. Attrition: How Much is too Much?" *The Chronicle of Higher Education*. July 1, 2013. https://www.chronicle.com/article/PhD-Attrition-How-Much-Is/140045.

Cazan, Ana-Maria, and Laura Elena Năstasă. 2015. "Emotional Intelligence, Satisfaction with Life and Burnout Among University Students." *Social and Behavioral Sciences* 180, no. 1 (May): 1574–1578. https://doi.org/10.1016/j.sbspro.2015.02.309.

Chang, Eunbi, Ahram Lee, Eunji Byeon, Hyunmo Seong, and Sang Min Lee. 2016. "The Mediating Effect of Motivational Types in the Relationship Between Perfectionism and Academic Burnout." *Personality and Individual Differences* 89, no. 1 (January): 202–210. https://doi.org/10.1016/j.paid.2015.10.010.

Coltrin, Sally, and William F. Glueck. 1977. "The Effect of Leadership Roles on the Satisfaction and Productivity of University Research Professors." *The Academy of Management Journal* 20, no. 1 (November): 101–116. https://doi.org/10.5465/255465.

Coolidge, Harold J., and Robert H. Lord, eds. 1932. *Archibal Cary Coolidge. Life and Letters*. Boston and New York: Houghton Mifflin.

Corrigan, Patrick W., Dinesh Mittal, Christina M. Reaves, Tiffany F. Haynes, Xiaotong Han, Scott Morris, and Greer Sullivan. 2014. "Mental Health Stigma and Primary Health Care Decisions." *Psychiatry Research* 218, no. 1–2 (August): 35–38. https://doi.org/10.1016/j.psychres.2014.04.028.

Cresswell, Scott L., and Robert C. Eklund. 2006. "The Nature of Player Burnout in Rugby: Key Characteristics and Attributions." *Journal of Applied Sport Psychology* 18, no. 3 (February): 219–239. https://doi.org/10.1080/10413200600830299.

Currie, Graeme, and Andrew D. Brown. 2003. "A Narratological Approach to Understanding Processes of Organizing in a UK Hospital." *Human Relations* 56, no. 1 (May): 563–586. https://doi.org/10.1177/0018726703056005003.

Duke University. n.d. "About Us". DuWell. Accessed March 26, 2020. https://studentaffairs.duke.edu/duwell.

Dyrbye, Liselotte N., Anne Eacker, Steven J. Durning, Chantal Brazeau, Christine Moutier, F. Stanford Massie, Daniel Satele, Jeff A. Sloan, and Tait D. Shanafelt. 2015. "The Impact of Stigma and Personal Experiences on The Help-Seeking Behaviors of Medical Students with Burnout." *Academic Medicine* 90, no. 7 (July): 961–969. https://doi.org/10.1097/ACM.0000000000000655.

Dyrbye, Liselotte N., Matthew R. Thomas, F. Stanford Massie, David V Power, Anne Eacker, William Harper, Steven Durning, Christine Moutier, Daniel W. Szydlo, Paul J. Novotny, Jeff A. Sloan, and Tait D. Shanafelt. 2008. "Burnout and Suicidal Ideation Among U.S. Medical Students." *Annals of Internal Medicine* 149, no. 5 (September): 334–41. https://doi.org/10.7326/0003-4819-149-5-200809020-00008.

Dyrbye, Liselotte N., Colin P. West, Daniel Satele, Sonja Boone, Litjen Tan, Jeff Sloan, and Tait D. Shanafelt. 2014. "Burnout Among U.S. Medical Students, Residents, and Early Career Physicians Relative to the General U.S. Population." *Academic Medicine* 89, no. 3 (March): 443–451. https://doi.org/10.1097/ACM.0000000000000134.

Endriulaitienė, Auksė, R. Markšaitytė, K. Žardeckaitė-Matulaitienė, Aistė Pranckevičienė, Doug R. Tillman, and David D. Hof. 2016. "Burnout and Stigma of Seeking Help in Lithuanian Mental Health Care Professionals." *The European Proceedings of Social and Behavioural Sciences*: 254–265. https://doi.org/10.15405/EPSBS.2016.07.02.25.

Eva, Amy L. 2019. "How Colleges Today are Supporting Student Mental Health." Greater Good Science Center at UC Berkeley. January 11, 2019. https://greatergood.berkeley.edu/article/item/how_colleges_today_are_supporting_student_mental_health.

Evans, Teresa M., Lindsay Bira, Jazmin Beltran Gastelum, L. Todd Weiss, and Nathan L. Vanderford. 2018. "Evidence for a Mental Health Crisis in Graduate Education." *Nature Biotechnology* 36, no. 3 (March): 282–284. https://doi.org/doi:10.1038/nbt.4089.

Farmer, Blake. 2018. "When Doctors Struggle with Suicide, Their Profession Often Fails Them." *NPR Morning Edition*. Aired July 31, 2018. https://www.npr.org/sections/health-shots/2018/07/31/634217947/to-prevent-doctor-suicides-medical-industry-rethinks-how-doctors-work.

Fore, Cecil, Christopher Martin, and William N. Bender. 2002. "Teacher Burnout in Special Education: The Causes and Recommended Solutions." *The High School Journal* 86, no. 1 (October): 36–44.

Fowler, Sean. 2015. "Burnout and Depression in Academia: A Look at the Discourse of the University." *Empedocles: European Journal for the Philosophy of Communication* 6, no. 2 (October): 155–167. https://doi.org/10.1386/ejpc.6.2.155_1.

Fyfe, Aileen, Kelly Coate, Stephen Curry, Stuart Lawson, Noah Moxham, and Camilla Mørk Røstvik. 2017. "Untangling Academic Publishing: A History of the Relationship Between Commercial Interests, Academic Prestige and the Circulation of Research." Accessed March 26, 2020. https://researchrepository.standrews.ac.uk/bitstream/handle/10023/10884/Fyfe_etal_UntanglingAcPub_CC.pdf?sequence=1.

Goffman, Ervin. 1986. *Stigma: Notes on the Management of Spoiled Identity*. New York City: Touchstone.

Golkar, Armita, Emilia Johansson, Maki Kasahara, Walter Osika, Aleksander Perski, and Ivanka Savic. 2014. "The Influence of Work-Related Chronic Stress on the Regulation of Emotion and on Functional Connectivity in the Brain." *PLoS ONE* 9, no. 9 (September): e104550. https://doi.org/10.1371/journal.pone.0104550.

Goodboy, Alan, Matthew Martin, and Zac Johnson. 2015. "The Relationships Between Workplace Bullying by Graduate Faculty with Graduate Students' Burnout and Organizational Citizenship Behaviors." *Communication Research Reports* 32, no. 3 (July): 272–280. https://doi.org/10.1080/08824096.2015.1052904.

Gradfutures. 2020. "Teaching and Mentoring." Accessed March 26, 2020. https://gradfutures.princeton.edu/competencies/teaching-and-mentoring.

The Graduate Assembly. 2016. "Graduate Student Happiness and Well-Neing Report." *UC Berkeley*. http://ga.berkeley.edu/wellbeingreport.

Griffith, Erin. 2019. "Why are Young People Pretending to Love Work?" *New York Times*. January 26, 2019. https://www.nytimes.com/2019/01/26/business/against-hustle-culture-rise-and-grind-tgim.html.

Hill, Andrew P., and Thomas Curran. 2015. "Multidimensional Perfectionism and Burnout: A Meta-Analysis." *Personality and Social Psychology Review* 20, no. 3 (July): 269–288. https://doi.org/ 10.1177/1088868315596286.

Holton, Susan A., and Gerald Phillips. 1995. "Can't Live with Them, Can't Live Without Them: Faculty and Administrators in Conflict." *New Directions for Higher Education* 92, no. 1 (Winter): 43–50.

Karimi, Yusef, Mehrab Bashirpur, Mahmoud Khabbaz, and Ali Asghar Hedayati. 2014. "Comparison Between Perfectionism and Social Support Dimensions and Academic Burnout in Students." *Social and Behavioral Sciences* 159, no. 1 (December): 57–63. https://doi.org/10.1016/j.sbspro.2014.12.328.

Kjeldstadli, Kari, Reidar Tyssen, Arnstein Finset, Erlend Hem, Tore Gude, Nina T. Gronvold, Oivind Ekeberg, and Per Vaglum. 2006. "Life Satisfaction and Resilience in Medical School—a Six-Year Longitudinal, Nationwide and Comparative Study." *BMC Medical Education* 6, no. 1 (September): 48–51. https://doi.org/10.1186/1472-6920-6-48.

Kognito. n.d. "About." Accessed March 26, 2020. https://kognito.com/about.

Kumar, Payal, and Manish Singhal. 2012. "Reducing Change Management Complexity: Aligning Change Recipient Sensemaking to Change Agent

Sensegiving." *International Journal Learning and Change* 6, no. 3–4 (December): 138–155. https://doi.org/ 10.1504/IJLC.2012.050855.

Lackritz, James R. 2004. "Exploring Burnout Among University Faculty: Incidence, Performance, and Demographic Issues." *Teaching and Teacher Education* 20, no. 7 (October): 713–729. https://doi.org/10.1016/j.tate.2004.07.002.

Lehmann-Willenbrock, Nale, Joseph A. Allen, and Dain Belyeu. 2016. "Our Love/Hate Relationship with Meetings: Relating Good and Bad Meeting Behaviors to Meeting Outcomes, Engagement, and Exhaustion." *Management Research Review* 39, no. 10 (October): 1293–1312.

Lindlof, Thomas, R., and Taylor, Bryan C. 2017. *Qualitative Communication Research Methods.* Thousand Oaks, CA: Sage.

Luo, Yun, Wang, Zhenhong, Zhang, Hui, and Chen, Aihong. 2016. "The Influence of Family Socio-economic Status on Learning Burnout in Adolescents: Mediating and Moderating Effects." *Journal of Child and Family Studies* 25, no. 7 (March): 2111–2119. doi.org/10.1007/s10826-016-0400-2.

Mangan, Katherine. 2010. "Texas A&M's Bottom-Line Ratings of Professors Find That Most are Cost-Effective." *Chronicle of Higher Education.* September 15, 2010. https://www.chronicle.com/article/Texas-A-Ms-Bottom-Line/124451.

Mårtensson, Gunilla, J. Jaconsson, and Maria Engstrom. 2014. "Mental Health Nursing Staff's Attitudes Towards Mental Illness: An Analysis of Related Factors." *Journal of Psychiatric and Mental Health Nursing* 21, no. 1: 782–788. https://doi.org/ 10.1111/jpm.12145.

Maslach, Christina, and Susan E. Jackson. 1981. "The Measurement of Experienced Burnout." *Journal of Occupational Behavior* 2, no. 1: 99–113. doi.org/10.1002/job.4030020205.

Maslach, Christina, Susan E. Jackson, and Michael Leiter. 1996. *Maslach Burnout Inventory Manual.* Palo Alto, CA: Consulting Psychologists Press.

Mitake, Tomoe, Shinichi Iwasaki, Yasuhiko Deguchi, Tomoko Nitta, Yukako Nogi, Aya Kadowaki, Akihiro Niki, and Koki Inoue. 2019. "Relationship between Burnout and Mental-Illness-Related Stigma among Nonprofessional Occupational Mental Health Staff." *BioMed Research International.* https://doi.org/10.1155/2019/5921703.

Mojtabai, Ramin, Mark Olfson, and Beth Han. 2016. "National Trends in the Prevalence and Treatment of Depression in Adolescents and Young Adults." *Pediatrics* 138, no. 6: e20161878. https://doi.org/10.1542/peds.2016-1878.

Mompremier, LaNiña. 2009. "Socioeconomic Status and Higher Education Adjustment." *American Psychological Association.* April 2009. https://www.apa.org/pi/ses/resources/indicator/2009/04/adjustment.

Moore, Kathryn M., and Marilyn J. Amey. 1993. "Making Sense of the Dollars: The Costs and Uses of Faculty Compensation." *ASHE-ERIC Higher Education Report No. 5.* Washington, DC: The George Washington University, School of Education and Human Development. Accessed March 26, 2020.

Olwell, Russell. 2017. "Moving Beyond 2 Percent." *InsideHigherEd.* January 24, 2017. https://www.insidehighered.com/advice/2017/01/24/why-mentoring-students-so-low-faculty-agenda-and-what-can-be-done-about-it-essay.

Owen, William F. 1984. "Interpretive Themes in Relational Communication." *Quarterly Journal of Speech* 70, no. 3: 274–287. https://doi.org/10.1080/003356 38409383697.

Parker, Mitch L. 2018. "An Examination of the Differences in Doctoral Students' Levels of Life Stress, Burnout, and Resilience by Program Phase." PhD diss., Sam Houston State University. https://shsu-ir.tdl.org/bitstream/handle/20.500.11875/2 349/PARKER-DISSERTATION-2018.PDF?sequence=1&isAllowed=y.

Rahmati, Zeinab. 2014. "Study of Academic Burnout in Students with High and Low Level of Self-Efficacy." *Procedia - Social and Behavioral Science* 171, no. 1: 49–55. https://doi.org/10.1016/j.sbspro.2015.01.087.

Rawat, Seema, and Sanjay Meena. 2014. "Publish or Perish: Where Are We Heading?" *Journal of Research in Medical Sciences: The Official Journal of Isfahan University of Medical Sciences* 19, no. 2: 87–89.

Rom, Noa, and Ori Eyal. 2019. "Sensemaking, Sense-Breaking, Sense-Giving, and Sense-taking: How Educators Construct Meaning in Complex Policy Environments." *Teaching and Teacher Education* 78, no. 1: 62–74. https://doi.org /10.1016/j.tate.2018.11.008.

Salvagioni, Denise A. J., Francine N. Melanda, Arthur E. Mesas, Alberto D. Gonzales, Flavia L. Gabani, and Selma M. Andrade. 2017. "Physical, Psychological and Occupational Consequences of Job Burnout: A Systematic Review of Prospective Students." *PLoS One* 12, no. 10 (2017): 1–29. https://doi.org/10.1371/journal.pon e.0185781.

Schulze, Beate. 2007. "Stigma and Mental Health Professionals: A Review of the Evidence on an Intricate Relationship." *International Review of Psychiatry* 19, no. 2 (2007): 137–155. https://doi.org/10.1080/09540260701278929.

Shetty, Aditya, Shetty, Amrith, Hegde, Mithra N., Narasimhan, Dhanya, and Shetty, Shishir. "Stress and Burnout Assessment Among Post Graduate Dental Students." *Nitte University Journal of Health Science* 5, no. 1 (2015): 31–36.

Smith, Ezra, and Brooks, Zachary. "Graduate Student Mental Health." *National Association of Graduate-Professional Students, University of Arizona.* Last modified 2015. http://nagps.org/wordpress/wp-content/uploads/2015/06/NAGPS_Insti tute_mental_health_survey_report_2015.pdf.

Sontag-Padilla, Lisa, Dunbar, Michael S., Ye, Feifei, Kase, Courtney, Fein, Rebecca, Abelson, Sara, Seelam, Rachana, and Stein, Bradley D. "Strengthening College Students' Mental Health Knowledge, Awareness, and Helping Behaviors: The Impact of Active Minds, a Peer Mental Health Organization." *Journal of Child & Adolescent Psychiatry* 57, no. 7 (2018): 500–507. http://dx.doi.org/10.1016/j.jaac .2018.03.019.

Sowell, Robert, Zhang, Ting, Redd, Kenneth, and King, Margaret F. "Ph.D. Completion and Attrition: Analysis of Baseline Program Data from the Ph.D. Completion Project." *Council of Graduate Schools.* Last modified 2008. https://cg snet.org/sites/default/files/phd_completion_attrition_baseline_program_data.pdf.

Stoeber, Joachim, Childs, Julian H., Hayward, Jennifer A., and Feast, Alexander R. "Passion and Motivation for Studying: Predicting Academic Engagement and Burnout in University Students." *Educational Psychology: An International*

Journal of Experimental Educational Psychology 31, no. 4 (2010): 513–528. http://doi.org/10.1080/01443410.2011.570251.

"Student Health 101." Campus Well. Accessed March 26, 2020. https://campuswell.studenthealth101.com.

Suzuki, Eiko, Kanoya, Yuka, Katsuki, Takeshi, and Sato, Chifumi. "Assertiveness Affecting Burnout of Novice Nurses at University Hospitals." *Japan Journal of Nursing Science* 3, no. 1 (2006): 93–105. http://doi.org/10.1111/j.1742-7924.2006.00058.x.

Tachibana, Chris. "New Tools for Measuring Academic Performance." Last modified February 10, 2017. https://www.sciencemag.org/features/2017/02/new-tools-measuring-academic-performance.

Tierney, William G. "Organizational Socialization in Higher Education." *The Journal of Higher Education* 68, no. 1 (1997): 1–16. http://doi.org/10.1080/00221546.1997.11778975.

The Jed Foundation. 2019. "Who We Are." Accessed March 26, 2020. https://www.jedfoundation.org.

The Regents of the University of Michigan. 2020. "How to Mentor Graduate Students: A Guide for Faculty." *University of Michigan.* https://rackham.umich.edu/wp-content/uploads/2020/01/Fmentor.pdf.

Toker, Sharon, Samuel Melamed, Shlomo Berliner, David Zeltser, and Itzhak Shapira. 2012. "Burnout and Risk of Coronary Heart Disease: A Prospective Study of 8838 Employees." *Psychosomatic Medicine* 74, no. 1: 840–847. https://doi.org/10.1097/PSY.0b013e31826c3174.

Twenge, Jean M., A. Bell Cooper, Thomas E. Joiner, Mary E. Duffy, and Sarah G. Binau. 2019. "Age, Period, and Cohort Trends in Mood Disorder Indicators and Suicide-Related Outcomes in a Nationally Representative Dataset, 2005–2017." *Journal of Abnormal Psychology* 128, no. 3: 185–199. https://doi.org/10.1037/abn0000410.

Twenge, Jean M., Thomas E. Joiner, Megan L. Rogers, and Gabrielle N. Martin. 2018. "Increases in Depressive Symptoms, Suicide-Related Outcomes, and Suicide Rates Among U.S. Adolescents After 2010 and Links to Increased New Media Screen Time." *Clinical Psychological Science* 6, no. 1: 3–17. https://doi.org/doi.org/10.1177/2167702617723376.

University of Illinois. n.d. "Mentoring Graduate Students." Illinois Graduate College. Accessed March 26, 2020. https://grad.illinois.edu/faculty/mentoring.

Wallace, Jean E. 2012. "Mental Health and Stigma in the Medical Profession." *Health: An Interdisciplinary Journal for the Social Study of Health, Illness and Medicine* 16, no. 1: 3–18. https://doi.org/10.1177/1363459310371080.

Watts, Jenny, and Noelle Robertson. 2011. "Burnout in University Teaching Staff: A Systematic Literature Review." *Educational Research* 53, no. 1: 33–50. https://doi.org/10.1080/00131881.2011.552235.

Weick, Karl E. 1995. *Sensemaking in Organisations.* London, UK: Sage.

Weick, Karl E., Kathleen M. Sutcliffe, and David Obstfeld. 2005. "Organizing and the Process of Sensemaking." *Organization Science* 16, no. 4: 409–421. https://doi.org/10.1287/orsc.1050.0133.

West Texas A&M University. n.d. "College Mentoring Program." *West Texas A&M University.* Accessed March 26, 2020. https://www.wtamu.edu/fye/college-mentoring-program.aspx.

WHO. 2019. "Burn-out an 'Occupational Phenomenon': International Classification of Diseases." *World Health Organization.* May 28, 2019. https://www.who.int/mental_health/evidence/burn-out/en/.

Yu, Ji Hye, Sun Jin Chae, and Ki Hong Chang. 2016. "The Relationship Among Self-Efficacy, Perfectionism and Academic Burnout in Medical School Students." *Korean Journal of Medical Education* 28, no. 1: 49–55. https://doi.org/10.3946/kjme.2016.9.

APPENDIX A

Academic Demographics:

1. What is your discipline?
2. Do you feel pressure to: (Check all that apply)
   a. Publish.
   b. Join committees.
   c. Teach.
   d. Volunteer. (for the department, university, or in the community)
   e. Network. (the action or process of interacting with others to exchange information and develop professional or social contacts)
3. How long is your degree program?
4. What best describes your final piece of work?
5. Do you work with a mentor?
6. Are you a teaching assistant/instructor of record?
7. (Burnout defined—exhaustion of physical or emotional strength or motivation usually as a result of prolonged stress, frustration, overwork or overuse)—Likert/Sliding Scale 1 to 7: Does this apply to you?

General Questions:

RQ1: How do graduate students sensemake burnout?
1. Have you heard of burnout?
   a. Yes
   b. No
   c. Not sure
2. On a scale of 1 to 7, how often do you experience . . .
   a. Headaches
   b. Aggression

      c. Anxiety
      d. Chronic fatigue
      e. Forgetfulness
      f. Lack of motivation
      g. Cognitive problems/Difficulty concentrating
      h. Not taking care of yourself
      i. Isolation
      j. Loss of enjoyment
      k. Hopelessness/Helplessness
      l. Detachment
      m. Loss of purpose
      n. Lack of productivity or poor performance
3. What causes you stress in your degree program? (Select all that apply)
4. Teaching
5. Instructors
6. Research
7. Taking classes yourself
8. Time management
9. Social life
10. Publishing
11. Networking
12. Extracurricular activities
13. Building a CV
14. Plans for the future (career path)
15. Other:
16. How is your personal life impacted by pursuing a graduate degree?
17. Do you believe (a) peer(s) have experienced burnout?
18. Has a mentor/or close professor experienced burnout
    a. Yes, please elaborate
       How did they cope with the burnout?
       How did watching the experience of burnout influence you?
    b. No, skip to next question
    c. Not sure.
19. Have you ever experienced burnout?
    a. Yes, please elaborate
    b. No, skip to next question.
    c. Not sure. Please explain.
20. Do you think that burnout is stigmatized?
    a. Yes, please elaborate
    b. No, skip to next question.
    c. Not sure. Please explain.

21. What are the resources to which you have that help in overcoming burnout?
    a. What resources would you like provided?

RQ2: How does the characterization of academia impact graduate students' career paths and perceived burnout?

1. How would you characterize academia?
2. How would you characterize the culture of academia?
3. How is the academy characterized by professors to prospective graduate students?
4. How is mental health characterized in academia?
   a. Is it frowned upon?
   b. Is it glorified?
5. Do you feel supported by your department?
   a. If Yes, please elaborate.
   b. If No, please elaborate.
6. Is there conversation in your department about burnout?
   a. If Yes (Check all that apply).
      i. I talk to my peers about stress/burnout
      ii. I talk to my professors about stress/burnout
      iii. I talk to my mentor about stress/burnout
   b. If No, please elaborate.
7. Have you ever considered quitting your degree program because of burnout?
8. How does the impact of potential burnout influence your desire to continue in academia?
9. Have you considered other career paths other than academia? Why or why not?

RQ3: How do graduate students cope with graduate school burnout and with the knowledge of the likely future of tenure burnout

1. What level of stress did you expect when starting your graduate degree?
   a. Were your expectations met?
2. Did you experience more or less stress than expected?
3. How does your stress level compare with that of your colleagues?
   a. Do you talk about stress?
   b. What do you talk about?
4. Do you think feeling stressed and overwhelmed is stigmatized in academia?

5. What are some of the measures you take to counter feelings of stress/burnout?
6. What are your perceived incentives to continuing your career in the academia?
7. Do you believe you will experience burnout in the future? Why or why not?
    a. How will you deal with future symptoms of burnout?
8. What do you think would help decrease burnouts for people working in academia?
9. What else would you like to share today?

Part 2

INTERSECTIONS OF MENTAL HEALTH AND MARGINALIZED ACADEMIC POPULATIONS

CULTURAL REPRESENTATIONS AND INSTITUTIONAL CLIMATES

Chapter 5

Effects of Chronic Exposure to Invalidation on People of Color in Academia

An Exploratory Study

Juan S. Muhamad, Jessica Wendorf Muhamad, and Maria Elena Villar

INTRODUCTION

Racial microaggression is an umbrella term for a series of ambiguous and racially motivated remarks, subjugations, or invalidations (Franklin and Boyd-Franklin 2000). These communications can be verbal or non-verbal, but all share the characteristic of hostility toward people of color (POC) (Sue 2010). Sue et al. (2007) refined the microaggression concept to include three key components: *microassaults* (i.e., racial name-calling); *microinsults* (i.e., delegitimizing POC); and *microinvalidation* (i.e., scenarios in which a POC feels ignored or obviated). Today, ample evidence suggests that microaggressions—as a form of racism—detrimentally affect the well-being of POC. Therefore, this chapter explores the effects of invalidation as a form of systemic racism and microaggression on the mental well-being of academics who are also POC.

A significant knowledge gap exists about how POC in academic institutions engage in sensemaking with their individual-level concerns, such as adapting to a new situation within the job environment or balancing work and life responsibilities, while carrying out their professional roles and responsibilities. It is important to note that individual-level concerns are not directly related to performing essential tasks at work, but to salient aspects of the individual's identity. Several studies (Maitlis and Sonenshein 2010; Weick 1995) have explored the role of sensemaking and crisis environments (high reliability organizations) in health contexts. However, the higher education context has been largely omitted from this conversation because colleges and universities are not conceptualized as high-risk organizations and/or environments. Risk, ambiguity, and sensemaking are normative parts of occupational assimilation and socialization in high reliability organizations (HROs), but risk in this type of occupational environment is often characterized by situational dangers that may cause immediate danger to someone's life or health. Unknown effects of health-related issues tend to focus more on long-term illnesses or health consequences and may appear in ambiguous, unpredictable, and/or probabilistic situations.

Research on microaggression across racial and ethnic minority groups suggests associations with negative mental health outcomes, including depression and negative affect (Nadal et al. 2014a), low self-esteem (Nadal et al. 2014b), and even increased risk of suicide (O'Keefe, Wingate, Cole, Hollingsworth, and Tucker 2015). Given the risk of danger(s) to psychological well-being for POC in academia (Harrell 2000; Pittman 2012; DeCuir-Gunby 2020), this chapter considers how the lived experiences of academics of color in primarily white institutions (PWIs) share many similarities with people in HROs. Further, we unpack the unfolding socio-material practices that are barriers and/or opportunities for POC in academia.

Specifically, this chapter highlights the ways that POC in academia, who are systemically socialized to accept invalidation (e.g., regularize atypical actions), might mistakenly normalize such actions' risk to help retain organizational and social reliability while fulfilling essential job tasks and organizational-level goals (i.e., tenure and promotion). We discuss role-related uncertainty studies that address information avoidance or information-seeking as a coping strategy. Building on the previous research, our study also examines how POC in academia use sensemaking (or filling the cognitive gap) to manage situations where they experience invalidation. Additionally, we identify emergent themes from our data analysis as evidence of how POC in academia engage in sensemaking of their group experience(s) of risky behaviors on and off the job. Our results document how these behaviors create or protect POC's possible shared understanding (collaborative sensemaking) of their experience as POC who navigate a white academic environment. Collaborative sensemaking might help mitigate the effects on mental well-being of constantly having to make sense of ambiguous information (microaggressions as information), which is often unclear and can be interpreted in different ways by different people (Reddy 2010).

MICROAGGRESSION

As previously mentioned, *racial microaggression* refers to a form of systemic racial discrimination that occurs in everyday life and places POC in the margins of the social environment. Microaggression can be expressed verbally and non-verbally and constitute assaults that are often subtle, automatic, and usually unconscious. These types of aggressions might have a layered form given the presence of race and its intersection with other minority status markers (e.g., gender, class, sexual orientation, and country of origin) (Kohli and Solórzano 2012; Pérez Huber and Solorzano 2015). The subtlety of microaggressions does not diminish their negative effects as experienced by POC. Cumulative exposure to microaggression can lead to further marginalization, especially considering that this abuse is continually experienced in many POC's everyday lives. Microinsults and microinvalidations might be considered non-injurious when the single interactions are viewed in isolation, but microaggressions take a cumulative emotional and psychological toll on a person (Pierce 1970). Pérez Huber and Solorzano (2015) assert that microaggressions mirror systemic and cultural understandings that are racist. However, Pérez Huber and Solorzano (2015) also suggest that the aggressions are much larger than individuals and originate from wider organizational culture.

Understanding microaggressions, and their impact and presence in social environments, is incredibly difficult, because they occur in everyday interactions and usually manifest in subtle or even imperceptible ways. Sue et al. (2007) classify microaggressions into three categories (microassaults, microinvalidations, and microinsults) to make these daily interactions more salient, perceptible, and quantifiable.

Microassault

Microassaults are a type of microaggression with explicit racial aspersion. The racial denigration can be verbal (i.e., racial epithets), non-verbal (behavioral discrimination), or environmental abuse (offensive visual displays). These racist attacks are deliberate and intentional acts directed at a minority (Dovidio and Gaertner 2000). Microassaults often include overt aggressions such as directly calling someone a racial slur. Because microassaults are not subtle and interpretative in nature, they are not this chapter's focus.

Microinsult

Microinsults are often unintentional attacks that manifest unconsciously, and thus do not deliberately attempt to cause harm. Given their unconscious nature, microinsults might reflect implicit racist attitudes and beliefs embedded in social discourse (Banaji 2001; DeVos and Banaji 2005). A microinsult occurs only if the recipient perceives that a comment or action is such, even though the perpetrator might not intend to commit an aggression. Microinsults are often received as rude, demeaning, or insensitive comments and actions related to race, identity, and/or heritage. Given that microinsults are unconscious and subtle attacks unknown to the perpetrator, the recipient uses processing and decoding to interpret the behavior (Sue et al. 2007).

Microinvalidation

Microinvalidations are also unconscious actions, remarks, and comments that represent a negative experience for the recipient, regardless of whether the perpetrator does them unconsciously. Microinvalidations exclude, negate, or nullify POC's experiences, thoughts, and/or feelings. As the most common form of microaggression, microinvalidations often result from a colorblind approach to racial relations. Recently, police in the town of Tiburon, California, interrogated an African-American business owner (Woodrow 2020). The questioning occurred because the man was inside the store after business hours. The officer reassured the man that he was not being profiled, but rather that the officer wanted to ensure that he was the business owner. His argument was based on the fact that it seemed unusual that somebody was inside the store at night. Yet, after the man informed the officer repeatedly that he was the owner of the store, the officer was not convinced until a white older man specified that, in fact, the African-American man was the owner of the store. At that point, the officer left. Colorblindness usually invalidates POC's lived experiences by negating the differences that exist in the experiential realities of individuals with different races (Sue et al. 2007). In the case above, the officer maintained that his questioning had nothing to do with race, yet race played a part in diffusing the situation. People's inability to talk about and process the uncertainty that results from their exposure to microaggressions might increase their chances of experiencing negative psychological consequences, such as anxiety and post-traumatic stress disorder (Liu et al. 2019).

POC IN ACADEMIA

POC in academia represent 21 percent of all faculty (or 7 percent Black, 7 percent Asian, 5 percent Hispanic, and 1 percent American Indian and Alaska Native) (Hoffman, Snyder, and Sonnenberg 1992; Snyder and Dillow 2013) Although these low numbers reflect double the number of POC faculty from thirty years ago, POC are still underrepresented in higher education. Faculty representation by race across all institutional types shows that white people comprise at least 80 percent of all faculty, thus indicating that faculty of color only increased by 9 percent over the past thirty years (Martinez, Chang, and Welton 2017). Given POC's presence in a white-dominated ecology, in academic settings they constantly battle to retain cultural identity, while attempting to uphold values, norms, and ways of interacting that are normative in the academic environment but often contrast their own (Martinez, Chang, and Welton 2017).

In light of how the academic setting is an adverse social environment for many POC, researchers have identified factors that can help them integrate into this type of setting. Singh, Shaffer, and Selvarajan (2018) identify how having social support from organizations is crucial for a person's sense of psychological safety. Psychological safety helps a person integrate into the organizational environment. Psychological safety can also help one process the uncertainty arising from needing to breach the cognitive gap in cultural differences and minority status. Hobfoll (2001) suggests that a person needs social support to achieve individual-level goals (i.e., health, relationships, finances) in various domains of life, including the workplace (i.e., promotion, relationships, schedule). In addition, Hobfoll (2001) points out that social support helps prevent burnout such as emotional exhaustion and depersonalization, which can occur when a person is not able to fit within an organization where they experience constant exposure to microaggression.

THEORETICAL FOUNDATIONS

Sensemaking, or bridging the cognitive gap, is the process in which individuals negotiate or rationalize their actions or experiences by constructing a narrative they can understand (e.g., Maitlis and Christianson 2014; Weick, Sutcliffe, and Obstfeld 2005; Webb and Weick 1979). Within organizational contexts, sensemaking is often described as both an individual (e.g., Klein, Moon, and Hoffman 2006) and social process (e.g., Maitlis and Christianson 2014; Weick, Sutcliffe, and Obstfeld 2005; Weick 1995). Sensemaking can be activated when individuals are confronted with new, confusing, or surprising events. Crisis situations meet these criteria and therefore invoke sensemaking (Livingston 2016). For example, Blatt et al. (2006) found that when medical students were faced with a critical moment, or a moment when they could alter or mitigate a lapse in patient care, many students chose to remain silent. For these students, the sensemaking process included two components: confidence in their understanding of the situation and the nature (positive or negative) of their relationship with the actor in charge. Silence resulted from low confidence and a negatively perceived relationship with others (Blatt et al. 2006). These findings are critical for our study because POC experience invalidation more often than their white counterparts (Torres-Harding and Turner 2015), and POC are often socialized to accept silence as a suitable response. However, POC's chronic exposure to microaggressions, which can be invisible and undetectable to others, can have lasting effects on psychological well-being. Moreover, our findings suggest that using self-silencing as a coping mechanism, or being silenced by others, might lead a person to internalize negative self-concepts that directly affect their mental well-being.

Existing studies largely focus on uncertainty reduction (e.g., Brashers, Goldsmith, and Hsieh 2002) or uncertainty management (Brashers 2001) as opposed to sensemaking. Although some studies examine the integration of sensemaking as normative to HRO members, little research covers sensemaking's relationship to organizational culture and occupational risk. More significantly, no research addresses the potential impact of organizational culture (as a product of socialization) and what is necessary for sustained reliability within HROs that might impact wellness factors such as the mental health at the individual level. Additionally, few studies have directly applied the theory to observable behaviors. Such studies (Bird 2007; Dulini and Patriotta 2020) focus on theoretical abstraction, with varying conceptualization of sensemaking. However, they fail to demonstrate how sensemaking might manifest in particular environments with certain risks as opposed to during transitional periods (i.e., layovers, change in leadership).

Given the findings and knowledge gaps in the existing research, our chapter explores the following research questions:

RQ1: How do POC in academia normalize the risk of invalidation in their effort to retain organizational and social reliability?

RQ2: What are the perceived effects of invalidation on mental health/psychological well-being among POC in academia?

METHODS

We conducted narrative interviews (NIs) with a convenience sample of participants ($N = 22$) who identify as POC in academia until we reached saturation ($N = 20$). We used NIs instead of the standard question-answer structure because they provide a holistic understanding of experiences by reconstructing psychosocial events from the individual's perspective. NIs encourage participants to share stories of events that significantly impact their lives. In this way, NIs enable researchers to "reconstruct social events from the perspective of the informant as much as possible" (Jovchelovitch and Bauer 1996, 3).

Each semi-structured interview lasted approximately forty-five minutes. NIs were analyzed for emergent themes using *NVivo* along with a systematic literature review and relevant statistics. After we thematically categorized all responses, two independent coders determined which response categories were most common in response to the interview prompts below.

1. What are your thoughts about being a member of academia?
2. What is your impression of academia?
3. Do you have relationships with others in academia?
4. How do you relate to them?
5. Have you ever found yourself in situations that made you *uncomfortable* within the academic setting?
   I. If so, could you please share the story of event
   II. In moments you have felt uncomfortable, what has been your response?
      i. Could you have done anything different?
      ii. Have you ever questioned your response to an uncomfortable situation?
   III. Thinking back on this uncomfortable event, what would it have meant to handle the situation differently?
      i. What would be the barriers, consequences, or opportunities of taking a different approach?
   IV. Do you believe that others have a similar experience?
      i. If so, who would be likely to have a similar uncomfortable experience?
6. *If the event shared above did not include POC identity this would be follow-up:* Have you ever found yourself in situations that made you *uncomfortable* within the academic setting that you felt was due to being a person of color?
   I. If so, could you please share the story of event
   II. In moments you have felt uncomfortable, what has been your response?
      i. Could you have done anything different?
      ii. Have you ever questioned your response to an uncomfortable situation?
   III. Thinking back on this uncomfortable event what would it have meant to handle the situation differently?
      i. What would be the barriers, consequences, or opportunities of taking a different approach?
   IV. Do you believe that others have similar experience?
      i. If so, who would be likely to have a similar uncomfortable experience?
7. Have you ever found yourself in situations that made you *very comfortable* within the academic setting?
   I. If so, could you please share the story of event
   II. Do you believe that others have had a similar experience?
      i. If so, who would be likely to have a similar, uncomfortable experience?
8. Do you want to add anything?

After determining which categories shared properties (Lindlof and Taylor 2017), coders then collapsed them into major themes. We used this constant comparative method (Strauss and Corbin 1990) until saturation was reached.

Inclusion criteria included people in academia who self-identified as POC and from different faculty ranks of assistant professor, associate professor, full professor, and specialized faculty (i.e., lecturer, adjunct, visiting scholar, teaching instructor).

Study participants were recruited via snowball sampling, the most commonly adopted sampling method in qualitative research (Patton 1990), with members of different academic departments from a major university in the Southeastern region of the United States. To help include diverse voices and experiences within the boundaries of a defined population (Ritchie and Lewis 2003), we asked interviewees to introduce other participants to the study. We sent interview requests via email, with follow-up emails sent depending on response rate. Methodological triangulation helped us converge research direction from more than one source (Lindlof and Taylor 2002).

FINDINGS

Among organizational factors, two main themes emerged: collective sensemaking and hierarchical information dissemination/diffusion cognitive gaps. Collective sensemaking manifested in conversations where participants shared that they felt uncertain about the adverse effects of systemic and continuous invalidation. For example, one participant stated, "At the end of the day we need to be productive and have a million responsibilities. I know it affects me, but I don't have time and space in my mind to sit with it." Additionally, it was unclear to participants whether they as a group had the ability to perform corrective actions to reduce their risk.

Our findings suggest that hierarchical information dissemination/diffusion cognitive gaps manifest in communicative interactions with senior faculty, directors, and supervisors that appear unclear and/or aggressive (do not equate to any culturally appropriate and/or positive recognized interactions). However, within these interactions, hierarchical positionality, coupled with minority status, seemed to prevent study participants from seeking clarification and/or expressing inconformity. Because participants did not see ways to formally and/or informally organize collectively, they did not pursue them. The resulting gap in understanding forced participants to internally and individually make sense of situations that are uncomfortable and/or perceived negatively, while simultaneously performing their academic and social roles.

Collective Sensemaking

Most participants identified and described experiences of participating in academic environments where diversity is considered important. Participants explained how a constant focus on diversity amplified people's awareness of perceived difference, specifically in PWIs (i.e., constantly having to talk about race and inclusion). Given the racial imbalance in the academic setting, participants recounted how a constant focus on diverse voices, inclusion, and equality led to them constantly feeling pressured to avoid fitting into negative racial stereotypes. For example, one participant said, "I try to answer questions without pressing the issue. How do you answer the question without pressing the issue? I am still trying to figure that out, but I am very cognizant of being a little bit softer, a little bit gentler, a little bit . . . not less educated, but a little less obviously woke." This inconsistency resulted in interviewees needing to adopt certain behaviors or demeanor to avoid reflecting a stereotype or being misunderstood. As another participant said, "I am a major reader, I am an introvert, I am quiet, I am not super expressive, but I also don't want to be thought of as a phony white woman. So, it is definitely a part of my everyday interactions, put on a happy face, which is really not who I am. I feel as though I need to make sure that I do not embody any negative stereotypes. I do find myself pepping it up a bit, cracking more jokes, 'Let's go for coffee!' things that if you knew me well . . . are not me." Another participant mentioned that "there is definitely a front of the mind awareness of my demeanor, more so than, I think, I had before [academia], when I think I was judged more by just, she does the work."

Participants described how too often they felt they had to over-explain (behaviors and thoughts). For example, stated one participant, "I said to her [colleague], 'I need to talk to you.' I feel as though, I can't remember exactly what it was . . . like, you are not talking with us, you are not communicating with us, and I remember her telling me, 'Well you always seem angry,' and I said, 'What do you mean?' 'Well, you seem angry and unhappy all the time,' and I said 'Do I seem unhappy now?'"

Participants said that they felt they had to represent their pertinent ethnic/racial group. A participant said, "People often assume things about you. So, for instance, he's Black, so perhaps he has an opinion about this. And I don't think that is necessarily malicious in any respect, but it was like, hey . . . let's ask him what he thinks, but I wonder if [race] would have been a topic of conversation with anyone else that just started a few days ago." Participants also described how often they found themselves consistently validating/reassuring others (whites) about their racial awareness. For instance, stated one participant, "They [the university] created their mascot after the Confederate South. From the pants, the Confederate uniform of the Union, they even used the rebel yell, which was the war cry of the Confederate army, and I was a little taken aback, but people kept wanting to talk to me about it, they wanted to know my opinion. I often reserve my opinion until I have more information, but they seem to be uncomfortable with that, they wanted to dialogue to make sure that I understood that they didn't agree with . . . or they were not ok with what was going on." Additionally, POCs frequently felt they had to carry the responsibility for fulfilling unclear expectations while needing to understand/accept ambiguous interactions (sensemaking). To this end, one participant noted, "In one situation I didn't know what I was expected to say, but I was aware that I wasn't going to go too in depth with it and possibly fall into other possible tropes of Black women around the world."

Hierarchical Information Dissemination/Diffusion Cognitive Gaps

Our participants' responses suggested how the ways in which information is communicated in PWIs might be causing greater cognitive gaps. For example, participants described unclear hierarchical structures in their departments and their colleagues' egalitarian way of interacting. They said that the subtle expressions of hierarchy and power distressed them.

Participants described how the pressure to fulfill work responsibilities while dealing with academic pressures (i.e., conducting research, publishing, and service to the university) was already challenging and/or stressful enough. On top of this, trying to understand unclear expectations from administrators in faculty colleagues, and especially from higher in the academic hierarchy, led participants to feel misunderstood and invalidated in their individual experiences. Participants described the impact of hierarchical structures in academic organizations, specifically in how they favor Eurocentric attitudes and behaviors, and how this might present a barrier to information flow. For instance, a participant said, "Email communication is at times difficult to deal with. I get emails that include charged language and where people are copied up the chain of command for no reason. I often feel that I am in trouble and that I have to respond very soon, but very carefully. I have been told by white colleagues that copying literally everyone is normal and that I am reading too much into it."

Emergent themes from the participant interviews included knowledge gaps about organizational structures and whether current organizational processes adequately disseminate the information needed to make mental health–related decisions. For example, participants discussed how some colleagues used their higher ranks to disregard conversation, opinions, and even reject relevant information from their colleagues who are POC. One participant explained, "Sometimes it seems as if though I am imagining . . . . I shared ideas for a symposium and felt ignored during the meeting. Then I found out an established professor [present at the meeting] was leading a 'similar' symposium and was getting a lot of attention." Although this finding might not be dissimilar for white academics, the participants who are POC described feeling invalidated in these situations. They especially felt invalidated given the constantly changing and unclear dynamics that they experienced when interacting with colleagues in the hierarchical environment. For example, one participant said, "At times participation and sharing my perspective is welcomed and encouraged; other times it seems that I am overstepping and feel shut down."

Overall, our observations and interviews reflected the participants' sensemaking in relation to occupational risk for decreased mental wellness. Our results indicate that POC in academia (faculty members, administrators, graduate students) recognized existing tension between occupational and social health–related (mental) sensemaking. Importantly, although POC in academia appear to realize they are at risk, they are not sure what to do about these risks. For example, one participant stated that uncertainty played a role in his not communicating with other POC in the department to discuss events or decisions that occurred or engaging in collective sensemaking. This response echoed that of others who chose to self-silence during situations such as meetings, where they were either silent or agreed with the consensus to avoid conflict. Stated one participant about this type of situation: "She [director] often interrupts me. So, I am here going like, ok .... I am no longer talking in meetings, I am no longer sharing my ideas, because it makes no sense, but you can imagine how hard those meetings are."

Clearly, POC in academia normalize the risk of invalidation by self-silencing, as well as acculturating to everyday workplace practices and academic socialization regardless of their awareness of the negative impact on their mental health and well-being. Although our study's participants are clearly aware of their experiences of invalidation, ambiguity, and uncertainty, given their minority status, it is unclear what measures might help mitigate the negative impact of constantly being self-aware of their race/ethnicity, as well as constantly needing to adapt or adopt behaviors to avoid being perceived negatively. As our findings demonstrate, POC understand that there are negative effects to their mental health/psychological well-being. However, they lack clarity about how these effects manifest long term, and what the implications of prolonged exposure to invalidation might be.

DISCUSSION

This chapter is a first step in investigating the ways that sensemaking regarding invalidation—as a form of microaggression—manifests among POC in academia, as well as possible consequences of socialization processes that normalize risky, uncertain, or chaotic situations. To begin to address the lack of knowledge in these general areas, this chapter explored how academics who are POC make sense of the risk to their mental well-being as a result of fulfilling their occupational roles and responsibilities within PWIs. The chapter also examines how these sensemaking behaviors are tied to the socialization process.

Our research contributes to scholarly understanding of how the culture of PWIs normalizes responses to risky, chaotic, or uncertain situations for POC and interacts with occupational hazards (mental well-being) to produce sensemaking responses related to health. Within HROs, members engage in socialization processes that result in trust, which is essential for individuals to perform job functions within this context (Muhamad, Harrison, and Yang 2019). Similar to HROs, POC individuals are exposed to mental health risk within PWIs, yet the absence of a framework that supports socialization and normalization processes to mitigate risk to mental well-being is common. Our interviews with POC demonstrate that they are aware that their socialization processes and position in academic culture might negatively impact their mental health. One participant stated, "I do not know how to compensate or to adjust in this situation [micro-aggression] so it doesn't get ugly, so I basically just have to say, 'This comes from a place of love,' because I see her [director] brace herself when I am about to speak. It has come to the point where I feel, well, I am not going to try anymore and just move on." However, academics of color are unclear about how to address and/or counteract the effects of constantly needing to engage in sensemaking in the face of ambiguity. Moreover, they are unclear about what resources are available to address invalidation, uncertainty, and/or risky situations, and/or how to counteract the negative effects of performing in academic culture while meeting their job's social and academic expectations. Additionally, academics who are POC are unclear what the ultimate effects of long-term exposure to invalidation and uncertain situations have on their mental health and overall well-being.

Given the results presented in this chapter, academic institutions should address normative practices that prevent true integration of POC into their academic cultures. To counterbalance the psychological and emotional burdens that academics of color experience, institutions should attempt to understand existing practices related to white, Eurocentric culture. Currently, some college campuses engage faculty, staff, and students in conversations about equality, inclusion, diversity, and racism to promote greater understanding (Stallings, Iyer, and Hernandez 2018). These often occur as workshops that encourage participation while focusing on interpersonal interactions that might negatively affect POCs in the academic environment. Although well intentioned, conversations about racism within a white academic environment often activate the same biases being combated in the first place (Sue et al. 2010; Sue et al. 2009a; Sue et al. 2009b).

Studies (Sue et al. 2010; Williams 2019) indicate how white individuals' experience of the academic environment within their own culture explains their inability to identify racial microaggressions because they are unintentionally delivered from their vantage point. From their position, it is argued that microaggressions can be reduced to minor mistakes that do not deserve addressing or correcting. Further, Sue and colleagues (2009) explain that when conversations about race aim for greater/deeper understanding of the experiences of POCs, white individuals might hesitate to openly share for fear of appearing racist or insensitive. Sue et al. (2009) also point out that white people may not engage in these discussions because they resist acknowledging their own bias/racism or dislike being confronted with the concept of white privilege.

Even though presenting information and encouraging conversation is an important first step, it is clearly not enough. Berk (2017) recommends following workshops with programs designed to ensure accountability by supporting POCs in reporting instances of micro-aggression. Evidently, for POCs to report, trust must be established between them and those tasked with supporting reporting efforts. Berk (2017) also suggests that workshops should be continuous throughout the academic year, at predetermined intervals, and should ensure monitoring of progress in reporting. Additionally, continuous adjustment to the programming is recommended to ensure possible decrease in racial incidents.

Miller and Donner (2000) suggest that conversations encompass social constructs and ideologies that inform stereotypes and biases. It is challenging for individuals to be socialized into a different cultural group that differs from their cultural group of origin. Therefore, academic institutions must highlight cultural humility and transparency by naming whiteness as a culture and a racial group (rather than the norm) from the onset of program implementation. Doing so might open the conversation between white individuals and other groups about behavior, perception, expectations, and difference. This conversation creates an opportunity to mitigate the risk of not being able to fulfill job responsibilities or making sense of unclear and ambiguous situations. Although researchers (Kennedy, Middleton, and Ratcliff 2020; Bohonos 2019) document that white people often do not identify as a racial group, having this conversation would help institutions examine the individual and collective roles that white academics play in subtly perpetuating racism and difference on their campuses.

This conversational approach might be a crucial first step to creating spaces where new ways of interacting and sharing information are possible. Engaging in conversation might lead institutions and their employees to acknowledge the prevalent, dominant, and normalized white culture that is forced, mostly unwillingly, upon minorities, and negatively affects their psychological well-being, while rendering real inclusion and diversity impossible. By addressing normativity, the burden to acculturate for academics of color can be lifted and replaced with environments with real inclusion where everyone can impact, contribute, and collaborate.

REFERENCES

Banaji, Mahzarin R. 2001. "Implicit Attitudes Can Be Measured." *The Nature of Remembering: Essays in Honor of Robert G. Crowder.* Edited by Henry L. Roedeger III, James S. Nairne, Ian Neath, Aimeé M. Suprenant, 117–150. American Psychological Association.

Blatt, Ruth, Marlys K. Christianson, Kathleen M. Sutcliffe, and Marilynn M. Rosenthal. 2006. "A Sensemaking Lens on Reliability." *Journal of Organizational Behavior: The International Journal of Industrial, Occupational and Organizational Psychology and Behavior* 27, no. 7 (November): 897–917. https://doi.org/10.1002/job.392.

Brashers, Dale E. 2001. "Communication and Uncertainty Management." *Journal of Communication* 51, no. 3: 477–497. https://doi.org/10.1111/j.1460-2466.2001.tb02892.x.

Brashers, Dale E., Daena J. Goldsmith, and Elaine Hsieh. 2002. "Information Seeking and Avoiding in Health Contexts." *Human Communication Research* 28, no. 2 (April): 258–271. https://doi.org/10.1111/j.1468-2958.2002.tb00807.x.

Bohonos, Jeremy W. 2019. "Including Critical Whiteness Studies in the Critical Human Resource Development Family: A Proposed Theoretical Framework." *Adult Education Quarterly* 69, no. 4: 315–337. https://doi.org/10.1177/0741713619858131.

Carmer, Erin. 2020. "Rhetorics of Whiteness: Postracial Hauntings in Popular Culture, Social Media, and Education." *Rhetoric Review* 39, no. 1: 118–119. https://doi.org/10.1080/07350198.2020.1686596.

Devos, Thierry, and Mahzarin R. Banaji. 2005. "American=White?" *Journal of Personality and Social Psychology* 88, no. 3: 447–466. https://doi.org/10.1037/0022-3514.88.3.447.

Franklin, Anderson J., and Nancy Boyd-Franklin. 2000. "Invisibility Syndrome: A Clinical Model of the Effects of Racism on African-American Males." *American Journal of Orthopsychiatry* 70, no. 1: 33–41. https://doi.org/10.1037/h0087691.

Jovchelovitch, Sandra, and Martin W. Bauer. 2000. "Narrative Interviewing." In *Qualitative Researching with Text, Image and Sound.* Edited by Martin W. Bauer and George Gaskell, 57–74. Thousand Oaks, CA: Sage.

Hobfoll, Stevan E. 2001. "The Influence of Culture, Community, and the Nested-Self in the Stress Process: Advancing Conservation of Resources Theory." *Applied Psychology* 50, no. 3: 337–421. https://doi.org/10.1111/1464-0597.00062.

Hoffman, Charlene, Thomas D. Snyder, and Bill Sonnenberg. *Historically Black Colleges and Universities, 1976-1990*. US Department of Education, Office of Educational Research and Improvement, National Center for Education Statistics, 1992.

Klein, Gary, Brian Moon, and Robert R. Hoffman. 2006. "Making Sense of Sensemaking 1: Alternative Perspectives." *IEEE Intelligent Systems* 21, no. 4 (July-August): 70–73. https://doi.org/ 10.1109/MIS.2006.75.

Kohli, Rita, and Daniel G. Solórzano. 2012. "Teachers, Please Learn Our Names!: Racial Microaggressions and the K-12 classroom." *Race Ethnicity and Education* 15, no. 4: 441–462. https://doi.org/10.1080/13613324.2012.674026.

Lindlof, Thomas R., and Bryan C. Taylor. 2017. *Qualitative Communication Research Methods*. Thousand Oaks, CA: Sage.

Liu, William Ming, Rossina Zamora Liu, Yunkyoung Loh Garrison, Ji Youn Cindy Kim, Laurence Chan, Yu Ho, and Chi W. Yeung. 2019. "Racial Trauma, Microaggressions, and Becoming Racially Innocuous: The Role of Acculturation and White Supremacist Ideology." *American Psychologist* 74, no. 1: 143–155. http://dx.doi.org/10.1037/amp0000368.

Livingston, Mark A. 2016. "Senior Leadership Response to Organizational Crises: Exploring the Relationship between Sensemaking and Organizational Resiliency." PhD diss., University of Maryland University College.

Maitlis, Sally, and Marlys Christianson. 2014. "Sensemaking in Organizations: Taking Stock and Moving Forward." *Academy of Management Annals* 8, no. 1: 57–125. https://doi.org/10.5465/19416520.2014.873177.

Maitlis, Sally, and Scott Sonenshein. "Sensemaking in Crisis and Change: Inspiration and Insights from Weick (1988)." *Journal of management studies* 47, no. 3 (2010): 551–580.

Martinez, Melissa A., Aurora Chang, and Anjalé D. Welton. 2017. "Assistant Professors of Color Confront the Inequitable Terrain of Academia: A Community Cultural Wealth Perspective." *Race Ethnicity and Education* 20, no. 5: 696–710. https://doi.org/10.1080/13613324.2016.1150826.

Muhamad, Jessica Wendorf, Tyler R. Harrison, and Fan Yang. 2019. "Organizational Communication: Theory and Practice." In *An Integrated Approach to Communication Theory and Research*, 3rd ed., 359–374. New York: Taylor and Francis.

Nadal, Kevin L., Katie E. Griffin, Yinglee Wong, Sahran Hamit, and Morgan Rasmus. 2014. "The Impact of Racial Microaggressions on Mental Health: Counseling Implications for Clients of Color." *Journal of Counseling & Development* 92, no. 1: 57–66. https://doi.org/10.1002/j.1556-6676.2014.00130.x.

Nadal, Kevin L., Yinglee Wong, Katie E. Griffin, Kristin Davidoff, and Julie Sriken. 2014. "The Adverse Impact of Racial Microaggressions on College Students' Self-esteem." *Journal of College Student Development* 55, no. 5: 461–474. https://doi.org/10.1353/csd.2014.0051.

Pérez Huber, Lindsay, and Daniel G. Solorzano. 2015. "Racial Microaggressions as a Tool for Critical Race Research." *Race Ethnicity and Education* 18, no. 3: 297–320. https://doi.org/10.1080/13613324.2014.994173.

Pierce, Chester. 1970. "Offensive Mechanisms." In *The Black Seventies*. Edited by Floyd B. Barbour, 265–282. Boston: Porter Sargent.

Paul, Sharoda A., and Madhu C. Reddy. 2010. "Understanding Together: Sensemaking in Collaborative Information Seeking." In *Proceedings of the 2010 ACM Conference on Computer Supported Cooperative Work*, 321–330.

Singh, Barjinder, Margaret A. Shaffer, and T. T. Selvarajan. 2018. "Antecedents of Organizational and Community Embeddedness: The Roles of Support, Psychological Safety, and Need to Belong." *Journal of Organizational Behavior* 39, no. 3 (March): 339–354. https://doi.org/10.1002/job.2223.

Snyder, Thomas D., and Sally A. Dillow. 2013. "Digest of Education Statistics, 2012. NCES 2014-015." *National Center for Education Statistics*. https://nces.ed.gov/pubs2014/2014015.pdf.

Stallings, Dontarie, Srikant Iyer, and Rigoberto Hernandez. 2018. "National Diversity Equity Workshops: Advancing Diversity in Academia." In *National Diversity Equity Workshops in Chemical Sciences (2011-2017)*, 1–19. ACS Symposium Series Vol. 1277. American Chemical Society. https://doi.org/10.1021/bk-2018-1277.ch001.

Strauss, Anselm, and Juliet Corbin. *Basics of Qualitative Research*. Thousand Oaks, CA: Sage.

Sue, Derald Wing, Jennifer Bucceri, Annie I. Lin, Kevin L. Nadal, and Gina C. Torino. 2007. "Racial Microaggressions and the Asian American Experience." *Cultural Diversity and Ethnic Minority Psychology* 13, no. 1: 72–81. https://doi.org/10.1037/1099-9809.13.1.72.

Sue, Derald Wing, Annie I. Lin, Gina C. Torino, Christina M. Capodilupo, and David P. Rivera. 2009a. "Racial Microaggressions and Difficult Dialogues on Race in the Classroom." *Cultural Diversity and Ethnic Minority Psychology* 15, no. 2: 183–190. https://doi.org/10.1037/a0014191.

Sue, Derald Wing, Jennifer Bucceri, Annie I. Lin, Kevin L. Nadal, and Gina C. Torino. 2009b. "Racial Microaggressions and the Asian American Experience." *Asian American Journal of Psychology* Vol S, no. 1 (August): 88–101.

Sue, Derald Wing. 2010. *Microaggressions in Everyday Life: Race, Gender, and Sexual Orientation*. Hoboken, NJ: John Wiley & Sons.

Weick, Karl E., Kathleen M. Sutcliffe, and David Obstfeld. 2005. "Organizing and the Process of Sensemaking." *Organization Science* 16, no. 4: 327–451. https://doi.org/10.1287/orsc.1050.0133.

Weick, Karl E. 1995. *Sensemaking in Organizations*. Vol. 3. Thousand Oaks, CA: Sage.

Webb, Eugene, and Karl E. Weick. 1979. "Unobtrusive Measures in Organizational Theory: A Reminder." *Administrative Science Quarterly* 24, no. 4: 650–659. https://doi.org/10.2307/2392370.

Woodrow, Melanie. 2020. "'Show Me That It's Your Store': Tiburon Police Demand Black Business Owner Prove Who He Is." ABC7 San Francisco. KGO-TV, August 26, 2020. https://abc7news.com/yema-tiburon-police-news-racial-profiling/6388570/.

Chapter 6

First-Generation Graduate and Professional Students in the United States

A Critical Narrative Review

Erinn C. Cameron

Robust evidence indicates that first-generation college students (FGCS) often face significant challenges in accessing post-secondary education, succeeding academically, and completing a degree. When demographic, educational, and economic factors are controlled for, first-generation students are still less likely to pursue graduate school, especially doctoral programs, due, in part, to the same challenges they encounter during the undergraduate experience (Engle 2007). FGCS are disproportionately underrepresented at the graduate level, as only 4 percent of first-generation college graduates go on to enroll in a graduate or professional program as compared to 10 percent of graduates whose parents attended or graduated from college, and only 3 percent will earn a master's degree or higher (Redford and Hoyer 2017).

This chapter's review of the extant literature indicates a significant lack of research regarding FGCS in higher education beyond the undergraduate years. However, this review posits that evidence suggests that the significant barriers faced by first-generation students do not diminish upon completion of the undergraduate degree, but rather persist in the pursuit of a graduate or professional degree, especially the doctoral degree. Institutions of higher education should be cautious when assuming that all students enrolled in graduate or professional degree programs have the skills and tools required to be successful (Gardner and Holley 2011). While a first-generation student may have successfully completed an undergraduate degree, this experience does not automatically ensure that the same student can transfer specialized knowledge and skills to the graduate or professional school experience.

Additionally, the existing research on FGCS has identified significant barriers faced by first-generation students, which likely remain in effect while in pursuit of graduate or professional degrees. For example, at the graduate level, academic barriers may translate to lack of access to study materials and preparation programs for graduate and professional school entrance exams, or a lack of research experience in STEM subjects, and first-generation students are more likely to have lower GPAs (Choy 2001; Engle 2007; Holmes and Slate 2017; Piat et al. 2019). Further, studies have shown that FGCS have lower median household incomes than their peers, come from lower socioeconomic status (SES) backgrounds, and are more likely to face significant additional financial barriers than their continuing-generation peers (Allan et al. 2015; Bauer et al. 2019; Piat et al. 2019; PPNI 2020; Unverferth, Talbert-Johnson, and Bogard et al. 2012). Additionally, when attending graduate and professional training, first-generation students must continue to navigate the challenging nuances and intense pressure that can result from the intersectional identities of competing sociocultural dimensions. We further posit that the barriers faced by first-generation graduate students should be examined within an intersectional framework, and through the lens of accompanying psychological considerations.

Future research is needed to ameliorate barriers that have led to the disproportionate underrepresentation of first-generation students at the graduate and professional levels. Disproportionate representation in graduate and professional programs means that first-generation students have less career mobility and total earning power in the job sector. This phenomenon further exacerbates the structural inequalities that first-generation students inherently face. This critical narrative review of the extant literature regarding first-generation graduate students provides a foundation for informing future research and policy recommendations at the personal, collegial, societal, and governmental levels.

FIRST-GENERATION DEFINED

First, what is meant by the *first-generation* designation must be defined. It may appear that the definition of first-generation status would simply be *college students or graduate students whose parents did not graduate from college*. However, this simple definition overlooks the diverse and intersecting identities of this population and has been heavily debated, and differences in this definition have many implications, including empirical, personal, theoretical, and policy. Research has shown that the definition of first-generation varies widely, both across and within academic and governmental institutions, as well as with educational funding bodies. Toutkoushian (2018) noted eight distinct and commonly used definitions of first-generation. Further, the U.S. Department of Education has three working definitions of first-generation: a) the legislative definition where no parent in the household has a bachelor's degree; and the two definitions used for research: b) no parent has any education beyond high school, and c) no parent has a degree beyond a high school diploma (Cataldi, Bennett, and Chen 2018).

Despite these governmental standards, other definitions are still commonly used among colleges, universities, and other educational bodies. For example, different conceptualizations of first-generation graduate students include someone whose parents did not obtain a college degree at all; someone whose parents have an undergraduate degree but not a graduate or professional degree; or a student whose parents have an associate degree and not a four-year undergraduate degree. The precise definition of FGCS can have far-reaching consequences across several domains.

Due to the competing definitions of the term *first-generation*, institutions need to reconsider how the concept is best defined and how it should be used in practice to best serve those whom it defines. As part of this process, institutions must clarify their goals regarding the first-generation designation. Varying and unpredictable definitions for first-generation student status may devalue or ignore the realities and barriers that students with intersecting identities may face. While defining first-generation is complicated and finely nuanced, it is crucial to highlight why such a precisely defined definition is necessary. Because identification as an FGCS is most often self-reported without defining guidelines, gaps in collected data are often unavoidable.

Moreover, not having a precisely operationalized definition makes it challenging to generalize research and survey results. Without such a definition, institutions are unable to accurately track student experiences, thereby making it hard to qualify and quantify student needs in comparison to other groups. Adding to this problem, students whose parent(s) have a college degree are often referred to as *continuing generation*, a definition that also varies across settings. The absence of a clearly operationalized definition for the first-generation designation may have contributed to the gaps in the literature regarding this population in graduate and professional school settings.

Additionally, studies regarding students with marginalized identities have primarily focused on one specific marginalized identity at a time, and the term *first-generation* is often conflated with working-class, minority, and low SES identities. However, first-generation students may embody one, or all, of these identities, and perhaps new identities as well. Some scholars have begun examining first-generation students from a framework of intersecting marginalities (Housel 2019). An intersectional framework allows for exploration and understanding of students with multiple identities, many of which may be marginalized.

FIRST-GENERATION STUDENTS IN THE UNITED STATES

In the United States, only 20 percent of first-generation students earn a bachelor's degree as compared to 42 percent of students whose parents have bachelor's degrees (Callan 2001). Additionally, first-generation students are disproportionately underrepresented in certain areas of American higher education, with first-generation students far less likely to attend any type of graduate program as compared to their peers (Callan 2001; Gardner and Holley 2011; Mullen, Goyette, and Soares 2003; Redford and Hoyer 2017), with first-generation students enrolling in graduate programs at a rate of 41 percent compared to 46 percent of those whose parents hold a degree (Cataldi, Bennett, and Chen 2018). Further, first-generation students are also applying to graduate and professional programs less frequently than continuing-generation peers (Gardner and Holley 2011), which indicates that the discrepancy is not merely one of first-generation students being accepted to such programs at lower rates.

Furthermore, studies have found no effect of level of parent education on entrance into MBA programs but have found a significant effect on entry into doctoral and professional degree programs (Mullen, Goyette, and Soares 2003). This evidence suggests that the effect of first-generation status is not a significant factor when considering lower levels of post-baccalaureate education but is intensified when considering higher levels of graduate and professional education that call for more support and resources across several personal, academic, and financial domains (Mullen, Goyette, and Soares 2003). This phenomenon may be perpetuating an economic disadvantage for first-generation students who also may never attain the higher paying careers that often accompany graduate and professional school degrees (Carlton 2015).

Valletta and colleagues (2015) reported that the earnings advantage gained by receiving a college degree versus a high school diploma increased only 6 percent from 2000 to 2013 as compared to a 17 percent increase in earnings for those with a graduate or professional degree. In 2012, among women aged forty to sixty-five, those with a master's, doctoral, or professional degree earned median salaries 25 percent, 60 percent, and 108 percent greater than women who had only obtained a bachelor's degree. Among men of the same age range, the benefits of having earned an advanced degree as compared to an undergraduate degree for median salaries were 17 percent, 30 percent, and 100 percent, respectively (NSF 2013). Further, Torpey and colleagues (2018) posited that employment requiring an advanced degree is projected to increase by 17 percent (master's level) and by 13 percent (doctoral and professional levels) through 2026.

Additionally, the growth in employment opportunities that require a graduate or professional degree is expected to exceed the growth for those jobs requiring only a bachelor's degree (Torpey 2018). To meet the national hiring demands for highly skilled workers, social justice–oriented policies and interventions are needed to support individuals from all sectors of American society, specifically those that have historically faced underrepresentation in graduate and professional education, such as first-generation students. Further, first-generation students are more likely to be underrepresented in society with respect to other demographics, such as class and race, as they are more likely to come from minority and/or working-class families. All aspects of the U.S. job sector are in need of increased diverse representation that better reflects the face of American society.

POTENTIAL BARRIERS TO FIRST-GENERATION STUDENT SUCCESS

Past studies indicate that first-generation students face significant challenges concerning college enrollment at any level (Carlton 2015; Choy 2011). Additionally, many characteristics of the FGCS population are the same as those that have been identified in students who are more likely to drop out of a doctoral degree program in general (Council of Graduate Schools 2004). Here, this chapter examines selected barriers for FGCS within an intersectional framework of diverse and competing identities and highlight how these barriers continue through graduate and professional training. The discussion also highlights how these factors may be associated with poor mental health in first-generation graduate and professional students. Finally, recommendations for providing support across multiple dimensions and platforms will be discussed.

Sociocultural Considerations

The impact of societal and structural inequality on marginalized populations has often been overlooked in psychology's propensity for focusing on the individual. Pierre Bourdieu posited that cultural capital is a crucial determinant of educational success, and that familiarity with dominant cultural codes is integral to student achievement because educators often equate it with intelligence (Jaeger 2017). Further, individuals with more social capital often come from backgrounds of higher SES, which contributes to the continuation of their privileged status within the context of higher education.

However, first-generation graduate students have reported that they experience a kind of cultural dissonance regarding social constructs such as accents, attire, food, and acceptable practices for socializing both in and out of the academic environment, indicating likely deficits in social capital (Hirudayaraj 2019). Stephens et al. (2012) found that such cultural dissonance persisted throughout the undergraduate experience and was still present at graduation, indicating that FGCS likely carry it through to graduate and professional school. This cultural dissonance, or mismatch, has been associated with poorer academic outcomes and overall well-being for first-generation students (Stephens et al. 2012).

FGCS face complex issues of identity that may become intensified when faced with the additional new identities of entering graduate and professional training programs. We posit that marginality increases upon entering this unfamiliar realm where the costs and consequences of cultural dissonance may be even more profound than in the undergraduate experience. The social and professional cultural expectations of degree programs that lead to professional careers such as in law, medicine, STEM, or higher education, have been shown to be largely unfamiliar to the majority of first-generation students. Additionally, studies have indicated that the most common aspect of marginality for first-generation students is their unfamiliarity with middle- and upper- class academic culture (Nguyen and Nguyen 2018).

Studies have also indicated that first-generation students may experience a form of classism that is unique to higher education, as many of these students come from backgrounds that are traditionally underrepresented in higher education (Allan, Garriott, and Keene 2016; Rubin 2013; Thompson and Subich 2013). Further, classism in the academic environment can have a significant effect on overall student success and satisfaction with the higher education experience and may contribute to poor mental health and higher attrition rates (Allan, Garriott, and Keene 2016; Becerra 2017; Cattaneo et al. 2019). Additionally, FGCS report high levels of stress associated with the transition from a working-class social environment to a middle-class higher education social environment (Stephens et al. 2012). Their identities clash as they struggle to be successful in a new social class while holding onto their old identities in an attempt to still identify with their families and associations outside the higher education environment.

Some researchers have noted that sociocultural factors, while highly impactful, are less detrimental to overall first-generation student success than how well the student was able to integrate and engage in academic and campus life while in college (House, Neal, and Kolb 2019). We argue that sociocultural factors are at the very core of an individual's ability to integrate into graduate and professional school environments. Studies indicate that first-generation students report struggles with belonging and feelings of being excluded in the college setting, which can have implications on well-being and mental health (Allan, Garriott, and Keene 2016; Stebleton, Soria, and Huesman Jr. 2014; Stephens et al. 2015). Research also suggests that a stronger sense of belonging among college students in their chosen higher education environment is associated with the level of confidence in academic abilities, more motivation for studies, better overall academic adjustment, higher levels of achievement, greater persistence, higher GPAs, and higher retention rates (Murphy and Zirkel 2015; Strayhorn 2018; Walton and Cohen 2011). Sociocultural factors and matters of identity not only contribute to poor educational success, but also contribute to mental health problems for first-generation graduate students and should be addressed as part of all levels of intervention.

Socioeconomic Status

According to the Postsecondary National Policy Institute (PNPI 2020), FGCS disproportionately come from lower SES backgrounds, with 27 percent coming from households with an annual income of $20,000 or less, as compared to only 6 percent of continuing-generation students. Additionally, low SES students are underrepresented in higher education (Hearn and Rosinger 2014) and hold an identity that is likely a deeply ingrained component of the self, that serves as a constant reminder of how they are different than their higher SES peers. Data shows that SES continues to have an effect on achievement and graduation rates once a student enters higher education (OECD 2014) and that students from lower SES backgrounds perceive less familial support as compared to students from higher SES backgrounds (Jenkins et al. 2013). Additionally, FGCS from lower SES backgrounds are four times more likely to quit after their first year of college, work more hours while also attending school, and borrow more money, which further contributes to attrition rates and an unsatisfactory work–life balance (PNPI 2020). These identified barriers, as well as the difficulties that are inherent in pursuing graduate and professional education, contribute to poor mental health for first-generation graduate students.

MENTAL HEALTH

Research has indicated that FGCS are largely underprepared psychologically for post-secondary pursuits (Pelco, Ball, and Lockeman 2014), with first-generation students reporting higher overall levels of depression and anxiety (Stebleton Soria, and Huesman Jr. 2014) and lower levels of well-being than their peers (Jenkins et al. 2013). Additionally, research has broadly shown that a significant number of graduate students experience symptoms of burnout, anxiety, and depression, which are likely exacerbated in populations with known vulnerabilities such as with first-generation students. Several studies have indicated that graduate students experience higher levels of stress than undergraduate students (Eleftheriades, Fiala, and Pasic 2020), and data demonstrate that graduate and professional students are more than six times as likely as the general American population to experience depression and anxiety (Evans et al. 2018), with data indicating prevalence rates of 18–47 percent for depression among doctoral students (Bairrera, Basilico, and Bolotnyy 2018; University of California, Berkley 2018), and the prevalence of suicide attempts among graduate and professional students at nearly 10 percent (University of California, Berkley 2018).

Another recent study noted that, despite high prevalence rates of mental health problems among graduate students, only 12 percent of surveyed students reported seeking help for anxiety and depression related to their graduate training programs (Woolston 2017). The most commonly identified student concerns across studies were mentor/advisor relationships, career prospects, personal finances, personal health, living conditions, and personal sense of value and inclusion (Bira, Evans, and Vanderford 2019), which are similar factors to those that have been associated with poor mental health in FGCS. In addition to the vulnerabilities already explored, research indicates that female graduate students who identify as gender non-conforming or transgender are significantly more likely to experience anxiety and depression than male graduate students (Evans et al. 2018).

It is broadly understood that graduate and professional training can be intensely demanding and stressful, and data suggest that graduate students are at higher risk for suicide attempts than undergraduates (Mortier et al. 2018). Further, suicide completion in graduate students is more often associated with academic stressors than other life circumstances. However, despite what is currently known regarding graduate student mental health, there is a paucity of studies regarding these issues, and future research in this area is urgently needed. Additionally, no current research focuses on suicide ideation in first-generation graduate and professional students.

Imposter Syndrome

First-generation students are more likely to report imposter syndrome and high levels of guilt regarding their educational achievements relative to those of family members (Covarrubias and Fryberg 2015; Gardner and Holley 2011; Ramsey and Brown 2018). *Imposter syndrome* is a psychological term that refers to a pattern of behavior wherein, despite adequate external evidence of success, individuals have an inability to internalize that success, and therefore doubt their abilities, which leads to a fear of not belonging (Clance and Imes 1978). Additionally, McGregor and colleagues (2008) noted that imposter syndrome was associated with higher levels of depression and anxiety in a cohort of doctoral students. Imposter syndrome in first-generation students may be driven by low academic self-concept, which undermines a sense of belonging. This imbalance may be related to feeling like an imposter due to a lack of majority representation in the group and thinking that one does not belong in a group that appears to exceed the level of their abilities.

Dasgupta (2011) noted that individuals who are underrepresented in their fields were more likely to experience imposter syndrome than those who were not and that self-esteem was directly correlated with performance. Also, when first-generation students do not have mentors who followed a similar path to theirs, they are less likely to be able to see themselves belonging to that particular group or obtaining similar roles after graduation (Holley and Gardner 2012). Further, during times of elevated stress, such as when an individual is in the minority, they may choose to abandon their group because they feel unworthy of belonging, which may contribute to attrition rates of first-generation students in graduate and professional programs. This inequality between achievement and self-efficacy, that a first-generation graduate student would abandon a chosen group when their abilities are equal to the rest of the group, is not well understood or represented in the literature. Future research is needed to better inform how improving self-efficacy should be incorporated into intervention and support programs for first-generation graduate and professional students.

RECOMMENDATIONS

Many colleges, universities, and educational agencies have implemented programs intended to improve the success and retention of first-generation undergraduate students. However, similar programs for first-generation graduate students are scarce, often leaving students to navigate the many challenges inherent to graduate and professional studies without guidance, including often overlooked variables such as significant cultural transitions and marginalization based on sociocultural factors. Earlier, this chapter argued the significant benefits of clarifying the definition of first-generation within a framework of intersecting identities. However, while highly beneficial, this one recommendation is not sufficient to the cause. While there is a considerable paucity of literature on this topic, there is research to support specific areas that may support the success and mental health of first-generation graduate students.

Self-Efficacy and Resiliency

Research has indicated that emotional support from friends and family and supportive relationships with faculty are two common factors that contribute to the resiliency of FGCS (Azmitia et al. 2018). Aspelmeier et al. (2012) noted that lower self-esteem or an external locus of control might directly influence how well first-generation students adjust when faced with graduate or professional school. While studies have investigated academic hardiness and self-efficacy in relation to the ability to cope with the many stressors that are inherent in graduate school, none of these studies has specifically addressed the experience of first-generation graduate students. One study, however, addressed self-efficacy in an academic context by noting that perceived ability to conduct graduate-level research was a significant predictor of graduate school enrollment for first-generation students (Tate et al. 2014).

Academic self-efficacy must be fully implemented into the undergraduate experience of students across all disciplines. Determining the factors that contribute to building resilience and self-efficacy in first-generation graduate students will contribute to targeted intervention programs and is an integral approach to ensuring improved mental health outcomes and success in this student population. However, future research is needed to achieve these goals, as there is not currently a robust body of literature from which to draw.

Faculty Mentorship

Ecker (2020) found that having an assigned faculty mentor increased first-generation student success in PhD programs, while Piat et al. (2020) reported that faculty mentoring and research involvement are associated with motivating first-generation student enrollment in graduate STEM programs, especially if those first-generation students were underrepresented in other areas such as race and class. Further, Lee and Kramer (2013) noted that faculty mentors are key to facilitating academic and social integration into the chosen discipline for doctoral students. These indications further support the importance of meaningful relationships between students and faculty that were previously identified as contributing to resilience in FGCS (Azmitia et al. 2018). However, Evans et al. (2018) noted that, among graduate students with mental health problems, approximately 50 percent reported that their immediate faculty mentor provided no actual mentorship, nor did they feel valued by their mentors.

These data emphasize the significant correlation between supportive mentoring relationships and first-generation and graduate student mental health. In support of improved and sustained mental health and overall success of first-generation graduate and professional students, institutions of higher education should implement mandatory faculty-student mentoring programs across all disciplines. All efforts should be made to partner students with faculty mentors who were also first-generation students. Such pairings would further work to mitigate the development of imposter syndrome, which could also contribute to a reduction in attrition rates among first-generation graduate students.

Mental Health Support

Alarmingly high rates of mental health problems across all graduate and professional student populations further highlight the need for establishing or expanding the social, professional, and familial support systems of first-generation graduate students. More robust attention is needed regarding the implementation of campus mental health programs, diverse career development guidance, training of faculty mentors, support for identity development, and broad changes to the overall culture of academia at the graduate and professional levels. Special mental health outreach efforts are indicated for first-generation students as the stigma associated with seeking care may limit help-seeking behaviors. In general, studies pertaining to graduate and professional student mental health are lacking, which justifies further research and policy analysis in order to meet the diverse and changing needs of first-generation students as they move from undergraduate to graduate and professional degree programs. Future studies should be approached with a multicultural lens.

LIMITATIONS

Varying definitions of the first-generation designation make it challenging to generalize and compare data and qualitative reports across first-generation student populations. An additional limitation is that studies have mostly used self-report surveys and assessments, and students may have been inaccurate in their reporting, or unwilling to admit to the severity of mental health symptoms or other problems and barriers due to stigma or fear of retribution. In addition, our review did not include studies or data from countries outside the United States. A more comprehensive and inclusive review is needed to better understand and conceptualize the global experience of first-generation graduate and professional students within an intersectional framework.

DISCUSSION

This chapter has highlighted the lack of literature regarding all aspects of the first-generation graduate and professional student experience. Studies have indicated that the challenges faced by first-generation graduate students do not end upon the completion of the undergraduate degree. Data suggests that the pursuit of graduate or professional studies may bring a host of additional challenges that may adversely affect the overall success and mental health of this student population. These challenges are in addition to those obstacles already faced by first-generation students, such as those identified across personal, sociocultural, academic, financial, and professional dimensions.

The poor mental health outcomes identified in graduate and professional student populations are especially alarming, and current data has demonstrated a critical need for further studies that investigate intervention strategies addressing this growing mental health crisis. There is an urgent need to inform institutions of higher education regarding the finely nuanced and oft-overlooked intersectionality of identity and sociocultural factors of first-generation students in graduate and professional training settings. Additionally, campus mental health practitioners must be trained in multicultural assessment and practice.

Higher education, and especially a graduate or professional degree, remains a significant indicator of upward socioeconomic mobility. However, the achievement gap between first-generation and continuing-generation students may indicate that the American dream is unattainable for many first-generation students. Significant and meaningful contributions to society may be lost if this underrepresented population is not successfully integrated into systems of higher education and, subsequently, the global workforce. Currently, few studies have tracked the global effects of the generational status of graduate and professional students in any context, especially at the doctoral level. Additionally, no literature was found regarding the transition of first-generation college students to graduate and professional programs, or subsequently, into the global job sector. Understanding the drivers of these huge achievement gaps and challenging transitional experiences is essential for informing social justice-oriented policies and interventions for first-generation graduate students who are disproportionately underrepresented in higher education and often represent historically marginalized groups.

REFERENCES

Allen, Jill M., Gregg A. Muragishi, Jessi L. Smith, Dustin B. Thoman, and Elizabeth R. Brown. 2015. "To Grab and to Hold: Cultivating Communal Goals to Overcome Cultural and Structural Barriers in First-generation College Students' Science Interest." *Translational Issues in Psychological Science* 1, no. 4, 331–341. https:/doi.org/10.1037/tps0000046.

Allan, Blake A., Patton O. Garriott, and Chesleigh N. Keene. 2016. "Outcomes of Social Class and Classism in First-and continuing-generation College Students." *Journal of Counseling Psychology* 63, no. 4: 487. https://doi.org/10.1037/cou0000160.

Aspelmeier, Jeffery E., Michael M. Love, Lauren A. McGill, Ann N. Elliott and Thomas W. Pierce. 2012. "Self-esteem, Locus of Control, College Adjustment, and GPA among First-and Continuing-generation Students: A Moderator Model of Generational Status." *Research in Higher Education* 53, no. 7: 755–781. https://doi.org/10.1007/s11162-011-9252-1.

Azmitia, Margarita, Grace Sumabat-Estrada, Yeram Cheong, Rebecca Covarrubias. 2018. ""Dropping Out is Not an Option": How Educationally Resilient First-Generation Students See the Future." *New Directions for Child and Adolescent Development* 2018, no. 160: 89–100. https://doi.org/10.1002/cad.20240.

Barreira, Paul, Matthew Basilico, and Valentin Bolotnyy. 2018. "Graduate Student Mental Health: Lessons from American Economics Departments." *Harvard University*. https://scholar.harvard.edu/bolotnyy/publications/graduate-student-mental-health-lessons-american-economics-departments.

Bauer, Hope H., Hope H. Bauer, Carter B. Anderson, Kelly Hirko, Andrea Wendling. 2019. "Barriers to College and Health Care Careers among US Students from a Rural Community." *PRiMER: Peer-Review Reports in Medical Education Research* 3, no. 10. https://doi.org./ 10.22454/PRiMER.2019.828405.

Becerra, Melissa. 2017. "Mental Health and Academic Performance of First-generation College Students and Continuing-generation College Students." https://escholarship.org/uc/item/4691k02z.

Bira, Lindsay, Teresa Evans, and Nathan Vanderford. 2019. "Mental Health in Academia: An Invisible Crisis." *Physiology News Magazine* 115 (Summer): 32–35. https://doi.org/10.36866/pn.115.32.

Callan, P. M. 2001. "Reframing Access and Opportunity: Problematic State and Federal Higher Education Policy in the 1990s." In *The States and Public Higher Education Policy: Affordability, Access and Accountability*. Edited by D. E. Heller, 83–99. Baltimore, MD: The John Hopkins University Press.

Carlton, Morgan T. 2015. "First Generation Students and Post-Undergraduate Aspirations." *SAGE Open* 5, no. 4 (October-December): 1–8. https://doi.org/10.1177/2158244015618433.

Cataldi, Emily Forrest, Christopher T. Bennett, and Xianglei Chen. 2018. *First-Generation Students: College Access, Persistence, and Postbachelor's Outcomes*. Stats in Brief. NCES 2018-421. National Center for Education Statistics. https://nces.ed.gov/pubs2018/2018421.pdf.

Cattaneo, Lauren B., Wing Yi Chan, Rachel Shor, Kris T. Gebhard, Nour H. Elshabassi. 2019. "Elaborating the Connection between Social Class and Classism in College." *American Journal of Community Psychology* 63, no. 3–4 (June): 476–486. https://doi.org/10.1002/ajcp.12322.

Cheng, Ying-Hsueh, Chin-Chung Tsai, and Jyh-Chong Liang. 2019. "Academic Hardiness and Academic Self-efficacy in Graduate Studies." *Higher Education*

Research & Development 38, no. 5 (June): 907–921. https://doi.org/10.1080/0 7294360.2019.1612858.

Choy, S. 2001. *Students Whose Parents Did Not Go to College: Postsecondary Access, Persistence, and Attainment.* Findings from the Condition of Education 2001. (Report No. NCES-2001-126). Washington, DC: National Center for Education Statistics. https://nces.ed.gov/pubs2001/2001126.pdf.

Clance, Pauline R., and Suzanne A. Imes. 1978. "The Imposter Phenomenon in High Achieving Women: Dynamics and Therapeutic Intervention." *Psychotherapy: Theory, Research & Practice* 15, no. 3: 241–247. https://doi.org/10.1037/h0086006.

Covarrubias, Rebecca, and Stephanie A. Fryberg. 2015. "Movin' on Up (To College): First-Generation College Students' Experiences with Family Achievement Guilt." *Cultural Diversity and Ethnic Minority Psychology* 21, no. 3: 420. https://doi.org /10.1037/a0037844.

Dasgupta, Nilanjana. 2011. "Ingroup Experts and Peers as Social Vaccines Who Inoculate the Self-Concept: The Stereotype Inoculation Model." *Psychological Inquiry* 22, no. 4, 231–246. https://doi.org/10.1080/1047840x.2011.607313.

Ecker, R. 2020. "Still On the Margins: Programs Aimed at Opening up a Conversation on the Invisible Issue of Social Class in Doctoral Programs." In *On the Borders of the Academy.* Edited by A. R. Standlee, 127–142. New York: Graduate School Press of Syracuse University.

Eleftheriades, Renee, Clare Fiala, and Maria D. Pasic. 2020. "The Challenges and Mental Health Issues of Academic Trainees." *F1000Research* 9, no. 104. https:// doi.org/10.12688/f1000research.21066.1.

Engle, Jennifer. 2007. "Postsecondary Access and Success for First-generation College Students." *American Academic* 3, no. 1: 25–48. http://hdl.voced.edu.au /10707/328327.

Evans, Teresa M., Lindsay Bira, Jazmin B. Gastelum, L. T. Weiss, and Nathan L. Vanderford. 2018. "Evidence for a Mental Health Crisis in Graduate Education." *Nature Biotechnology* 36, no. 3: 282–284. https://doi.org/10.1038/nbt.4089.

Gardner, Susan K., and Karri A. Holley. 2011. ""Those Invisible Barriers are Real": The Progression of First-Generation Students through Doctoral Education." *Equity & Excellence in Education* 44, no. 1: 77–92. https://doi.org/10.1080/10665684.20 11.529791.

Hearn, James C., and Kelly Ochs Rosinger. 2014. "Socioeconomic Diversity in Selective Private Colleges: An Organizational Analysis." *The Review of Higher Education* 38, no. 1 (Fall): 71–104. https://doi.org/10.1353/rhe.2014.0043.

House, Lisa A., Chelsea Neal, and Jason Kolb. 2019. "Supporting the Mental Health Needs of First Generation College Students." *Journal of College Student Psychotherapy* 34, no. 2: 157–167. https://doi.org/10.1080/87568225.2019.15 78940.

Housel, Teresa Heinz, ed. 2019. *First-Generation College Student Experiences of Intersecting Marginalities.* New York: Peter Lang.

Jæger, Mads Meier, and Stine Møllegaard. 2017. "Cultural Capital, Teacher Bias, and Educational Success: New Evidence from Monozygotic Twins." *Social Science Research* 65 (July): 130–144. https://doi.org/10.1016/j.ssresearch.2017.04.003.

Jenkins, Sharon R., Aimee Belanger, Melissa L. Connally, Adriel Boals, and Kelly M. Durón. 2013. "First-Generation Undergraduate Students' Social Support, Depression, and Life Satisfaction." *Journal of College Counseling* 16, no. 2: 129–142. https://doi.org:10.1002/j.2161-1882.2013.00032.x.

Lee, Elizabeth M., and Rory Kramer. 2013. "Out with the Old, In with the New? Habitus and Social Mobility at Selective Colleges." *Sociology of Education* 86, no. 1: 18–35. https://doi.org/10.1177/0038040712445519.

Lunceford, Brett. 2011. "When First-generation Students go to Graduate School." *New Directions for Teaching and Learning* 2011, no. 127: 13–20. https://doi.org/10.1002/tl.453.

McGregor, Loretta Neal, Damon E. Gee, and K. Elizabeth Posey. 2008. "I Feel Like a Fraud and It Depresses Me: The Relation between the Imposter Phenomenon and Depression." *Social Behavior and Personality: An International Journal* 36, no. 1: 43–48. https://doi.org/10.2224/sbp.2008.36.1.43.

Mortier, Philippe, P. Cuijpers, G. Kiekens, R. P. Auerbach, K. Demyttenaere, J. G. Green, R. C. Kessler, M. K. Nock, R. Bruffaerts. 2018. "The Prevalence of Suicidal Thoughts and Behaviours among College Students: A Meta-analysis." *Psychological Medicine* 48, no. 4: 554–565. https://doi.org/10.1017/S0033291717002215.

Mullen, A. L., K. A. Goyette, and J. A. Soares. 2003. "Who Goes to Graduate School? Social and Academic Correlates of Educational Continuation after College." *Sociology of Education* 76, no. 2 (April): 143–169. https://doi.org/10.2307/3090274.

Murphy, M. C., and S. Zirkel. 2015. "Race and Belonging in School: How Anticipated and Experienced Belonging Affect Choice, Persistence, and Performance." *Teachers College Record* 117, no. 12: 1–40.

Nguyen, Thai-Huy, and Bach Mai Dolly Nguyen. 2018. "Is the "First-generation Student" Term Useful for Understanding Inequality? The Role of Intersectionality in Illuminating the Implications of an Accepted—Yet Unchallenged—Term." *Review of Research in Education* 42, no. 1: 146–176. https://doi.org/10.3102/0091732X18759280.

NSF (National Science Foundation). 2013. National Survey of College Graduates. Washington, DC: National Science Foundation.

OECD. "World Bank (2014)." *Global Value Chains: Challenges, Opportunities and Implications for Policy*. July 19, 2014. G20 Taskforce.

Pelco, Lynn E., Christopher T. Ball, and Kelly Lockeman. 2014. "Student Growth from Service-Learning: A Comparison of First-generation and Non-First-Generation College Students." *Journal of Higher Education Outreach and Engagement* 18, no. 2: 49–66. https://files.eric.ed.gov/fulltext/EJ1029848.pdf.

Piatt, Elizabeth, Elizabeth Piatt, David Merolla, Eboni Pringle and Richard T. Serpe. 2019. "The Role of Science Identity Salience in Graduate School Enrollment for First-generation, Low-income, Underrepresented Students." *The Journal of Negro Education* 88, no. 3 (Summer): 269–280. https://doi.org/10.7709/jnegroeducation.88.3.0269.

Post-Secondary National Policy Institute (PPNI). 2020. *Factsheets: First-generation Students*. https://pnpi.org/first-generation-students/.

Ramsey, Elizabeth, and Deana Brown. 2018. "Feeling Like a Fraud: Helping Students Renegotiate their Academic Identities." *College & Undergraduate Libraries* 25, no. 1: 86–90. https://doi.org/10.1080/10691316.2017.1364080.

Redford, J., and K. Mulvaney Hoyer. 2017. *First Generation and Continuing-Generation College Students: A Comparison of High School and Postsecondary Experiences.* September. U.S. Department of Education. NCES 2018–009. https://uc.uiowa.edu/sites/uc.uiowa.edu/files/nces_study_of_first-generation_college_students.pdf.

Rubin, Mark. 2012. "Social Class Differences in Social Integration among Students in Higher Education: A Meta-Analysis and Recommendations for Future Research." *Journal of Diversity in Higher Education* 5, no. 1: 22–38. https://doi.org/10.1037/a0026162.

Stebleton, Michael J., Krista M. Soria, and Ronald L. Huesman Jr. 2014. "First-generation Students' Sense of Belonging, Mental Health, and Use of Counseling Services at Public Research Universities." *Journal of College Counseling* 17, no. 1: 6–20. https://doi.org/10.1002/j.2161-1882.2014.00044.x.

Stephens, Nicole, Sarah Townsend, Hazel Markus, and Taylor Phillips. 2012. "A Cultural Mismatch: Independent Cultural Norms Produce Greater Increases in Cortisol and More Negative Emotions among First-Generation College Students." *Journal of Experimental Social Psychology* 48, no. 6: 1389–1393. https://doi.org/10.1016/j.jesp.2012.07.008.

Stephens, N. M., Tiffany N. Brannon, Hazel Rose Markus, Jessica E. Nelson. 2015. "Feeling at Home in College: Fortifying School-Relevant Selves to Reduce Social Class Disparities in Higher Education." *Social Issues and Policy Review* 9, no. 1: 1–24. https://doi.org/10.1111/sipr.12008.

Stephens, Nicole M., M. Hamedani, and Sarah S. M. Townsend. 2019. "Difference-education: Improving Disadvantaged Students' Academic Outcomes by Changing their Theory of Differences." In *Handbook of Wise Interventions: How Social-Psychological Insights Can Help Solve Problems.* Edited by Gregory M. Walton and Alia J. Crum, 126–147. New York: Guilford Press.

Strayhorn, T. L. 2018. "Sense of Belonging and Graduate Students." In *College Students' Sense of Belonging,* 124–139. New York: Routledge. https://doi.org/10.4324/9781315297293-9.

Toutkoushian, Robert K., Robert A. Stollberg, and Kelly A. Slaton. 2018. "Talking'Bout My Generation: Defining 'First-Generation College Students' in Higher Education Research." *Teachers College Record* 120, no. 4: 1–38.

Tate, Kevin A., Nadya A. Fouad, Laura Reid Marks, Gary Young, Eddie Guzman, and Eric G. Williams. 2012. "Underrepresented First-generation, Low-income College Students' Pursuit of a Graduate Education." *Journal of Career Assessment* 23, no. 3: 427–441. https://doi.org/10.1177/1069072714547498.

Thompson, Mindi N., and Linda M. Subich. 2013. "Development and Exploration of the Experiences with Classism Scale." *Journal of Career Assessment* 21, no. 1: 139–158. https://doi.org/10.1177/1069072712450494.

Torpey, Elka. 2018. *Employment Outlook for Graduate-Level Occupations: Career Outlook*. August. Bureau of Labor Statistics. https://www.bls.gov/careeroutlook/2018/article/pdf/ graduate-degree-outlook.pdf.

University of California, Berkeley. 2018. *Graduate Student Happiness and Well-Being Report*. http://ga.berkeley.edu/wellbeingreport/631.

Unverferth, Anthony Richard, Carolyn Talbert-Johnson, and Treavor Bogard. "Perceived Barriers for First-generation Students: Reforms to Level the Terrain." *International Journal of Educational Reform* 21, no. 4: 238–252. https://doi.org/10.1177/105678791202100402.

Valletta, Rob. 2015. "Higher Education, Wages, and Polarization." *FRBSF ECONOMIC LETTER*. September 12, 2015. https://www.frbsf.org/economic-research/files/el2015-02.pdf.

Vuong, Mui, Sharon Brown-Welty, and Susan Tracz. 2010. "The Effects of Self-efficacy on Academic Success of First-generation College Sophomore Students." *Journal of College Student Development* 51, no. 1: 50–64. https://doi.org/10.1353/csd.0.0109.

Walton, G. M., and Cohen, G. L. 2011. "A Brief Social-belonging Intervention Improves Academic and Health Outcomes of Minority Students." *Science* 331, no. 6023: 1447–1451. https://doi.org/10.1126/science.1198364.

Woolston, Chris. 2017. "Graduate Survey: A Love–hurt Relationship." *Nature* 550, no. 7677: 549–552. https://doi.org/10.1038/nj7677-549a.

Chapter 7

Give and Take

Exploring the Role of Confidants When Friends Disclose Chronic and/or Mental Health–Related Information

Robert D. Hall

Approximately one out of six adults in the United States is affected by a mental health issue (National Institute for Mental Health 2017). According to the National Center for Chronic Disease Prevention and Health Promotion (2019), approximately six out of every ten adults in the United States has a chronic health issue. People who experience chronic health issues are also likely to have mental health issues (Raphael et al. 2006) and vice versa (National Institute for Mental Health 2015). These adjoining factors are known as comorbidities. This is particularly alarming because people affected by mental health conditions are likely to die sooner than the general population (Hayes et al. 2015).

Nonetheless, individuals experiencing these conditions are likely to seek social support from others (Koetsenruijter et al. 2016; Naslund et al. 2016). Obtaining support for such conditions is inherently an interpersonal issue (Ackerson and Viswanath 2009) and yet, support is not forthcoming until members of a person's social network receive a disclosure of the illness (Horan et al. 2009). It is thus important to understand the transactional process of interpersonal disclosure when discussing chronic and mental health information (CMHI).

Many scholars have examined the role of chronic and mental health communication in interpersonal and family contexts. Researchers suggest that people affected by CMHI seek out friends and family for social support (Venetis, Chernichky-Karcher, and Gettings 2018; Segrin and Flora 2017). Additionally, family members often influence a person's choices to receive medical care (Dean and Rauscher 2018). The dynamic of revealing and concealing private information encapsulates sender, receiver, social networks, and contextual information (Petronio 2002). Because most researchers focus on the *sender* of CMHI, very little scholarly attention examines the *receiver* of CMHI.

Building on a growing body of literature that examines the pivotal role of friends in CMHI disclosures (Basel 2018; Venetis, Chernichky-Karcher, and Gettings 2018), this chapter examines the confidant's role in CMHI disclosures. In doing so, I use Petronio's (2002) conceptualization and categorization of confidants as conceptualized in communication privacy management theory (CPM). Namely, through interpretive inquiry, I examine deliberate, inferential, and reluctant confidants who receive CMHI disclosures. To carry out this study, I first describe friends as a pivotal communicative relationship, then investigate stigma and CMHI, and finally analyze confidants through CPM. Drawing from my analysis, I make conclusions about undergraduate college students who receive CMHI from their friend and propose future research.

FRIENDSHIP AND COMMUNICATION

Despite friendship's pivotal role in shaping the idea of self (Anthony and McCabe 2015), communication scholars have not given much attention to friendship's role. People often cite friendship as the main type of love they experience (Fehr and Russell 1991). What communication scholars know about friendship is largely developmental and definitional. By the time people reach adolescence, Rawlins (1992) argues that they understand the "voluntary, mutually accomplished, ongoing personal attachment" aspects of friendship (59). By young adulthood, friends begin to influence people's identity, career, dating life, community, and leisurely activities (Rawlins 1992, 103). Friendships are typically defined by equality, no blood relation or sexual intimacy, enjoyment, trustworthiness, and similar age range (Fehr 1996). However, friends may also play a pivotal role in shaping people's health.

Previous scholars noted that friendship differs from other close relationships because it is inherently voluntary (Dainton, Zelley, and Langan 2003). Braithwaite et al. (2010) explore this difference in that voluntary kinship relationships may be perceived as closer than familial ties, yet absence of blood relation or legal obligation removes them from consideration of *traditional* familial relationships. While Braithwaite et al. (2010) noted that voluntary kin sometimes come into one's life as a form of support, Carr and Wilder (2016) found that friendships may provide support differently than family relationships (i.e., siblings) when experiencing an avoidant attachment style. However, Carr and Wilder (2016) did not examine specific stressors such as CMHI in their discussion of close relational differences.

Friends are a pivotal relationship that offers people social support (Bliezner and Adams 1992; Fehr 1996; Rawlins 1992, 2008). When considering the societal stigma around mental illness (Corrigan 2006), the friendship relationship may become an even more important area of inquiry. Vangelisti (2009) found that social support can moderate the effects of mental health, yet prior studies have largely disregarded the specific relationship of friendship. Venetis, Chernichky-Karcher, and Gettings (2018) noted that college-aged young adults disclose their mental illness status to friends. These researchers found that, although a friend's openness may lead directly to disclosing mental illness concerns, assessment of mental illness information (e.g., stigma) was mediated by a participant's assessment of their friend's ability to receive such information. However, as previously noted, these scholars suggest that those receiving health disclosures must remain open and willing to discuss private health information with their friend. More information is needed to understand friendship's role in receiving CMHI disclosures, particularly from the confidant's perspective. Therefore, I will examine stigma and CMHI to better understand the central role of communication in CMHI disclosures.

STIGMA AND CMHI

Broadly conceptualized, stigma is an undesired trait that separates a person from societal acceptance (Goffman 1963). Smith (2011) discussed how stigma is inherently a communicative issue that can be identified through marks, labels, responsibility, and peril. She noted that these aspects of stigma, particularly in discussing chronic and mental health, "are formed, sustained, and socialized through communication" (Smith 2011, 459). As Smith (2011) explained, close relational partners to the stigmatized individual may increase stigma or stigma burden through avoidant communication, ignoring the stigma, or enhancing the stigma. Corrigan, Druss, and Perlick (2014) reiterated this sentiment by providing evidence that health campaigns should target close relational partners such as friends to enhance confidants' willingness to become a support system for mental health disclosures. Their assertion supports my goal in this chapter to examine the disclosure process of CMHI between friends to better understand this type of disclosure.

Mental health is a highly nuanced and pressing issue in academia. Among emerging adult and undergraduate populations, researchers consistently reported an increase in mental illness symptomology (Auerbach et al. 2018; Lipson et al. 2015; Prince 2015). Although researchers described how these increases could result from inadequate university resources, Eisenberg (2019) noted that universities are now addressing mental health issues among undergraduates. At the same time, mental health issues are sharply increasing among graduate students and faculty because of different factors: a lack of university resources, a publish-or-perish culture, and academic staff's reluctance to share mental health information because of fears of being perceived as mentally weak (Evans et al. 2018; Price et al. 2017; Wedemeyer-Strombel 2019). Therefore, while undergraduate students may have access to mental health resources and be more open to discussing mental health issues, their instructors and mentors do not necessarily have the same social or institutional support.

Chronic and mental health–related issues may be pathologically different, but both may manifest as invisible illnesses, or illness that is not readily detectible in a person (Kundrat and Nussbaum 2003). Invisible illnesses are inherently a communicative concern because they are not known until the person with the illness or another informed individual discloses this information to the confidant (Horan et al. 2009). Knowing this, individuals who face stigma because of an invisible illness may withhold disclosure to avoid "discriminatory cultural attitudes" (Cardillo 2010, 536) and/or isolation from such disclosure (Smith 2011). As such, non-disclosure burdens the stigmatized individual (Persson, Pfaus, and Ryder 2015), but receiving the disclosure of CMHI may also burden the confidant (Harvey et al. 2017).

Because of these known barriers to disclosure, researchers have placed the burden of acceptance on confidants to be more *open* and *accepting* of such disclosures (Basel 2018; Corrigan, Druss, and Perlick 2014; Smith 2011; Venetis, Chernichky-Karcher, and Gettings 2018). However, disclosure is not a one-sided issue, and the confidant's role should be further considered as an area of inquiry because recommendations for openness could have limitations (Iedema et al. 2009). As such, I use communication privacy management theory (CPM) in this chapter as the guiding theoretical framework to better understand the confidant's forgotten role in receiving CMHI disclosures.

COMMUNICATION PRIVACY MANAGEMENT THEORY

Petronio (2002, 2010, 2018; Petronio and Durham 2015) created CPM through inquiries into private information's role in the tension between a person's desire to reveal and/or conceal private information (e.g., Petronio 1991). As previously explained in this chapter's stigma section, the interpersonal contexts of invisible illness have this inherent dynamic tension. However, Petronio (2002) discussed how multiple people (the sender and the receiver, or confidant, and collective networks) are involved in disclosure. Through the theoretical lens of CPM, Petronio (2002) conceptualized confidants into three main categories: inferential (expects to hear private information), deliberate (asks for private information), and reluctant (does not want to receive private information) confidants.

All three types of confidants receive private information, but how the confidant elicits and/or responds to the disclosure determines their category. Primarily, an inferential confidant is one that would expect to receive private information (Petronio 2002). As McBride and Bergen (2008) suggest, friends tend to fall within the inferential confidant role because of the "implicit expectations of friendship" (52). Second, a deliberate confidant, or one who asks for private information, would ask a friend directly about their CMHI. The third category, or the reluctant confidant, may perhaps be the rarest or most infrequent type of confidant (McBride and Bergen 2008). A confidant is categorized as reluctant when they did not desire or expect to receive the private information (O'Mara and Schrodt 2017; Petronio 2002). Most researchers framed their studies within these three categories despite the fact that some asserted that these categories need to be expanded (see Basel 2018).

In research that discusses health-related disclosures, researchers have not often examined friends as confidants despite the fact that friends are often sought out as significant relationships for social support (Bliezner and Adams 1992; Fehr 1996; Rawlins 1992, 2008), and particularly within CMHI domains (e.g., Venetis, Chernichky-Karcher, and Gettings 2018). McBride and Bergen (2008) noted that friends span all three categories of confidants when receiving various types of information, including health-related information such as sex, traumatic life events, and addiction. Therefore, the purpose of the study in this chapter is to understand what happens between friends when a CMHI is disclosed, particularly from the confidant's perspective. Specifically, I ask the following research question:

RQ: How do friends navigate the role of the confidant in receiving CMHI?

METHOD

I situated my study in the interpretive paradigm to fully explore the firsthand, lived experiences of individuals receiving CMHI. As such, I further gained access to the local knowledge (Baxter and Babbie 2004) of the participants to better understand their lived experiences in receiving a CMHI. I interviewed thirteen participants using a semi-structured format (Appendix A), which is an interview strategy that allows for flexibility to adapt and adjust the interview guide so that each participant can best recount their experience (Lindlof and Taylor 2018). I used CPM as a guiding theoretical framework for constructing the interview protocol (Creswell 2016) to best understand the confidant's role in receiving CMHI from a friend, which is the study's central phenomenon. To test the interview guide's flow and effectiveness, I pilot interviewed a scholarly colleague (Creswell and Poth 2018).

Procedures

Prior to interviewing, I obtained approval from the university's IRB. I used criterion sampling to ensure that participants fit within the goal of the project's inquiry (Lindlof and Taylor 2018). To that end, participants should be at least nineteen years old and should have received CMHI from a friend. I recruited participants who fit the study's criteria through social media (Facebook), a communication listserv, an online research board, and campus flyers. I interviewed all participants face-to-face. Participants received and agreed to an informed consent prior to study participation. Students received compensation from their professors in the form of research credit for participating in the study. I audio recorded each interview and used the fully encrypted transcription service www.temi.com to aid in the transcription process. Interviews lasted from approximately twenty-five to fifty-six minutes ($M = 34.23$).

In the interviews, I asked participants to discuss their experience of receiving a CMHI disclosure from a friend. Part of the interview consisted of co-creating a brochure with the participants. For this part of the interview, I shared a brochure template and writing utensil with the participants and led them through designing the brochure, as seen at the end of the semi-structured interview guide (Appendix A). After I asked a participant each question, they responded to the question. After discussing their response, I asked them to place the shared information where they felt it belonged. Each participant filled out a template in this manner.

Participants

I interviewed thirteen participants for this study. The participants' ages ranged between nineteen and twenty-three years old ($M = 20.15$) and included undergraduate college students. They mostly self-identified as female ($n = 10$) compared to male ($n = 3$), and as Caucasian ($n = 10$) compared to other ethnicities (Asian, $n = 1$; Filipino, $n = 1$; Hispanic, $n = 1$). I asked each participant to provide the demographic information for the friendship relationship that they discussed during the interviews. The participants described their friends as slightly younger (ages eighteen to twenty-two, $M = 19.23$), more often female ($n = 7$) than male ($n = 6$), and mostly Caucasian ($n = 12$; Hispanic, $n = 1$). Almost all participants described receiving a mental illness disclosure from their friend ($n = 12$) as opposed to a chronic illness disclosure ($n = 1$).

Data Analysis

I used Braun and Clarke's (2006) thematic analysis as an analytical guide to understanding the experiences of receiving CMHI through a CPM lens. I initially uploaded the audio recordings to www.temi.com to aid in the transcription process. To familiarize myself with these transcripts, I examined the transcriptions while listening to the audio recording, to make changes for accuracy. Second, to generate initial findings, I used Owen's (1984) criteria for inclusion: recurrence (similarity across data); repetition (similarity of words/phrases across data); and forcefulness (participant emphasis). Because I used CPM as a sensitizing theoretical framework to understand the confidant's role (Bowen 2006; Brinkmann and Kvale 2015), CPM guided my thematic development from the participants' experiences.

Regarding the brochure, I also thematized it using a modification of Braun and Clarke's (2006) thematic analysis for produced texts during the interview. For the purposes of this study, I will refer to this thematic approach as Talk & Text Thematic Analysis (3TA) that I developed for this study. Using a hermeneutical perspective of textual analysis (see Brinkmann and Kvale 2015), I studied themes produced not only during the *talk* recorded during the brochure's construction, but also the *text* of the brochure. I used Owen's (1984) criteria for including data in the final brochure. The ultimate goal of 3TA is to produce a single, translational object for dissemination. I first analyzed the brochure's *talk* and *text* separately for themes, and then comparatively analyzed themes across the transcript and brochure data. After this comparison, I created a final brochure (Appendix B) based on the participants' data.

For verification, I performed a data conference (Braithwaite, Allen, and Moore 2017) with scholarly colleagues in my doctoral seminar on interpretive research methods to defend the data's interpretive themes. In conducting this data conference, I presented my initial results to my doctorate-level interpretive methodology class. I discussed my findings with the class, providing justification for the themes. Based on their feedback, I modified the findings as needed for coherence. After my data conference, I wrote my results based on my analysis and data conference discussion.

RESULTS

Generally speaking, all participants experienced receiving some type of CMHI disclosure. After receiving the disclosure, most participants noted that their relationship with their friend grew closer. If their relationship grew apart, participants stated that this was due to a factor not related to CMHI. All participants also discussed some aspect of their health with their friend at some point during their relationship.

Regarding the study's research question, I found two overarching themes through my analysis: types of confidants and privacy boundary coordination. Within these main themes, I identified subthemes within each. For types of confidants, I found inferential, deliberate, and reluctant confidants. For privacy boundary coordination, I found implicit and explicit boundary coordination. In analyzing the brochure co-creation data, I will explain the final product thematically through an overarching theme of importance. Within the theme of importance, I found two subthemes of placement and content. I will first examine the types of confidants in order of inferential confidants, deliberate confidants, and reluctant confidants.

Types of Confidants

As noted earlier, Petronio (2002) described confidants generally as individuals who receive private information disclosure. She categorizes confidants into inferential, deliberate, and reluctant types.

Inferential Confidants

The most common type of confidant present in the interviews was the inferential confidant ($n = 10$). I conceptualized this category using Petronio's (2002) description as someone who expects to receive private information from their relational other. Participants noted that the nature of the friendship meant that receiving a CMHI disclosure may be shocking but not detrimental to the friendship. For example, one participant said:

> Part of having, like, real friendships with people is going through the rougher parts with them. Whether there's a conflict between the two of you or they're having a conflict somewhere else in their life and they're coming to you for help or just, like, a place to let things out. (1: 97–100)[1]

Other participants stated that, based on the nature of their friendship, they felt like they were worthy candidates of the CMHI disclosure because of the trust they had built with their friend. Participants in the inferential confidant category commonly cited trust as a reason they believed they received such a disclosure. For example:

> She knows that I'm not going to judge her. She knows that we kind of have a trusting relationship. Um, I'm not going to tell other people . . . . [I'm] just someone to talk to about it, I think beyond her family. (3: 628–630)

Not only did participants state that they expected to receive this information, but they also wanted to do more for their friend after receiving the disclosure.

However, participants described how they did not know what to say, how to help, or how to ask for more information to be a better confidant for their friend. The following participants exemplified this experience:

> I didn't know what to say. I had to think about what I wrote back 'cause I wanted to be supportive of her, but also, like, I needed to understand what she had, and I had to be conscious of what I was saying to her. (4: 856–858)

> I would have loved to know all that was going on. And he said he was embarrassed, and, um, he, uh, he just didn't know what to do. And I'm, like, well, you could always talk to me like, you know, I'm here for you always. (8: 2004–2006)

Overall, those in the inferential confidant category expressed that, due to the nature of friendship, they expected to be there for their friend and felt like the trust built within the friendship served as a motivator for receiving the disclosure. However, they were unsure how to be even more supportive or helpful in navigating their role as an inferential confidant. These participants often expressed shock or surprise at learning about their friends' condition but noted that, despite the uncertainty, they did not think any less of their friendship. Instead, they wanted to do more to continue developing their friendship.

Deliberate Confidants

The second most common type of confidant was the deliberate confidant ($n = 2$). Although Petronio (2002) noted that a deliberate confidant is someone who will solicit private information, she also noted that self-disclosure may be a deliberate method for soliciting private information. Both conceptualizations appeared in my data. First, one participant demonstrated the deliberate confidant subtheme through deliberately asking for the disclosure after noticing changes in her roommate's behavior:

> She was my roommate, and she would lie to me about her eating. Then she just got so weak at one point that I was like, "What's wrong?" But she still wouldn't say anything ... after we didn't eat for a whole week together, I knew I had to keep asking. (2: 353–357)

Another participant deliberately sought out her friend's mental health disclosure through disclosing her own circumstances. In her interview, she says:

> She felt it was important to explain her past a little bit more [after I told her that I have depression].... So we both went through our entire backstory and stayed up really late and sat there and cried for hours. It was one of those things where

we were able to really connect and bond based off of our past experiences. (7: 1712–1718)

Given the increase of access and discussion opportunities for undergraduate students, it comes as little surprise that confidants would be willing to elicit these disclosures from their friends. This study's deliberate confidants sought out the disclosure from their friend regarding their CMHI. Although the actual process for doing so differed for each participant, each of them felt a stronger bond with their friend after the disclosure occurred. The participants still wanted to hear their friend's disclosures like that of the inferential confidant, but, through a more deliberate method, sought out the disclosure to either understand changes in behavior or seeking support from their friend in similar circumstances.

Reluctant Confidant

The least common type of confidant was the reluctant confidant ($n = 1$). This participant did not want to receive the disclosure of CMHI, which is an aspect of Petronio's (2002) definition of the *reluctant confidant*. This participant described what it was like to receive the CMHI:

> Just seeing something like that was . . . like you wouldn't think that his family, who was very well off, that you wouldn't think someone would be depressed. . . we just didn't know if he was like being serious or if it was just you're trying to get attention or something. (13: 3335–3339)

Here, the participant noted that he did not believe his friend was disclosing an actual condition, but was just seeking attention. Later in the interview, however, this participant described how he felt about this reaction at the time of the interview, ten years after he first heard the disclosure:

> I wasn't even sad [at the time] 'cause I just didn't know what was going on. So, for me, it was just kinda, like, I don't know, it made me, it was kinda like I was an ass. That's the best way to phrase it. (13: 3354–3356)

In asking what, if anything, he wish had been different about this situation, this participant explained:

> I wish I kind of, like, took more of his words to heart and kind of, like, really talked to him about it, or just really gave him a little bit more guidance than just saying, you know, take that stuff to your parents. (13: 3377–3379)

Although this participant noted that he was initially a reluctant confidant, he wished that he had the capacity to be more of either an inferential or deliberate confidant to better support his friend. However, just because the friends disclosed their CMHI does not mean they always clearly communicated the expectations of this information.

Boundary Coordination Processes

Petronio (2002) suggested that, when discussing private information, the information's original owner is likely to create stricter rules about more sensitive private information. The participants' friends coordinated boundaries in two ways: implicit and explicit boundaries. Even though implicit and explicit boundary coordination occurred between friends to not further reveal the information, all participants stated that they told at least one other individual about their friend's CMHI, usually someone of authority (i.e., parent or teacher), out of concern of the participant or their friend. Nonetheless, both boundary coordination processes held expectations for how the participant should handle the information as the information's co-owner.

Educators and administrators across higher education in recent years have called for reducing mental health stigma in classrooms (Goldman 2018; Smith and Applegate 2018). White and LaBelle (2019) found that instructors are discussing mental health–related issues frequently and openly in college and university classrooms. None of this study's participants, who were all undergraduate students, reported the role of the instructor or collegiate classroom environment in their conversations. These conversations could have happened with a peer in the classroom, but this was not mentioned. Despite the growing trend in classrooms to be more cognizant of mental health issues among undergraduates, the following disclosures, whether implicit or explicit, seemingly remained between friends.

Implicit Boundaries

Participants described implied boundaries as the most common boundary when receiving CMHI ($n = 8$). These participants reported that their friend did not explicitly place boundaries around the private CMHI once shared. Despite the lack of a defined boundary surrounding the CMHI, the participants described their responsibility to not further disclose the CMHI to others. For example:

> She's never been, she's never said to me, "Don't tell anybody. . . ." I feel like she knows with our friendship, like, I'm not going to just go and tell the whole world. (1: 139–143)

> Um, I don't think it was super explicitly said, like, "Hey, don't tell anyone about this." But that's something that I feel like most people just know. You don't just

talk about [it] with random people. You kind of keep that private because it's not your life story to share someone else's. (7: 1763–1765)

These participants demonstrated how, by the nature of their friendship relationship, they knew that this information should not be shared further outside this dyad. However, some participants who described implicit boundaries discussed how their observations of the discloser's revelation process led to keeping the information between friends:

I think it was more so implied that it wasn't information that I should just go [share] .... Because just based on how she had taken time to tell people slowly, one at a time, it obviously wasn't my right to go tell everyone. (3:695–699)

Even though the discloser did not frame expectations of a boundary, the participants still felt like a boundary existed due to either the nature of the friendship or observations of the discloser's previous disclosure behavior. Thus, they did not feel that an explicit boundary was necessary.

Explicit Boundaries

These participants ($n = 5$) experienced their friend telling them what they could or could not do with the information. Often, this was because the friend wanted to disclose the information to other people, not that they were afraid of others finding out. For example:

She told me that I couldn't tell anyone else because she wanted to tell them herself. (2: 406)

She told me not to tell him [our mutual friend] because she wanted to tell him. (4: 897–898)

He wanted to keep it between ... us for at least a while until he felt comfortable enough sharing it on his own. (7: 1222–1223)

She told me, "I'm really private about it right now," and she didn't exactly want everyone to know. (9: 2354–2355)

The participants who experienced explicit boundaries reported having less dialogue than those participants experiencing implicit boundary coordination. This suggests perhaps that the cultural expectation for boundary coordination lies within explicit coordination and implicit coordination. No matter the type of confidant or boundary experienced, all participants said that they did not know how to properly receive or respond to their friend's CMHI as well as they wished.

People such as instructors who have authoritative positions in higher education may have little to no option for boundary coordination with a discloser. For example, White and LaBelle (2019) found that college instructors often have a role that is more of a listener, first responder, and/or bystander because they feel unqualified to offer further support. When facing a lack of empathy in initial disclosure with instructors, however, college students may withhold future disclosures of mental health and illness with faculty (Meluch and Starcher 2020). Institutional policies may mandate instructors to report mental health–related disclosures to university officials when a student is at-risk for the harm of themselves or others, as legal action may be taken against the university should the university fail to provide proper care for this individual (The Jed Foundation 2008). This dimension of instructors as confidants could be a reason why this study's participants did not mention instructors in conversations about mental health.

Brochure Report

Appendix B includes the final sample of the co-constructed brochure from the results of the 3TA. As previously noted, all participants said they wished they had more information or knew how to better communicate with a friend who told them about CMHI. All participants accepted the option to co-construct the brochure. Through my analysis of the transcripts and the brochures, I found importance as the main theme. With regard to importance, the sub-themes of (a) placement and (b) content were the brochure's most prevalent aspects.

Placement

Although not directly asked throughout the brochure's co-creation, participants described information placement as a key factor in the brochure. Participants described placement as important because, with their previous experience receiving brochures, they identified certain panels that would be more accessible for where the most important information should be:

> I think I would put it somewhere on the inside 'cause I would want something that would give people information on the title soon within it. (8: 2142–2143)

> Um, honestly, like, whenever I look at brochures, I, I read them like a book. I don't know how other people do it, but it's just, like, how I'll only look at the parts that seem really interesting unless I'm completely dedicated to reading the

whole thing. So, I mean actually maybe that should go in the middle. That's one of the first things you'll see. (10: 2833-2836)

Participants also discussed placement regarding where the brochure should be distributed. They said that brochures with this information should be put up/ distributed in busy places both on campus (e.g., union, dining halls) and off campus (e.g., grocery stores, gas stations). They also suggested junior high and high school counseling offices, residence halls, medical doctor's offices, and therapeutic offices as key places where this brochure should be made available. They suggested that this content is especially important for people from junior high up through the age of thirty.

Content

Participants described the content as an important brochure feature. Although question prompts asked for certain information (see Appendix A), the participants' insights were the main focus of the brochure co-creation part of the study. For example, the participants often described resources in the brochure for anyone who may need them:

> Um, as a student you could put [insert the university's counseling services] . . . and the student health center. . . so obviously, like, the professionals that are on campus that we have available to us . . . and if you don't want to go on campus, you can go to like a private practice or have mental health hotlines. (1: 245-252)

The participants often described the various resources they would want to see in a brochure regarding CMHI. While creating the brochure, I found the contact information for various local and national resources they wanted to see in the brochure. I repeated this process with the CMHI data panel. With the other content, however, the participants' interviews informed these panels of the brochure. The participants described how they wanted to see pictures that were not overly sad or overly happy with two individuals talking and a column for actual advice. Finally, the title for the brochure is a quotation from a participant that encapsulated the theme of the brochure.

Overall, the participants' experiences suggested that college-age students discuss CMHI, but are unsure of how to do so in the best manner possible with their friends. The participants described that they wished they had resources available in order to better ameliorate their uncertainty. Through the various confidants, the privacy coordination, and the brochure co-creation, it is clear that this population merits special attention in the discussion of CMHI.

Additionally, the co-constructed brochure provides a firsthand look at the lived, local knowledge of undergraduate students regarding conversations of CMHI. Providing such information to our collegiate instructors could help create classroom environments that support students with CMHI conditions or concerns. Perhaps instructors could pass out similar pamphlets at the beginning of the semester, post a pamphlet or poster on their office door, or make them available another way, such as on a course website. As Goldman (2018) suggested, discussing or implementing supportive CMHI information could assist college instructors in creating a positive classroom environment, reduce mental health stigma, and allow students to receive the necessary accommodations and/or support for their struggles. In answering his call to "promptly act upon best practices and innovative pedagogical strategies to improve learning conditions for all our students," the co-constructed brochure could be a starting point for normalizing CMHI in classrooms (Goldman 2018, 403). Until then, students may be left to fill roles as unprepared confidants for their friends in need.

DISCUSSION

Through the study in this chapter, I sought to better understand how individuals navigate the confidant's role in experiencing CMHI disclosure from a friend. I focused on friends due to their unique relational communicative features in our lives (Rawlins 2008), and confidants because of their under-represented presence in the literature, yet critical role in CMHI disclosure (Venetis, Chernichky-Karcher, and Gettings 2018). Because of the invisible stigma surrounding CMHI, changes in the self, other, and relational unit do not occur until the affected person reveals such an illness (Cardillo 2010; Horan et al. 2009). The theoretical implications of the findings have translational implications and limitations, but also yield opportunities for future research.

Summary and Theoretical Implications of the Findings

As I described throughout my results, participants demonstrated experiences of types of confidants and privacy coordination processes. In discussing the types of confidants as conceptualized by Petronio (2002), I identified participants as inferential, deliberate, and reluctant confidants. When receiving CMHI as a friend, the inferential confidant was the most common type of confidant identified. This may be rather unsurprising given that friendships are a key relationship for which people seek social support (Rawlins 2008). Previous researchers also found that inferential confidants are often the most common type of confidant experienced in sensitive friendship disclosures (McBride and Bergen 2008). Participants reflected this previous research finding in their interviews when they cited the nature of their friendships and the established trust as reasons why they *expected* their friend to reveal private information with them. However, not all participants experienced their friend coming to them first about their CMHI.

The participants identified as deliberate confidants *solicited* their friend's CMHI in one of two strategies: directly asking and disclosure. Although the directly asking method was rather straightforward, this participant made inquiries about their friend's CMHI due to their behavioral changes. In other words, the invisible CMHI became visible through critical changes in behavior, regardless of whether the revelation through the behavior was intentional (Goffman 1963). The other participant in this category used disclosure as a method for deliberately soliciting their friend's CMHI. Although Petronio (2002) described disclosure as a tactic through which deliberate confidants expect a reciprocal response from their relational other, she notes that "friends and family members who solicit private information often learn more than they want to know. This sometimes turns them into reluctant confidants" (114). However, this participant did not turn into a reluctant confidant, but rather wanted to learn more about their friend's experiences of CMHI. In fact, I only found one participant in my present study who demonstrated qualities of the reluctant confidant.

The participant who identified as a reluctant confidant stated that he did not want to initially hear his friend's CMHI disclosure. This may be unique, as Petronio (2002) originally conceptualized the reluctant confidant as someone "expected to attend to the problems and difficulties of people with whom they have no relationship" (117). Even though this participant did not ask for or want to receive the information, he still considered the discloser to be a friend to the present day. However, McBride and Bergen (2008) suggested that friends may become reluctant confidants in the face of CMHI-related disclosures (i.e., suicidal thoughts, addiction). My participant did not experience similar friendship effects from CMHI as reported in McBride and Bergen (2008). The participant reported that he wished he would have been more of an inferential confidant (or someone who *expects* the information and is supportive of their friend) in their retrospective telling of their story. Nonetheless, across all cases and types of confidants, the participants all experienced boundary coordination in two ways: implicit and explicit boundary coordination.

Petronio (2002) described implicit boundary coordination as those that occur through indirect methods of *hinting* (e.g., maybe this is a private topic) and *prompts* (e.g., What do you think we should do with this information?). She also notes, however, that implicit boundaries may also never be stated because the discloser feels that these rules are already so ingrained in their mind that boundaries may not need coordination. The confidant, however, may not be aware of these rules until they are broken. The participants identified more with the non-disclosed boundaries, as their friends did not communicate any boundary around the friendship. However, their experiences reflected Petronio's (2002) notion that the discloser likely already had made the rules surrounding the disclosure so stringent that the discloser did not feel a need to further limit the disclosure of CMHI.

Some participants, however, described explicit rules that are often communicated such that "the expectations for the way a confidant is to treat the information are unambiguous" (Petronio 2002, 77). Contrary to Petronio (2002), the participants did not report these explicit boundaries before the disclosure occurred. Petronio (2002) conceptualized explicit boundary coordination through disclosure warnings in which the discloser notes that, before they go any further in revealing private information, they communicate a desire for the information to stay between the discloser and the confidant. Although the participants' verbal content was similar to what Petronio (2002) described as disclosure warnings (i.e., "Don't tell anyone," 77), this did not occur until *after* the participant received their friend's disclosure. Thus, explicit boundary coordination conceptualization should not be limited to the idea of a cautionary phrase. In thinking about explicit boundary coordination post-disclosure, this could affect the discloser because supporting a close relational other could burden the confidant (Bailey and Grenyer 2014). In any case, all participants wanted to support their friends, but were unsure how to effectively perform this role.

Translational Implications of the Study

I planned this study to have a translational aspect in the brochure co-construction. Rubio et al. (2010) described how translational research can be done in three main domains in health-related studies: movement between patient and basic research, movement between patient and population research, and interaction between laboratory and population research. The authors mentioned that good research, particularly if medical in nature, must have a translational aspect. In conceptualizing CMHI alongside CPM, the study's aim to have a translational approach is theoretically important.

As mentioned earlier, this brochure is a resource for how friends can effectively have conversations around mental health. Because students may experience increased stigma from their friends' reactions (Moses 2010), having a tangible resource for better management could mitigate stigmatized reactions. Additionally, instructors and other campus staff can reference the brochure's information to better understand actual processes of disclosures of their students with one another. Many college instructors report that "they never received formal, university-sanctioned mental health training," (White and LaBelle 2019, 149) yet repeatedly manage student mental health concerns. Therefore, this brochure reflects how referential materials could inform those on the frontlines of mental health conversations (White and LaBelle 2019; see also Goldman 2018). The brochure resource could also help instructors maintain authority, while reducing the perception that receiving a student's mental health information would make them seem more like a friend (White and LaBelle 2019).

Theoretically, Petronio (2007) asserted that CPM may be particularly useful in conceptualizing studies with a translational goal. She noted that while some studies considering themselves *translational* may simply describe that the research problem could benefit from translational research, she emphasized that researchers using CPM should incorporate translational factors in their studies, such as adapting their findings into usable practices and collaborating with researchers trained in designing and implementing translational research objectives (Petronio 2007, 222). Therefore, throughout this chapter and in my study, I made sure to have a translational aim in developing a disseminatable communication material to benefit the target population using my findings (Petronio, 1999). Through theoretical development, local knowledge, and rigorous interpretive inquiry, I produced a working template that other mental health practitioners, instructors, campus advocates, and communication researchers could disseminate on campus. However, the brochure is a *working template* because its photos (stock images in the example) and information should be tailored for specific agency use.

The exercise of creating a translational piece (brochure) through local knowledge and a socially constructed, hermeneutical, and translational approach has further implications. Interacting with individuals from a marginalized population can reduce uncertainty and create better treatment for health-related conditions (Duggan and Bradshaw 2013). In fact, creating interventions from the targeted community's input can create more effective results than interventions based on observational data (Hecht and Krieger 2006). Therefore, I provide administrators and mental health professionals a tool kit for developing at translational product to assist people struggling with mental health.

Limitations and Future Research Possibilities

Although this chapter makes theoretical and translational contributions through its novel approach to CPM and translational research, its findings have key aspects that should be considered if translated into other contexts. First, the sample was from a Predominately White Institution (PWI) and inherently not diverse. This merits importance because we know that minority populations experience CMHI differently, and often with greater deficit in resource seeking, than the dominant white population (Shushansky 2017). Therefore, future inquiries into CMHI and CPM research must pay special attention to developing materials for minority populations, to not further isolate them from necessary CMHI care and support-seeking in interpersonal relationships.

Second, although I achieved theoretical saturation and verified my results through a data conference, this research cannot begin and end at thirteen participants. CMHI is a global issue spanning gender, race, and culture. The interview and brochure results need further verification through member reflections to effectively discuss the results with participants for critical reflection of their experiences in tandem with the final products a researcher presents to them (Tracy 2019). Third, this work also needs to be longitudinally tested to examine if receiving this brochure helps college students become more willing to discuss CMHI issues with a friend. Finally, collaborative work among chronic and mental health professionals is also needed to not only build interdisciplinary relationships, but also to improve the communicative process of CMHI disclosure with as many informed stakeholders as possible.

CONCLUSION

Throughout this chapter, I examined how friends communicate about CMHI through the lens of the confidant. Although this work is inherently limited, I provided insights about the understudied friendship relationship, filled gaps in CPM-related confidant studies, and developed a new translational, interpretive method (3TA) that pertains to CMHI. My goal in this chapter to better understand confidants' roles in discussing CMHI reflected how friendships are truly give and take. In order to be a friend, a person must meet others' expectations to commit to the relationship for better or worse, including in health or when disclosing CMHI.

NOTE

1. Numbers within parentheses following quotes represent participant number and line numbers within the main document of 154 pages of double-spaced transcripts.

REFERENCES

Ackerson, Lisa K., and K. Viswanath. 2009. "The Social Context of Interpersonal Communication and Health." *Journal of Health Communication* 58, no. 14 (May): 5–17. https://doi.org/10.1080/10810730902806836.

Anthony, Amanda K., and Janice McCabe. 2015. "Friendship Talk as Identity Work: Defining the Self through Friend Relationships." *Symbolic Interaction* 38, no. 1 (January): 64–82. https://doi.org/10.1002/symb.138.

Auerbach, Randy P., Philippe Mortier, Ronny Bruffaerts, Jordi Alonso, Corina Benjet, Pim Cuijpers, Koen Demyttenaere et al. 2016. "WHO World Mental Health Surveys International College Student Project: Prevalence and Distribution of Mental Disorders." *Journal of Abnormal Psychology* 127, no. 7 (October): 623–638. https://doi.org/10.1037/abn0000362.

Bailey, Rachel C., and Brin F. S. Grenyer. 2014. "Supporting a Person with Personality Disorder: A Study of Carer Burden and Well-being." *Journal of Personality Disorders* 28, no. 6 (December): 796–809. https://doi.org/10.1521/pedi_2014_28_136.

Basel, Sarah R. 2018. "The Confidant's Role in Managing Private Disclosures: An Analysis Using Communication Privacy Management Theory." PhD diss., Kent State University.

Bliezner, Rosemary, and Rebecca G. Adams. 1992. *Adult Friendship*. Newbury Park, CA: Sage.

Bowen, Glenn A. 2006. "Grounded Theory and Sensitizing Concepts." *International Journal of Qualitative Research Methods* 5, no. 3 (September): 12–23. https://doi.org/10.1177/160940690600500304.

Braithwaite, Dawn O., Jordan Allen, and Julia Moore. 2017. "Data Conferencing." In *The International Encyclopedia of Communication Research Methods*, edited by Jörg P. Matthes, Christine S. Davis, and Robert F. Potter. Hoboken, NJ: Wiley-Blackwell. https://doi.org/10.1002/9781118901731.iecrm0057.

Braithwaite, Dawn O., Betsy Wackernagel Bach, Leslie A. Baxter, Rebecca DiVerniero, Joshua R. Hammonds, Angela M. Hosek, Erin K. Willer, and Bianca M. Wolf. 2010. "Constructing Family: A Typology of Voluntary Lin." *Journal of Social and Personal Relationships* 27, no. 3 (April): 388–407. https://doi.org/10.1177/0265407510361615.

Braun, Virginia, and Victoria Clarke. 2006. "Using Thematic Analysis in Psychology." *Qualitative Research in Psychology* 3, no. 2 (July): 77–101. https://doi.org/10.1191/1478088706qp063oa.

Brinkmann, Svend, and Steinar Kvale. 2015. *InterViews: Learning the Craft of Qualitative Research Interviewing*. Thousand Oaks, CA: Sage.

Butler, Hannah. 2016. "College Students' Disclosure of Mental Health Counseling Utilization." *Iowa Journal of Communication* 48, no. 1–2 (Fall): 156–170. https://static1.squarespace.com/static/59e7a2c8d0e6285c031b4026/t/5bf4c79e4fa51adde979fd31/1542768543694/College+Students+Disclosure+of+Mental+Health+counseling+utilization.pdf.

Cardillo, Linda Wheeler. 2010. "Empowering Narratives: Making Sense of the Experience of Growing up with Chronic Illness or Disability." *Western Journal of Communication* 74, no. 5 (November): 525–546. https://doi.org/10.1080/10570314.2010.512280.

Carr, Kristen, and Sarah E. Wilder. 2016. "Attachment Style and the Risks of Seeking Social Support: Variations between Friends and Siblings." *Southern Communication Journal* 81, no. 5 (August): 316–329. https://doi.org/10.1080/1041794X.2016.1208266.

Corrigan, Patrick W., Benjamin G. Druss, and Deborah A. Perlick. 2014. "The Impact of Mental Illness Stigma on Seeking and Participating in Mental Health Care." *Psychological Science in the Public Interest* 15, no. 2 (September): 37–70. https://doi.org/10.1177/1529100614531398.

Creswell, John W. 2016. *30 Essential Skills for the Qualitative Researcher*. Thousand Oaks, CA: Sage.

Creswell, John W., and Cheryl N. Poth. 2018. *Qualitative Inquiry and Research Design: Choosing Among Five Approaches*. Thousand Oaks, CA: Sage.

Dainton, Marianne, Elaine Zelley, and Emily Langan. 2003. "Maintaining Friendships throughout the Lifespan." In *Maintaining Relationships through Communication: Relational, Contextual, and Cultural Variations*, edited by Daniel J. Canary and Marianne Dainton, 79–102. Mahwah, NJ: Lawrence Erlbaum.

Dean, Marleah, and Emily A. Rauscher. 2018. "Men's and Women's Approaches to Disclosure about BRCA-related Cancer Risks and Family Planning Decision-making." *Qualitative Health Research* 28, no. 14 (July): 2155–2168. https://doi.org/10.1177/1049732318788377.

Duggan, Ashley P., and Ylisabyth S. Bradshaw. 2013. "Shifting Communication Challenges to Education and Reflective Practice: Communication to Reduce Disparities toward Patients with Disabilities." In *Reducing Health Disparities: Communication Interventions*, edited by Mohan J. Dutta and Gary L. Kreps, 15–34. New York: Peter Lang.

Eisenberg, Daniel. 2019. "Countering the Troubling Increase in Mental Health Symptoms among U.S. College Students." *Journal of Adolescent Health* 65, no. 5 (November): 573–574. https://doi.org/10.1016/j.jadohealth.2019.08.003.

Evans, Teresa M., Lindsay Bira, Jazmin Beltran Gastelum, L. Todd Weiss, and Nathan L. Vanderford. 2018. "Evidence for a Mental Health Crisis in Graduate Education." *Nature Biotechnology* 36, no. 3 (March): 282–284. https://doi.org/10.1038/nbt.4089.

Fehr, Beverly. 1996. *Friendship Processes*. Thousand Oaks, CA: Sage

Fehr, Beverly, and James A. Russell. 1991. "The Concept of Love Viewed from a Prototype Perspective." *Journal of Personality and Social Psychology* 60, no. 3 (February): 425–438. https://doi.org/10.1037/0022-3514.60.3.425.

Goffman, Erving. 1963. *Stigma: Notes on the Management of Spoiled Identity*. Englewood Cliffs, NJ: Prentice Hall.

Goldman, Zachary W. 2018. "Responding to Mental Health Issues in the College Classroom." *Communication Education* 67, no. 3 (May): 399–404. https://doi.org/10.1080/03634523.2018.1465191.

Harvey, Jacquelyn, Elizabeth Sanders, Linda Ko, Valerie Manusov, and Jean Yi. 2017. "The Impact of Written Emotional Disclosure on Cancer Caregivers' Perceptions of Burden, Stress, and Depression: A Randomized Controlled Trial." *Health Communication* 33, no. 7 (May): 824–832. https://doi.org/10.1080/10410236.2017.1315677.

Hayes, J. F., J. Miles, K. Walters, M. King, and D. P. J. Osborn. 2015. "A Systematic Review and Meta-analysis of Premature Mortality in Bipolar Affective Disorder." *Acta Psychiatrica Scandinavica* 131, no. 6 (March): 417–425. https://doi.org/10.1111/acps.12408.

Hecht, Michael L., and Janice L. Raup Krieger. 2006. "The Principle of Cultural Grounding in School-based Substance Abuse Prevention." *Journal of Language and Social Psychology* 25, no. 3 (September): 301–319. https://doi.org/10.1177/0261927X06289476.

Horan, Sean M., Matthew M. Martin, Nicole Smith, Meghan Schoo, Mary Eidsness, and Angela Johnson. 2009. "Can we Talk? How Learning of an Invisible Illness Impacts Forecasted Relational Outcomes." *Communication Studies* 60, no. 1 (January): 66–81. https://doi.org/10.1080/10510970802623625.

Iedema, Rick, Christine Jorm, John Wakefield, Cherie Ryan, and Stewart Dunn. 2009. "Practising Open Disclosure: Clinical Incident Communication and Systems Improvement." *Sociology of Health & Illness* 31, no. 2 (February): 262–277. https://doi.org/10.1111/j.1467-9566.2008.01131.x.

Koetsenruijter, Jan, Nathalie van Eikelenboom, Jan van Lieshout, Ivo Vassilev, Christos Lionis, Elka Todorova, Mari Carmen Portillo et al. 2016. "Social Support and Self-management Capabilities in Diabetes Patients: An International Observational Study. *Patient Education and Counseling* 99, no. 4 (April): 638–643. https://doi.org/10.1016/j.pec.2015.10.029.

Kundrat, Amanda L., and John F. Nussbaum. 2003. "The Impact of Invisible Illness on Identity and Contextual Age across the Lifespan." *Health Communication* 15, no. 3: 331–347. https://doi.org/10.1207/S15327027HC1503_5.

Lindlof, Thomas R., and Bryan C. Taylor. 2018. *Qualitative Communication Research Methods*. Thousand Oaks, CA: Sage.

Lipson, Sarah Ketchen, S. Michael Gaddis, Justin Heinze, Kathryn Beck, and Daniel Eisenberg. 2015. "Variations in Student Mental Health and Treatment Utilization across US Colleges and Universities." *Journal of American College Health* 63, no. 6 (August): 388–396. https://doi.org/10.1080/07448481.2015.1040411.

McBride, M. Chad, and Karla Mason Bergen. 2008. "Becoming a Reluctant Confidant: Communication Privacy Management in Close Friendships." *Texas Speech Communication Journal* 33, no. 1: 50–61.

Meluch, Andrea L., and Shawn C. Starcher. 2020. "College Student Concealment and Disclosure of Mental Health Issues in the Classroom: Students' Perceptions of Risk and Use of Contextual Criteria." *Communication Studies* (June): 1–15. https://doi.org/10.1080/10510974.2020.1771392.

Moses, Tally. 2010. "Being Treated Differently: Stigma Experiences with Family, Peers, and School Staff among Adolescents with Mental Health Disorders." *Social Science & Medicine* 70, no. 7 (April): 985–993. https://doi.org/10.1016/j.socscimed.2009.12.022.

Naslund, J. A., K. A. Aschbrenner, L. A. Marsch, and S. J. Bartels. 2016. "The Future of Mental Health Care: Peer-to-peer Support and Social Media." *Epidemiology and Psychiatric Science* 26, no. 2 (April): 113-122. https://doi.org/10.1017/S2045796015001067.

National Center for Chronic Disease Prevention and Health Promotion. 2019. "Chronic diseases in America." Accessed August 9, 2020. https://www.cdc.gov/chronicdisease/resources/infographic/chronic-diseases.htm.

National Institute for Mental Health. 2015. "Chronic Illness and Mental Health." Accessed March 30, 2020. https://www.nimh.nih.gov/health/publications/chronic-illness-mental-health/index.shtml.

National Institute for Mental Health. 2017. "Mental Illness." Accessed March 30, 2020. https://www.nimh.nih.gov/health/statistics/mental-illness.shtml.

Owen, William Foster. 1984. "Interpretive Themes in Relational Communication." *Quarterly Journal of Speech* 70, no. 3: 274–287. https://doi.org/10.1080/003356 38409383697.
Persson, Tonje J., James G. Pfaus, and Andrew G. Ryder. 2015. "Explaining Mental Health Disparities for Non-monosexual Women: Abuse History and Risky Sex, or the Burdens of Non-Disclosure?" *Social Science & Medicine* 128 (March): 366–373. https://doi.org/10.1016/j.socscimed.2014.08.038.
Petronio, Sandra. 1999. "'Translating Scholarship into Practice': An Alternative Metaphor." *Journal of Applied Communication Research* 27, no. 2 (April): 87–91. https://doi.org/10.1080/00909889909365527.
Petronio, Sandra. 2002. *Boundaries of Privacy: Dialectics of Disclosure*. New York: New York University Press.
Petronio, Sandra. 2007. "Translational Research Endeavors and the Practices of Communication Privacy Management." *Journal of Applied Communication Research* 35, no. 3 (July): 218–222. https://doi.org/10.1080/00909880701422443.
Petronio, Sandra. 2010. "Communication Privacy Management Theory: What Do we Know about Family Privacy Regulation?" *Journal of Family Theory & Review* 2, no. 3 (August): 175–196. https://doi.org/10.1111/j.1756-2589.2010.00052.x.
Petronio, Sandra. 2018. "Communication Privacy Management Theory: Understanding Families." In *Engaging Theories in Family Communication: Multiple Perspectives*, edited by Dawn O. Braithwaite, Elizabeth A. Suter, and Kory Floyd, 87–98. New York: Routledge.
Petronio, Sandra, and Wesley T. Durham. 2015. "Communication Privacy Management Theory: Significance for Interpersonal Communication." In *Engaging Theories in Interpersonal Communication: Multiple Perspectives*, edited by Dawn O. Braithwaite and Paul Schrodt, 335–347. Thousand Oaks, CA: Sage.
Price, Margaret, Mark S. Salzer, Amber O'Shea, and Stephanie L. Kerschbaum. 2017. "Disclosure of Mental Disability by College and University Faculty: The Negotiation of Accommodations, Supports, and Barriers." *Disability Studies Quarterly* 37, no. 2. https://doi.org/10.18061/dsq.v37i2.5487.
Prince, Jeffrey P. 2015. "University Student Counseling and Mental Health in the United States: Trends and Challenges." *Mental Health & Prevention* 3, no. 1–2 (April): 5–10. https://doi.org/10.1016/j.mhp.2015.03.001.
Raphael, Karen G., Malvin N. Janal, Sangeetha Nayak, Joseph E. Schwartz, and Rollin M. Gallagher. 2006. "Psychiatric Comorbidities in a Community Sample of Women with Fibromyalgia." *Pain* 124, no. 1–2 (April): 117–125. https://doi.org/10 .1016/j.pain.2006.04.004.
Rawlins, William K. 1992. *Friendship Matters: Communication, Dialectics, and the Life Course*. New Brunswick, NJ: Transaction Publishers.
Rawlins, William K. 2008. *The Compass of Friendship: Narratives, Identities, and Dialogues*. Thousand Oaks, CA: Sage.
Rubio, Doris McGartland, Ellie E. Schoenbaum, Linda S. Lee, David E. Schteingart, Paul R. Marantz, Karl E. Anderson, Lauren Dewey Platt, Adriana Baez, and Karin Esposito. 2010. "Defining Translational Research: Implications for Training." *Academic Medicine* 85, no. 3 (March): 470–475. https://doi.org/ 10.1097/ACM.0b013e3181ccd618.

Segrin, Chris, and Jeanne Flora. 2017. "Family Conflict is Detrimental to Physical and Mental Health." In *Communicating Interpersonal Conflict in Close Relationships: Contexts, Challenges, and Opportunities,* edited by Jennifer A. Samp, 207–224. New York: Routledge.

Shushansky, Larry. 2017. "Disparities Within Minority Mental Health Care. Accessed March 30, 2020. https://www.nami.org/Blogs/NAMI-Blog/July-2017/Disparities-Within-Minority-Mental-Health-Care.

Smith, Rachel A. 2011. "Stigma, Communication, and Health." In *The Routledge Handbook of Health Communication*, edited by Teresa. L. Thompson, Roxanne Parrott, and John F. Nussbaum, 455–468. New York: Routledge.

Smith, Rachel A., and Amanda Applegate. 2018. "Mental Health Stigma and Communication and their Intersections with Education." *Communication Education* 67, no. 3 (May): 382–408. https://doi.org/ 10.1080/03634523.2018.1465988.

The Jed Foundation. 2008. "Student Mental Health and the Law: A Resource for Institutions of Higher Education." New York: The Jed Foundation. http://www.jedfoundation.org/wp-content/uploads/2016/07/student-mental-health-and-the-law-jed-NEW.pdf.

Tracy, Sarah J. 2019. *Qualitative Research Methods: Collecting Evidence, Crafting Analysis, Communicating Impact.* Hoboken, NJ: John Wiley and Sons.

Venetis, Maria K., Skye Chernichky-Karcher, and Patricia E. Gettings. 2018. "Disclosing Mental Illness Information to a Friend: Exploring how the Disclosure Decision-making Model Informs Strategy Selection." *Health Communication* 33, no. 6 (March): 653–663. https://doi.org/ 10.1080/10410236.2017.1294231.

Wedemeyer-Strombel, Kathryn R. 2019. "Why we Need to Talk more about Mental Health in Graduate School." *The Chronicle of Higher Education.* https://www.chronicle.com/article/Why-We-Need-to-Talk-More-About/247002.

White, Allie, and Sara LaBelle. 2019. "A Qualitative Investigation of Instructors' Perceived Communicative Roles in Students' Mental Health Management." *Communication Education* 68, no. 2 (January): 133–155. https://doi.org/10.1080/03634523.2019.1571620.

APPENDIX A

Interview Protocol

Before we begin with the open-ended questions, I would like to learn a bit about you.

1) Demographic Information:
   a. What is your age?
   b. What is your sex?
   c. What is your ethnicity?
   d. What is your religious affiliation?
   e. What is your highest level of education?

Now that I know a bit more about you, I'm going to ask you some questions regarding receiving chronic and/or mental health-related information from a friend. Prior to this interview, I asked you to reflect on your relationship with one particular friend who talked about their chronic and/or mental health-related information with you. I would like to know a little bit more about your relationship with them.

1) Friendship Information:
   a. When and where did you meet this friend?
   b. How long have you been friends with this person?
   c. What is this friend's...
      Sex?
      Age?
      Ethnicity?
      Religious affiliation?
      Highest level of education?
   d. What health condition(s) did your friend tell you they have?
   e. Approximately when do you recall your friend telling you their health-related information for the first time?
      Clarification, if needed: This can be month, year, and/or season. I'm basically trying to get an idea of how long it has been since you found out this information.
   f. How close would you say you are/were with this friend at the time of them first telling you this information about their health condition?
      How close would you say you are with this friend today?
2) Tell me the story about when your friend first told you about their health-related information. Describe, as best as you can recall, what you and your friend did and said in this situation.
   a. Probe on disclosure:
      Why do you think your friend chose you to tell you this information?
      How did your friend tell you? For example, was it in person, over the phone, texting, etc.?
      What was your immediate reaction to receiving this information from your friend? What did you do or say?
      1. How satisfied were you with your reaction?
      2. How comfortable did your friend seem to be with what you did or said after they told you about their health condition?
      How did you feel about receiving this information from your friend?

1. What emotions did you experience?
In many situations we can choose to receive information from another person or not. Thus,
   1. How much choice did you feel you had when your friend told you this information?
   2. What, if anything, do you wish had been different about this?
   b. What motivated you to receive this information?
   c. Probe on information management:
      1. Once your friend told you this information, what, if anything, did they tell you about what you could and couldn't do/say with the information they gave you?
         a. Please describe.
      2. How well did you follow their request about what to do or say?
         a. Probe:
            Who, if anyone, did you tell about your friend's health condition?
            1. Why did you decide to tell this person(s)?
3) How often have you and your friend discussed this information about their health condition since the first time they revealed their condition to you?
   a. How often do you talk about this?
   b. What have you discussed?
   c. Why have you two discussed this information?
   d. How, if at all, did any of the expectations change about what your friend wants you to say or do with this information?
      If so, why?
      If not, why?
   e. What personal, health-related information have you told your friend, if anything?
      1. Who discussed their health information first, and why?
      2. What motivated you to talk with your friend about your health condition?
      3. How do you believe this affected your friendship, if at all?

Now that I'm aware of a few of your experiences regarding your friendship, I'd like to ask you a few final questions on this topic.

1) How does a friendship differ from talking with family members or a partner when the topic is chronic and/or mental health-related information?
2) What advice, if any, would you give to another person if they are thinking about talking with a friend about their chronic and/or mental health-related information?
   a. Probe:
      Why (if needed)?
3) What advice, if any, would you give to another person receiving chronic and/or mental health-related information?
   a. Probe:
      Why (if needed)?

Based on your answers, I'd like to do an activity. Part of my interest in researching this topic is to improve the communication between friends regarding CMHI. In doing so, I am looking to develop materials for those who may be in similar situations as yours. In this stage of the research, my plan is to develop a brochure that one could pick up and/or download for accessible information about receiving chronic and/or mental health-related information from a friend. Would you mind participating in this activity with me?

1) If yes, go to Appendix A, then continue with the protocol.
2) If no, continue to the next question.

What else do you think I should know about receiving information from friends about chronic and/or mental health-related information?
   Thank you again for agreeing to participate in my study. The experiences you provided me with today will help shed light on the process of friends receiving information about various chronic and/or mental health issues. What other information would you like to add that I didn't address today would you like to add before we end?
   Thank you again for agreeing to participate in this study.

APPENDIX A: BROCHURE DESIGN PROMPTS

In this activity, we will construct a brochure so that others experiencing similar situations as you can have a resource for improving the communication between friends regarding chronic and/or mental health disclosures. In this activity, I will guide you through the creation of the brochure, but the information on the brochure will come primarily through you. I can certainly help with wording or small details, but the ideas and content will be completely your ideas. What questions do you have at this point?

1) Content.
   a. Based on our conversation from today, what are the three main takeaways you would want someone to know about receiving chronic and/or mental health-related information from a friend?

Please talk with me about why you chose the main points you did.
   b. Based on our conversation from today, what are the three main takeaways you would want someone to know about talking with a friend about chronic and/or mental health-related information?

Please discuss with me why you chose these main points.
   c. Based on our conversation today, what images come to mind that would represent friends discussing chronic and/or mental health-related information?

Please discuss with me why you chose these images.
   d. Based on our conversation from today, what would be the most important chronic and/or mental health-related information you would like to see on a brochure of this type?

Please talk with me about why this information would be important.
2) Title:
   a. Based on our conversation from today, what would be the best title for this brochure?

Please tell me why this title would be best.
3) Audience:
   a. In your opinion, who would be the best audience for this type of information?

Please tell me why you think this particular audience is best.
   b. Would you pick up this brochure and read it?

Please discuss why you would or wouldn't.
   c. Where do you think would be the best place to have this brochure available?

Give and Take 167

Please tell me why you think this is the best location.
   d. What would be your reaction to someone giving you this brochure?

Please tell me why you would react in such a way.
   e. What is the best way to get the information out about this information?

Please discuss why you think that this method is best.
Now go back to the questionnaire.

APPENDIX B

General Statistics

- Over half of all mental illness begins by age 14, and three-fourths begins by 24 (National Alliance on Mental Illness, 2019)

- Approximately one-quarter of all mental health conditions are in young adults (National Institute for Mental Health, 2019)

- 20% of all youth ages 13-18 live with a mental health condition (National Alliance on Mental Illness, 2019)

- Between 13-18% of all young adults have a chronic illness (Center for Disease Control and Prevention, 2009)

Key Resources

University Counseling/
Psychological Services:
(insert phone number)

National Suicide
Prevention Hotline:
1-800-273-8255

National Alliance on
Mental Health:
1-800-950-6264

Providing Access to
Help:
1-888-865-9903

Friends Don't Let
Friends Suffer
Alone

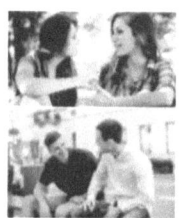

How To Talk About Mental and Chronic Health with Your Friends

Figure 7.1 Click here to enter text.

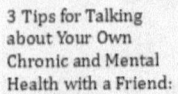

Figure 7.2 Click here to enter text.

Chapter 8

The Academic Amygdala
Tropes of PTSD in Higher Education News Coverage

Alena Amato Ruggerio and Erica Knotts

Post-Traumatic Stress Disorder (PTSD) is so ubiquitous that the term is now often used colloquially to refer to any haunted or distressed feeling: "Having to go to school in that awful uniform gave me PTSD." Yet, below this metaphorical usage lies a genuine clinical condition defined by the American Psychiatric Association's (APA) *Diagnostic Statistical Manual-5* and protected by the Americans with Disabilities Act (APA 2013).

Unfortunately, a majority of the population can expect to be directly exposed to or witness a life-threatening traumatic event such as rape or sexual abuse, motor vehicle accidents, war or terrorism, or natural disaster at some point in their lifetimes. In the typical brain, the small, almond-shaped amygdala located deep in the mammalian limbic system activates temporarily into self-protective high alert, to help the body cope with such traumas, and then subsides. However, in up to 10 percent of the population (U.S. Department of Veterans Affairs 2018), the amygdala, which renowned PTSD researcher Bessel van der Kolk refers to as the "smoke alarm of the brain" (2015), remains perpetually stuck in the state of activation following exposure to trauma, resulting in the condition now called PTSD, formerly known as shell shock or combat fatigue (APA 2013, 271). PTSD symptoms can include flashbacks and re-experiencing of the trauma, avoidance of cues to the trauma, negative changes in mood and thought, and increased arousal manifested as disordered sleep, hypervigilance, or irritability (271–272). The overwhelming majority of people with PTSD are non-violent, much more prone to the freeze response under stress than fight or flight (Mittal et al. 2013), and more likely to be the victims of violence than the perpetrators, counter to the damaging myth of PTSD instigating gunmen (gendered noun intentional) to massacre civilians—some on college campuses—with semi-automatic weapons.

In the United States, the stereotypical image of a person with PTSD is usually a white man who has been exposed to the acute trauma of military combat. There is an epidemic of PTSD in military contexts and an unacceptably high rate of veteran suicide, and this depiction is clearly incomplete. The trope of the white, male combat veteran as the only identity for PTSD extends into higher education, which heaps on a further reductive image that our white, male vet with PTSD is most likely an undergraduate student. In addition to silencing undergrads with PTSD who are not men or have not engaged in military service, this assumption negatively affects faculty, staff, administrators, and graduate assistants for whom academia is a workplace. This incomplete trope of the typical person with PTSD is based on assumptions constructed and reinforced rhetorically through mainstream news stories (Houston, Spialek, and Perreault 2016).

Is the academic press any different? This chapter offers a feminist rhetorical analysis of how news coverage in which the frame is limited exclusively to the academy not only perpetuates the same PTSD trope as the general press, but also adds a pernicious form of symbolic dissociation unique to academia's anxieties about the cognitive productivity of its workers. The Theory of Planned Behavior (TPB) offers insights from the health communication literature on interrupting these mental constructs to enact better mindsets and better policies about PTSD in higher education.

METHOD

The Chronicle of Higher Education is respected as the authoritative English-language news source focusing exclusively on academia. Reaching more than 300,000 readers, the *Chronicle* is required reading in print or web format on college and university campuses across the U.S. and beyond (The Editors of *Encyclopædia Britannica* 2017). The *Chronicle* itself promotes this positioning, referring to the publication on its website as "the unrivaled leader in higher education journalism" ("About Us" 2020). For this chapter, we identified all the news articles published in *The Chronicle of Higher Education* from 1995 to 2019 that mention the terms Post-Traumatic Stress Disorder or PTSD. This search of the ProQuest Central academic database yielded eighty-five articles. We discarded twenty-eight articles that referred to trauma only metaphorically, covered scientists developing new medical research and therapies, mentioned the disorder in a book recommendation, focused on animals and PTSD research, or merely listed a connection to PTSD in author credentials. We retained a total of fifty-seven articles as artifacts for feminist rhetorical criticism.

Despite the popular usage of *rhetoric* to indicate empty or flowery words, the rhetorical choices made by human beings who create meaning together through the exchange of verbal and non-verbal messages are symbolic actions with material consequences (Burke 1950, 43), especially for people from marginalized populations (Otis 2019). Among the multiplicity of approaches to feminist rhetorical criticism, ours conceptualizes culture as a kyriarchy, in which groups of people are assigned sociocultural marginalization or privilege (often some combination of both) based on an intersecting matrix of identities based on race, class, sexual orientation, gender performance, ability, nationality, age, and so on (Fiorenza 1992, 115–117). For instance, a woman of color who has a psychological disability such as PTSD would not only be under triple domination as a member of those identity groups, but would also experience a distinct, exponentially compounded form of domination living at the intersection of those identities (Crenshaw 1989). This process is established and maintained rhetorically, and can be revealed and ultimately resisted through feminist rhetorical criticism (Nudd and Whalen 2016). Feminist scholars practice self-reflexivity regarding their perspectives within the lived experiences of their own bodies, and value their feelings about their research topics (Bizzell 2000, 12–14). As the authors of this chapter, we endeavor to wield our privilege as cishet, white, highly educated American scholars to interrupt injustice. We simultaneously embody the intersecting dominations of feminine gender, psychological disability, and for one of us, contingent faculty status.

Feminist rhetorical critics analyze artifacts of public communication for their word selection, example narratives, discursive structure, and visual images to identify whether the message reinforces or disrupts (often some combination of both) the hegemonic power of kyriarchy, with the ultimate goals of liberation and justice (Foss 2018, 147). Dow (2016) asserts that "[R]hetorical critics, especially feminist ones, recognize that rhetoric is a political practice and performance through which power ebbs and flows" (67). Therefore, this chapter examines the rhetorical choices of *The Chronicle of Higher Education* artifacts with an eye toward the power relations made normative in the academic role, gender, military status, and race projected onto the identity of the typical person with PTSD.

The profound social stigma of psychological disabilities, and the potential for interruption of that stigma, is committed rhetorically, making rhetorical criticism an appropriate method of analysis. People with disabilities face "bias, prejudice, segregation and discrimination" (Knapp 2008, 108), which are all problems of attitude influenced by the collective social process of communication. This rhetorical construction of PTSD stigma then shapes public policy, research dollars, workplace conditions, and individual experiences (Houston, Spialek, and Perreault 2016, 240). Without a vociferous counter narrative about people with PTSD, this stigma and its material implications are unlikely to be eradicated, even via legal means.

ANALYSIS

Among the fifty-seven articles from *The Chronicle of Higher Education* depicting stories of members of campus communities who have PTSD, thirty mention active military or veterans. Nineteen articles acknowledge women with PTSD. Twenty-five mention students, whereas faculty or other non-undergraduate academic workers are featured in only eight articles. The racial identities of the people with PTSD go unmarked except in two.

Person with PTSD = Veteran

More than half the *Chronicle* articles equate PTSD with a military veteran. Some reporters offer extended narratives of vets in article-length coverage of trauma (Bartlett 2011; Goldberg 2011; Farrell 2005; Mangan 2009; Mangan 2008; Sander 2012). This acknowledgment of PTSD among veterans is not problematic; rather, the problem lies with the weight of the repeated rhetorical trope in the academic news coverage that implies developing PTSD from military service is inevitable, and that all those with PTSD are veterans. This study reveals myriad brief, offhand sentences in articles not otherwise about trauma equating PTSD with military identity as a fait accompli. For example:

> [An instructor of introductory psychology keeps his examples of psychological disorders short and relatable]: . . . a movie clip of Jack Nicholson obsessively washing his hands, or the story of a friend whose brother came home from Iraq with PTSD and subsequently killed himself. (McMurtrie 2018, para. 27)

> My dad was also a Vietnam vet, and he suffered from severe PTSD. The smell of the rich, moist dirt under the houses often gave him flashbacks. (Gifford 2015, para. 2)

> Working in small groups, first-year students role-play as doctors and consider the best course of action for a Pueblo man suffering from post-traumatic stress disorder after serving in the military. (Waitzkin 2011, para. 19)

> One section of the [art] show, "A Soldier's Heart," is dedicated to those wrestling with post-traumatic stress disorder. (Klein 2002, para. 22)

The three-dimensional virtual worlds . . . are now moving out of computer science research labs and into hospitals. They are being used to treat pain in burn patients and to help veterans overcome chronic post-traumatic stress disorder. (Olsen 2000, para. 2)

Over the next several years, Goerling attended trainings for cops and firefighters, interviewed military personnel and civilian first responders with post-traumatic stress disorder, and took Rogers to various police trainings, where the two talked to officers about building resilience. (Schimke 2017, para. 8)

The memetic proliferation of this trope in *The Chronicle of Higher Education* is not surprising, given that survivors of military combat do develop PTSD at a higher rate than civilians. The language of the diagnosis of PTSD originated within the military, and the U.S. Departments of Defense and Veterans Affairs provide millions of dollars for PTSD research annually (National Center for PTSD 2018). Purtle (2014) points out that the military origin (but not exclusively the incidence) of the PTSD diagnosis has colored federal policy, which has passed war-focused legislation out of proportion to the higher total numbers of PTSD cases in the civilian population.

Higher education is not immune to these military and linguistic influences, and carries the added consideration of funding dollars. American public institutions of higher education receive tuition payments from the federal government for accepting and supporting returning veterans into the classroom through the military's tuition assistance programs (Department of Defense 2018). This tempts some colleges and universities to prioritize their consciousness of PTSD among their veteran populations out of proportion with the numbers of affected civilians.

Person with PTSD = White Man

It follows in the popular misconception that if men are the great majority of soldiers, especially in combat specialties, and PTSD is ostensibly the inevitable result of military combat, then the typical person with PTSD must be male. Men with PTSD function as the default in *The Chronicle of Higher Education* articles, and only 33 percent of the articles mention women at all.

No people with PTSD who identify as non-binary or genderqueer appear in our data set. In part, this omission in the *Chronicle* coverage might be attributed to the institutional erasure of non-binary genders. For instance, an Oregon circuit court approved "non-binary" as a legally designated gender only as recently as 2016, in a case filed by an army veteran (Mele 2016). Under the Trump administration, people who are transgender are currently banned from military service (Cooper 2018, A14); thus, the conflation between PTSD, masculinity, and the armed forces is further reified as cismale.

Despite appearing in only one-third of the *Chronicle* artifacts, more women than men, of all races, suffer from PTSD (American Psychiatric Association 2013, 278); women are twice as likely to develop PTSD when exposed to trauma than men (Breslau and Anthony 1998; Kilpatrick et al. 2013); women can be more sensitive than men to developing PTSD following an initial traumatic event (Breslau and Anthony 2007; Rivollier et al. 2015); women tend to experience the symptoms of PTSD more severely (Tolin and Foa 2006); and women's symptoms are less likely to be validated with a PTSD diagnosis (U.S. Department of Defense 2007). Women's cases of PTSD tend to originate from intentional, personally intimate, sometimes ongoing abuse, whereas, for men, the traumas are more likely to be faceless, acute incidents. Dr. Ralph Ryback (2016), formerly of Harvard Medical School, reports that "women are more likely to develop PTSD due to sexual assault and child sexual abuse, whereas men are more likely to develop the disorder due to accidents, physical assault, natural disaster and combat." Even a female member of the U.S. military is just as likely to develop PTSD from a rape perpetrated by a person from within her own ranks than from battle ("When It Comes" 2010).

The *Chronicle* articles either group women together with men in discussions of their responses to natural disasters, campus massacres, and academic bullying (Audrey 2011; Fogg 2008), or signify women as deviants from the male default through stories drawing attention to their gender. In the latter case, the women who have PTSD are doubly marked for their gender difference by being portrayed primarily as survivors of some form of sexual violence. Take, for example, the following essay about sexual harassment against women in the academy:

> What I keep seeing is that women are getting hounded out of the academy, and we're losing their contributions, and that's a tragedy. Even if they stay in the academic world, their research has been compromised. They had to change advisers. They lost their funding because they had to move from one institution to another. They gave up a multiyear package. Even if they stay—so many tenured professors have contributed—they talk about their continuing PTSD, continuing depression, anxiety. So people are living emotionally compromised lives because of this. (Gluckman 2017, para. 21)

Or this one, in which the female author alludes to her sexual abuse:

> Beyond that single letter I wrote to my professor in grad school, I have never written or spoken publicly about the abuse I survived. I never told a single college professor about why I would disappear for weeks after being required to view or read narratives of violent sexual encounters. (Shaw-Thornburg 2014, para. 14)

This study finds no articles singling out men who developed PTSD after a traumatic experience motivated by misandry. Our analysis also did not find any mention of people who are non-binary or genderqueer.

Again, it is not inaccurate to report on the widespread incidence of PTSD among men, or to associate PTSD with sexual violence against women. However, it is inaccurate when the reporting stops there, failing to complicate the narrative with additional examples counter to the trope and more in proportion to the demographic realities of PTSD cases. The narrative should place additional emphasis on women of color. The *DSM-5* reports that "compared with U.S. non-Latino whites, higher rates of PTSD have been reported among U.S. Latinos, African Americans, and American Indians" (American Psychiatric Association 2013, 276). Recent research confirms that trauma such as the enslavement of African Americans and the genocide of Native Americans can be transmitted through epigenetic changes in the methylation of DNA in subsequent generations (Youssef et al. 2018). Yet, the image of the typical person with PTSD as white is so culturally ingrained that only two of the fifty-seven *Chronicle* articles analyzed comment on race at all. On both occasions, the person's deviation from assumed whiteness as a racial minority is directly connected to their PTSD (Valentine 2015; Waitzkin 2011), but in neither case is the generational and structural origins of trauma cited as a trigger.

Purtle (2014) asserts that American policymakers reify the trope of the white male veteran when passing PTSD legislation because advocating on behalf of the "low-income racial and ethnic minorities" who develop PTSD in larger numbers "could be seen as a politically risky maneuver with little payoff—especially if the voting public is unknowledgeable, or unconcerned about, the burden of PTSD among these segments of the civilian population" (506). Perceptions of lawmakers are also influenced by popular news coverage. Content analysis of news coverage in the *New York Times* finds a strong association between PTSD and military combat, to the exclusion of other events that traumatize larger numbers of people. This overrepresentation of combat trauma maps to historical spikes in the news coverage of PTSD during the events of wars in Bosnia, Iraq, and Afghanistan, and the terrorist attacks of September 11, 2001 (Houston, Spialek, and Perreault 2016, 245). In other words, the most common traumatic events that cause PTSD are ongoing childhood sexual abuse, rape, and domestic violence, not war. The largest affected demographic group is women. However, in a culture of intersecting dominations, these truths are too "dog bites man" to warrant much news coverage or supportive legislation. PTSD seems to only be worthy of notice when it happens to white men in combat. This expedient legislating and reductive reporting can have negative consequences, as those who do not fit the profile of the trope may question the legitimacy of their own symptoms and hesitate to ask for the accommodations to which they are legally entitled. These groups are further marginalized within the academy by the assumption that the typical person with PTSD is most likely an undergraduate student.

Person with PTSD = Student

Nearly 44 percent of the articles in *The Chronicle of Higher Education* linked coverage of PTSD with undergraduates. By contrast, a mere 14 percent referred to faculty or other academic workers such as staff, administrators, or graduate assistants. The *Chronicle* articles tell multiple stories of traumatized students who were the targets of sexual violence (Kipnis 2015; Schmidt 2015; Wilson 2015). Students with PTSD are sometimes framed in the current debate as the only ones who might benefit from the use of trigger warnings in the classroom (Schmidt 2015). The fact that faculty might struggle with course subject matter and might also be triggered in class, given their own histories of trauma, is frequently overlooked (for examples beyond the *Chronicle*, see "An Introduction to Content Warnings" 2017; Hanlon 2015).

Among the minority of coverage that features faculty, most noteworthy is "When the Professor's Trauma is an Open Book" (2016), describing R. M. Douglas's apprehension about returning to the classroom after the publication of his book disclosing his rape as a child by a priest. Even on the rare occasions when faculty publish in the *Chronicle* about their own traumatic experiences, they turn the disclosure to the purposes of urging more resources for their students or considering PTSD's impact on their professional careers, as does Douglas (2016):

> Still, the fact remains that when I next stand before a classroom in the autumn, the students facing me will know deeply personal things about me that, until 18 months ago, my wife didn't (para. 8). . . . My professorial persona, like that of nearly all academics I know, is based on a standpoint of critical separation from the things I teach and study. In their encounters with the records and controversies of the past, my students look to me, on the basis of my disciplinary and scholarly qualifications, to keep them on the right track (para. 9). What happens when that separation can no longer be taken for granted? (para. 10)

Largely missing from the articles linking faculty with PTSD is any expression of concern about their own mental health or quality of life. Academic workers who have PTSD are afforded little space to present themselves as fully human in the classroom or the conference room.

Faculty with psychological disabilities are under-acknowledged in comparison to students for several reasons. The laws that govern the universities' handling of faculty and student disabilities differ (Pryal 2017, 45–46); data on students who have disabilities is collected more regularly than that of faculty (Knapp 2008, 106); and disability resources on campus are designed to be found and used primarily by students (Pryal 2017, 47). Faculty with psychological disabilities, including PTSD, are likely to keep their conditions quiet, not only because of the professional stigma around mental health issues for intellectual laborers but also because they notice that more easily detectable disabilities are served but "invisible disabilities" such as their own are not (Price and Kerschbaum 2017, 7–8). It is no wonder students are more likely to disclose their condition and request accommodations than their professors (Brown and Leigh 2018, 986), reinforcing the trope that the typical person with PTSD on campus must be an undergraduate.

Everyone who has PTSD, academic workers included, copes with significant cultural stigma. However, for faculty, the stigma is unique and especially invidious due to the intellectual demands of the position. Disability Studies scholars point to the repulsion communicated to faculty with psychological disabilities, flowing from the academy's fear that the very organ most necessary to do their jobs has been compromised. In *Mad at School: Rhetorics of Mental Disability and Academic Life*, Price (2011, 8) puts it powerfully:

> Academic discourse operates not just to omit, but to abhor mental disability—to reject it, to stifle and expel it. For thousands of years academe has been understood as a bastion of reason, the place in which one's rational mind is one's instrument. But what does this mean for those of us with atypical (some would say "impaired" or "ill") minds who work, learn, and teach in this location?

Faculty who choose to disclose their psychological disabilities face the very real risk of a "presumption of incompetence," under which they are obligated to invest harder and longer work hours to prove their ability to do their jobs (Pryal 2017, 23). Brown and Leigh (2018) ascribe to academic workers a tendency to sacrifice their home lives in an attempt to countermand the presumption of professional incompetence: "Academics with disabilities or illness work hard to hold onto their academic work and identity while compromising other aspects of their life. In contrast, non-academic individuals with similar health challenges reported that work was the first thing they dropped to maintain their personal lives and relationships" (987). Faculty who are publicly out about their PTSD also open themselves up to the "bonus work" of mentoring students who seek an authority figure who understands their experiences of living with a traumatized brain (Pryal 2017, 138).

Price (2011) goes on to document not just the attitudinal barriers against faculty with psychological disabilities but also the structural ones, such as overstimulating academic conferences, high-pressure campus job interviews, and opaque tenure and promotion processes in which collegiality can be invoked against atypical cognitive and social behaviors. The pervasive pressure of job insecurity and untenable workloads has risen as "the share of faculty members nationwide who are off the tenure track has reached 73 percent" (Tugend 2019). The stress is likely to escalate in the coming decade as American higher education faces what is increasingly referred to as the immanent "apocalypse," in which analysts forecast a perfect storm of public disinvestment in college funding, a dramatic demographic drop off of traditional-aged college students, and a political environment hostile to the working-class students, students of color, and international students who otherwise might have filled the empty seats (Camera 2019; Reed 2019). These anxieties systematically disadvantage people with conditions such as PTSD, contribute to a dearth of empathy from colleagues, and explain the lag in institutional campus policies to support their needs. In the worst-case scenarios, faculty with PTSD are pushed out of higher education altogether.

Placing stigma on individuals in the academy who live with PTSD is to be expected, given neoliberalism's refashioning of higher education into a place where one's value is only as high as one's productivity and profitability. An economics-first academy obscures the structural sources of trauma and ignores in its calculus quality of life, contributions to the public sphere, and academic integrity (Fish 2009). In a leashless free-enterprise work environment in which academic labor must be ever more minutely quantified and measured (Ball 2012), and in which students are framed as consumers of a higher education commodity (Schwartzman 2017), the stage is thoroughly set for trauma in faculty and other academic workers, and for locating the consequences of that trauma on the workers themselves instead of on the system.

RECOMMENDATIONS

In an unintentional irony, the term *dissociation* is meaningful in both the spheres of trauma research and rhetoric. In the context of PTSD, dissociation is a symptomatic phenomenon in which the traumatized person feels numb or detached from their own body, moving through life feeling like an alien or a person trapped in an unreal dream (American Psychological Association 2013, 272). In the context of rhetoric, on the other hand, dissociation is a move in argumentation identified by Perelman and Olbrechts-Tyteca (1969), in which paired components are separated from each other as incompatible. Dissociated terms are defined by what they are *not,* and ranked on a hierarchy. A term higher on the hierarchy is valued as normative and uncoupled from the one that is not. The trope performed in *The Chronicle of Higher Education* equating PTSD with white male veteran undergraduate students serves to rhetorically dissociate psychological disability from the "normal" space of the academy.

This construction of reasoning dissociates the legitimacy of PTSD symptoms and the rights to accommodation from women and individuals who are genderqueer, people of color, those whose inciting traumas were not combat-related, and university faculty. Price (2011) argues that, despite the fact that academia is a stressful, high-pressure environment in which any worker could potentially manifest issues with their mental health—and therefore the need for support for everyone on campus with psychological disabilities should be institutionally anticipated and routinized—these disabilities are often treated, instead, as unexpected deviations from the norm that must be symbolically and materially separated out of the "safe zone" of the academy (22). From an epidemiological perspective, this dissociation is statistically inaccurate; from a feminist perspective, it reifies the domination of marginalized identity groups. How can this injustice be disrupted?

Currently, many of the recommendations made by disability studies scholars are policy changes (American Association of University Professors 2017; Knapp 2008; Price and Kerschbaum 2017). Price and Kerschbaum (2017) offer a resource guide for administrators to create a supportive academic environment which benefits faculty regardless of their mental health status. Their comprehensive guide addresses the importance of acknowledging and normalizing the conversation around those with mental disabilities, to counteract stigma. The guide also validates the reasons why faculty may choose to not speak up. When so many institutions are working proactively to support undergraduates and their mental health needs, they should also dedicate that same attention to those who work with those students every day. Price and Kerschbaum's (2017) recommendations in five areas of higher education are strong starting points for institutional transformation: 1) developing a culture of access; 2) promoting inclusive language; 3) managing accommodations; 4) recruitment, hiring, and sustaining employment; and 5) reconnecting after leave.

Another way institutions can normalize the campus conversation surrounding mental health is by providing resources to faculty and staff in a visible way via their websites. The University of Wisconsin-Milwaukee has devoted a web page to faculty and staff titled "Mental Health Resources." They not only address common concerns when working with students but also include sections titled, "I am concerned about my own mental health," "I am concerned about a UWM faculty or staff member," and "I want to stay mentally healthy." Each of these sections includes both campus and community resources through which faculty can seek support. This website manifests the institution's prioritization of the well-being of its entire campus population. The Wisconsin model demonstrates a simple change most institutions can make to start normalizing the conversation and offering support for mental health ("Mental Health Resources: Faculty and Students").

Both recommendations above share a common theme of shifting and normalizing the conversation surrounding mental health for faculty and staff. In an article about self-disclosure, Lee (2019) points out that one in five people report clinical symptoms of anxiety. Because of this alarming statistic, we need to "normalize the need for health" and "assume everyone can benefit from resources and treatment at every stage of life." Lee (2019) urges a change in the language to reframe these struggles from a "mental health condition" to a "human condition," and to diminish the damaging culture of stigma and silent suffering.

Although policy reform is necessary and appropriate to achieve greater equity for people with PTSD, no number of laws or rules can entirely overcome the problem of rhetorical dissociation marginalizing people with psychological disabilities in the academy. The first step is to complicate the reductive trope of the typical person with PTSD as a white male veteran undergraduate with counternarratives. Let us start with our own. Both the co-authors of this chapter—white, female civilians working as academic faculty—identify as people living with PTSD. One or both of us have survived traumatic experiences on or near campus, the disruption of being unintentionally triggered while teaching, and the distress of attempting to perform perfectly under threat of academic budget cuts and job insecurity. Even in the process of writing this chapter, both authors struggled with the ramifications of self-disclosing. While treating our mental health, we both have been recognized for teaching excellence, and participate effectively in the life of the university and our discipline. Revealing our own experiences of PTSD contradicts the dissociation of the academy from people whose identities are outside the trope, and forges rhetorical room for our trauma-affected amygdalae to inhabit the same university campus as the other people assumed to represent this disorder.

People with psychological disabilities should not have to shoulder the expectation of risking their own careers to effect change. We challenge the *Chronicle* and other newspapers to catch up with the epidemiological realities of PTSD. Writers publishing in the *Chronicle* should purposefully seek out examples of academics with PTSD who run counter to the incomplete picture of the white, male, veteran undergraduate, feature them as newsworthy, and contextualize them as everyday occurrences in the academy. According to Ajzen's (1991) popular health communication theory, the Theory of Planned Behavior (TPB, formerly known as the Theory of Reasoned Action), the intentions to change one's health behaviors are shaped by a multiplicity of factors including an individual's attitudes, social pressure and norms, and one's own perceived control. Each of these factors shapes the ability to enact a health behavior change. The TPB posits that when the *Chronicle* repeats the damaging tropes conflating PTSD with white, male, veteran undergraduates, it narrows institutions' understanding of what PTSD is and who PTSD affects, which in turn influences campus policies.

According to TPB, if we can disrupt or interrupt a person at any level of their health behavior, whether it be their personal attitude, social norms, or perceived control, we can alter that behavior. Therefore, we call for countertropes in which coverage in the *Chronicle* realistically represents the full variety of PTSD identities in higher education. From this shift in perception, institutions can begin to change their behavior, enabling a higher priority of care for academic workers impacted by PTSD.

We also challenge our institutions of higher education. Inspired by the work at the K-12 level, campuses across the United States are making promising progress in understanding and serving our traumatized students, such as through Adverse Childhood Experiences (ACEs) training (Blodgett and Lanigan 2018; Brogden and Gregory 2019; Windle et al. 2018). However, a truly trauma-informed campus would acknowledge that its workers—inclusive of all faculty, staff, administrators, and graduate assistants—also bring to campus their own brains potentially affected by PTSD. Initiatives to interrupt stigma, normalize accommodations, and cover the mental health needs of everyone who performs academic labor should come from all corners of campus.

PTSD would not be so culturally prevalent that it has generalized into a metaphor ("I think I have PTSD from having to grade all those papers") if the real traumatic events that overwhelm the amygdala were reduced. An end to sexual violence, an end to child abuse, and an end to armed combat are unattainable dreams. In the meantime, let us challenge rhetorical tropes that marginalize people with PTSD and other mental health conditions, and create university classrooms with people from many intersecting identities who can teach and learn together.

REFERENCES

"About Us." 2020. The Chronicle of Higher Education. Accessed Sept. 8, 2020. https://www.chronicle.com/page/about-us/.

Ajzen, Icek. 1991. "The Theory of Planned Behavior." *Organizational Behavior and Human Decision Processes* 50, no. 2: 179–211. https://doi.org/10.1016/0749-5978(91)90020-t.

"Accommodating Faculty Members Who Have Disabilities." 2017. American Association of University Professors. Accessed September 9, 2020. 1–6. https://www.aaup.org/report/accommodating-faculty-members-who-have-disabilities.

American Psychiatric Association. 2013. *Diagnostic and Statistical Manual of Mental Disorders: DSM-5* (5th ed.). Arlington, VA: American Psychiatric Association.

"An Introduction to Content Warnings and Trigger Warnings." LSA Inclusive Teaching Initiative, University of Michigan. Accessed Sept. 12, 2020. https://sites.lsa.umich.edu/inclusive-teaching/inclusive-classrooms/an-introduction-to-content-warnings-and-trigger-warnings/.

Ball, Stephen J. 2012. *Politics and Policy Making in Education: Explorations in Sociology*. London: Routledge.

Bartlett, Tom. 2011. "Psychologists Battle over Army's Optimism Training: Is New Army Psychology Program Simply a Shot in the Dark?" *The Chronicle of Higher Education*. Oct. 30, 2011. https://www.chronicle.com/article/soldiers-of-optimism/.

Bizzell, Patricia. 2000. "Feminist Methods of Research in the History of Rhetoric: What Difference do they Make?" *Rhetoric Society Quarterly* 30, no. 4 (Autumn): 5–17. https://doi.org/10.1080/02773940009391186.

Blodgett, Christopher, and Jane D. Lannigan. 2018. "The Association between Adverse Childhood Experience (ACE) and School Success in Elementary School Children." *School Psychology Quarterly* 33, no. 1: 137. https://doi.org/10.1037/spq0000256.

Breslau, Naomi, and James C. Anthony. 2007. "Gender Differences in the Sensitivity to Posttraumatic Stress Disorder: An Epidemiological Study of Urban Young Adults." *Journal of Abnormal Psychology* 116, no. 3: 607–611. https://doi.org/10.1037/0021-843X.116.3.607.

Breslau, Naomi, Ronald C. Kessler, Howard D. Chilcoat, Lonni R. Schultz, Glenn Craig Davis, and Patricia Andreski. 1998. "Trauma and Posttraumatic Stress Disorder in the Community: The 1996 Detroit Area Survey of Trauma." *Archives of General Psychiatry* 55, no. 7: 626–632. https://doi.org/10.1001/archpsyc.55.7.626.

Brogden, Laura, and Dennis E. Gregory. 2019. "Resilience in Community College Students with Adverse Childhood Experiences." *Community College Journal of Research and Practice* 43, no. 2: 94–108. https://doi.org/10.1080/10668926.2017.1418685.

Brown, Nicole, and Jennifer Leigh. 2018. "Ableism in Academia: Where Are the Disabled and Ill Academics?" *Disability & Society* 33, no. 6: 985–989. https://doi.org/10.1080/09687599.2018.1455627.

Burke, Kenneth. 1950. *A Rhetoric of Motives*. Berkeley, CA: University of California Press.

Camera, Lauren. 2019. "The Higher Education Apocalypse: A Steady Drip of Crises in Massachusetts and Across New England May just Signal its Arrival." *U.S. News and World Report*, March 22, 2019. https://www.usnews.com/news/education-news/articles/2019-03-22/college-closings-signal-start-of-a-crisis-in-higher-education.

Cooper, Helene. 2018. "Critics See Echoes of 'Don't Ask, Don't Tell' in Military Transgender Ban.'" *New York Times*, March 28, 2018. https://www.nytimes.com/2018/03/28/us/politics/pentagon-transgender-ban-legal-challenges.html.

Crenshaw, Kimberle. 1989. "Demarginalizing the Intersection of Race and Sex: A Black Feminist Critique of Antidiscrimination Doctrine, Feminist Theory and Antiracist Politics." *University of Chicago Legal Forum* Issue 1, Article 8: 139–167. https://chicagounbound.uchicago.edu/uclf/vol1989/iss1/8.

Douglas, R. M. 2016. "When the Professor's Trauma is an Open Book." *The Chronicle of Higher Education*. March 27, 2016. https://www.chronicle.com/article/when-the-professors-trauma-is-an-open-book/.

Dow, Bonnie J. 2016. "Authority, Invention, and Context in Feminist Rhetorical Criticism." *Review of Communication* 16, no. 1: 60–76. https://doi.org/10.1080/15358593.2016.1183878.

Farrell, Elizabeth F. 2005. "GI blues." *The Chronicle of Higher Education*. May 13, 2005. https://www.chronicle.com/article/gi-blues/.

Fiorenza, Elisabeth S. 1992. *But She Said: Feminist Practices of Biblical Interpretation*. Boston: Beacon Press.

Fish, Stanley. 2009. "Neoliberalism and Higher Education." *The New York Times*. March 8, 2009. https://opinionator.blogs.nytimes.com/2009/03/08/neoliberalism-and-higher-education/.

Fogg, Piper. 2008. "Academic Bullies." *The Chronicle of Higher Education*. Sept. 12, 2008. https://www.chronicle.com/article/academic-bullies/.

Foss, Sonja K. 2017. *Rhetorical Criticism: Exploration and Practice*. Long Grove, IL: Waveland Press.

Gifford, Justin. 2015. "The Ex-pimp Who Remade Black Culture." *The Chronicle of Higher Education*. July 24, 2015. https://www.chronicle.com/article/the-ex-pimp-who-remade-black-culture/#:~:text=My%20search%20for%20the,Microsoft%20and%20Starbucks%20changed%20everything.

Gluckman, Nell. 2017. "'A Complete Culture of Sexualization': 1,600 Stories of Harassment in Higher Ed." *The Chronicle of Higher Education*. December 12, 2017. https://www.chronicle.com/article/a-complete-culture-of-sexualization-1-600-stories-of-harassment-in-higher-ed/.

Goldberg, Joyce S. 2011. "Why I Can No Longer Teach U.S. Military History." *The Chronicle of Higher Education*. Sept. 18, 2011. https://www.chronicle.com/article/why-i-can-no-longer-teach-u-s-military-history/.

Hanlon, Aaron R. 2015. "My Students Need Trigger Warnings—and Professors Do, Too." *The New Republic* (blog). May 17, 2015. https://newrepublic.com/article/121820/my-students-need-trigger-warnings-and-professors-do-too.

Houston, J. Brian, Matthew L. Spialek, and Mildred F. Perreault. 2016. "Coverage of Posttraumatic Stress Disorder in the *New York Times*, 1950-2012." *Journal of Health Communication* no. 21: 240–248. https://doi.org/10.1080/10810730.2015.1058441.

June, Audrey Williams. 2011. "A Shattered Department Picks up the Pieces: A Year after their Colleagues were Shot, Professors in Huntsville, Alabama, Rebuild." *The Chronicle of Higher Education*. February 6, 2011. https://www.chronicle.com/article/in-huntsville-a-shattered-department-picks-up-the-pieces/.

Kilpatrick, Dean, Heidi S. Resnick, Melissa E. Milanak, Mark W. Miller, Katherine M. Keyes, and Matthew J. Friedman. 2013. "National Estimates of Exposure to

Traumatic Events and PTSD Prevalence Using DSM-IV and DSM-5 Criteria." *Journal of Traumatic Stress* 26, no. 5: 537–547. https://doi.org/10.1002/jts.21848.

Kipnis, Laura. 2015. "Sexual Paranoia Strikes Academe." *The Chronicle of Higher Education*. February 27, 2015. https://www.chronicle.com/article/sexual-paranoia-strikes-academe/.

Klein, Julia M. 2002. "Art That Defies Categories." *The Chronicle of Higher Education*. May 24, 2002. https://www.chronicle.com/article/art-that-defies-categories/.

Knapp, Sara D. 2008. "Why 'Diversity' Should Include 'Disability' with Practical Suggestions for Academic Unions." *American Academic* 4: 105–130. https://citeseerx.ist.psu.edu/viewdoc/download?doi=10.1.1.168.6633&rep=rep1&type=pdf

Lee, Kris. 2019. "Why I Openly Share My Own Mental Health Condition with my College Students." *Psychology Today*. March 31, 2019. https://www.psychologytoday.com/ca/blog/rethink-your-way-the-good-life/201903/why-i-share-my-own-mental-health-condition-my-students.

Mangan, Katherine. 2009. "Colleges Help Veterans Advance from Combat to Classroom." *The Chronicle of Higher Education*. October 18, 2009. https://www.chronicle.com/article/colleges-help-veterans-advance-from-combat-to-classroom/.

Mangan, Katherine. 2008. "Disabled Veterans Get Hands-on Training in the Art of Entrepreneurship." *The Chronicle of Higher Education*. September 5, 2008. https://www.chronicle.com/article/disabled-veterans-get-hands-on-training-in-the-art-of-entrepreneurship/.

McMurtrie, Beth. 2018. "The Hope and Hype of the Academic Innovation Center." *The Chronicle of Higher Education*. January 21, 2018. https://www.chronicle.com/article/the-hope-and-hype-of-the-academic-innovation-center.

Mele, Christopher. 2016. "Oregon Court Allows a Person to Choose Neither Sex." *New York Times*. June 13, 2016. https://www.nytimes.com/2016/06/14/us/oregon-nonbinary-transgender-sex-gender.html?partner=bloomberg.

"Mental Health Resources: Faculty and Students." University of Wisconsin-Milwaukee. Accessed Sept. 19, 2020. https://uwm.edu/mentalhealth/for-faculty-and-staff.

Mittal, Dinesh, Karen L. Drummond, Dean Blevins, Geoffrey Curran, Patrick Corrigan, Greer Sullivan. 2013. "Stigma Associated with PTSD: Perceptions of Treatment Seeking Combat Veterans." *Psychiatric Rehabilitation Journal* 36, no. 2: 86–92. https://doi.org/10.1037/h0094976.

National Center for PTSD. 2018. *Fiscal Year 2018 Funding*. National Center for PTSD. https://www.ptsd.va.gov/about/work/docs/annual_reports/2018/NCPTSD_2018_Annual_Report_AppendixC.pdf.

Nudd, D. M., and K. S. Whalen. 2016. "Feminist Analysis." In *Rhetorical Criticism: Perspectives in Action*, edited by J. Kuypers, 91–214. Lanham, MD: Rowman & Littlefield.

Olsen, Florence. 2000. "Scholars in Medicine and Psychology Explore Uses of Virtual Reality." *The Chronicle of Higher Education*. Sept. 22, 2000. https://ww

w.chronicle.com/article/scholars-in-medicine-and-psychology-explore-uses-of-virtual-reality/.
Otis, Hailey N. 2019. "Intersectional Rhetoric: Where Intersectionality as Analytic Sensibility and Embodied Rhetorical Praxis Converge." *Quarterly Journal of Speech* 105, no. 4: 369–389. https://doi.org/10.1080/00335630.2019.1664755.
Perelman, Chaim, and Lucie Olbrechts-Tyteca. 1969. *The New Rhetoric: A Treatise on Argumentation.* Translated by J. Wilkinson and P. Weaver. Notre Dame, IN: University of Notre Dame Press.
Price, Margaret. 2011. *Mad at School: Rhetorics of Mental Disability and Academic Life.* Ann Arbor, MI: University of Michigan Press.
Price, Margaret, and Stephanie L. Kerschbaum. 2017. *Promoting Supportive Academic Environments for Faculty with Mental Illnesses: Resource Guide and Suggestions for Practice.* Philadelphia, PA: Temple University Collaborative.
Pryal, Katie R. Guest. 2017. *Life of the Mind Interrupted: Essays on Mental Health and Disability in Higher Education.* Chapel Hill NC: Snowraven Books.
Purtle, Jonathon. 2014. "The Legislative Response to PTSD in the United States (1989-2009): A Content Analysis." *Journal of Traumatic Stress* 27, no. 5: 501–508. https://doi.org/10.1002/jts.21948.
Reed, Matt. 2019. "Hypothetically: Looking Back at the Present." *Inside Higher Ed.* October 9, 2019. https://www.insidehighered.com/blogs/confessions-community-college-dean/hypothetically%E2%80%A6-0.
Rivollier, Fabrice, Hugo Peyre, Nicolas Hoertel, Carlos Blanco, Frederic Limosin, and Richard Delorme. 2015. "Sex Differences in DSM-IV Posttraumatic Stress Disorder Symptoms Expression using Item Response Theory: A Population-based Study." *Journal of Affective Disorders* 187: 211–217. https://doi.org/10.1016/j.jad.2015.07.047.
Ryback, Ralph. 2016. "Five Myths about PTSD (and the Facts you Need to Know)." *Psychology Today.* Oct, 31, 2016. https://www.psychologytoday.com/us/blog/the-truisms-wellness/201610/5-myths-about-ptsd.
S. 3406-110th Congress: ADA Amendments Act of 2008. GovTrack.us. Accessed Sept. 15, 2020. https://www.govtrack.us/congress/bills/110/s3406.
Sander, Libby. 2012. "Female Veterans Can Be Hard to Spot, and to Help." *The Chronicle of Higher Education.* June 30, 2012. https://www.chronicle.com/article/female-veterans-on-campuses-can-be-hard-to-spot-and-to-help/.
Schimke, David. 2017. "Taking Mindfulness to the Streets: Neuroscientists Explore Whether Resilience Training Can Help Cops in Crisis." *The Chronicle of Higher Education.* Jan. 22, 2017. https://www.chronicle.com/article/taking-mindfulness-to-the-streets/.
Schmidt, Peter. 2015. "A Faculty's Stand on Trigger Warnings Stirs Fears Among Students." *The Chronicle of Higher Education.* Oct. 6, 2015. https://www.chronicle.com/article/a-facultys-stand-on-trigger-warnings-stirs-fears-among-students/.
Schwartzman, Roy. 2017. "Unma(s)king Education in the Image of Business: A Vivisection of Educational Consumerism." *Cultural Studies, Critical Methodologies* 17, no. 4: 333–346. https://doi.org/10.1177/1532708617706126.

Shaw-Thornburg, Angela. 2014. "This is a Trigger Warning." *The Chronicle of Higher Education*. June 16, 2014. https://www.chronicle.com/article/this-is-a-trigger-warning/.

The Editors of the Encylopædia Britannica. 2017. *"The Chronicle of Higher Education." Encyclopædia Britannica*. Encyclopædia Britannica, Inc. https://www.britannica.com/topic/The-Chronicle-of-Higher-Education.

Timberline Knolls Residential Treatment Center. 2010. "When it Comes to PTSD in the Military, Sexual Trauma Can Cause as Much Damage as Combat." Oct. 28, 2010. *PR Newswire*. https://www.prnewswire.com/news-releases/when-it-comes-to-ptsd-in-the-military-sexual-trauma-can-cause-as-much-damage-as-combat-106140808.html.

Tolin, David F., and Edna B. Foa. 2006. "Sex Differences in Trauma and Posttraumatic Stress Disorder: A Quantitative Review of 25 Years of Research." *Psychological Bulletin* 132: 959–992. https://doi.org/10.1037/0033-2909.132.6.959.

Tugend, Alina. 2019. "How Penn State Improved Conditions for Adjuncts." *The Chronicle of Higher Education*. Oct. 30, 2019. https://www.chronicle.com/article/how-penn-state-improved-conditions-for-adjuncts/.

U.S. Department of Defense. 2007. *An Achievable Vision: Report of the Department of Defense Task Force on Mental Health*. Falls Church, VA: Defense Health Board. https://apps.dtic.mil/dtic/tr/fulltext/u2/a469411.pdf.

U.S. Department of Defense. 2018. *Department of Defense Tuition Assistance Summary Data*. dodmou.com/tadecide.

U.S. Department of Veterans Affairs 2018. "How Common is PTSD in Adults?" https://www.ptsd.va.gov/understand/common/common_adults.asp.

Valentine, Sarah. 2015. "When I Was White." *The Chronicle of Higher Education*. July 6, 2015. https://www.chronicle.com/article/when-i-was-white/.

van der Kolk, Bessel A. 2015. *The Body Keeps the Score: Brain, Mind, and Body in the Healing of Trauma*. New York, NY: Penguin Books.

Waitzkin, Howard. 2011. "Strangers in Paradise: Reaching Out to Deprived Students." *The Chronicle of Higher Education*. Oct. 27, 2011. https://www.chronicle.com/article/strangers-in-paradise-reaching-out-to-deprived-students/.

Wilson, Robin. 2015. "An Epidemic of Anguish: Overwhelmed by Demand for Mental-health Care, Colleges Face Conflicts in Choosing How to Respond." *The Chronicle of Higher Education*. August 31, 2015. https://www.chronicle.com/article/an-epidemic-of-anguish/.

Windle, Michael, Regine Haardörfer, Beth Getachew, Jean Shah, Jackie Payne, Dina Pillai, and Carla Berg. 2018. "A Multivariate Analysis of Adverse Childhood Experiences and Health Behaviors and Outcomes Among College Students." *Journal of American College Health* 66, no. 4: 246–251. https://doi.org/10.1080/07448481.2018.1431892.

Youssef, Nagy A., Laura Lockwood, Shaoyong Su, Guang Hao, and Bart P. F. Rutten. 2018. "The Effects of Trauma, With or Without PTSD, on the Transgenerational DNA Methylation Alterations in Human Offsprings." *Brain Science* 8, no. 5: 83. https://doi.org/10.3390/brainsci8050083.

Part 3

INSTITUTIONAL POLICIES ON MENTAL HEALTH AND RECOMMENDATIONS FOR BEST PRACTICES

Chapter 9

Culturally Sensitive Mental Health Support for Higher Education Employees

Lukasz Swiatek and Ursula Edgington

INTRODUCTION

Over the past two decades, organizations in diverse sectors have increasingly realized that mental health support for individuals needs to be provided in culturally competent ways. The reasons for this are numerous. Ever-larger international migration flows have resulted in more culturally and linguistically diverse populations around the world. Within this globalized employment marketplace, migrants require varying mental health services, and for different reasons. The social stigma surrounding mental health needs in society generally has decreased in recent years, partly because of changes in government policies, but also due to increasing awareness of potential symptoms, more research, and the publicizing of available support by social media campaigns (such as #mentalhealthawareness). However, without culturally competent approaches, some individuals may not receive access to the information, and thus the appropriate forms of support, that they need. This is because social norms may lead to prejudice. Many barriers often prevent people from culturally and linguistically diverse backgrounds from accessing mental health support in timely ways. These barriers include stigma, interpretation and cultural differences, insensitive language or format, a lack of information about mental health service support formats (especially ones that are culturally safe and appropriate), and poor communication (Department of Health, UK and Department of Education, UK 2017; Long et al. 1999; Rickwood 2006).

Culturally competent mental health support can be provided in multiple ways. Being aware of potential social prejudices allows organizations to prevent unfair discrimination against individuals and groups. For instance, higher education institutions (HEIs) must be mindful of the potential harm of reinforcing common stereotypes that can further embed negative attitudes and stigma. Adopting a balanced approach through culturally sensitive language can increase understanding of mental ill-health (Mindframe 2020). Above all, strategies and policies must be holistic, so that the "development and provision of systems of care demonstrate an awareness and integration of the health-related beliefs and cultural values of diverse populations" (Bennett 2009, 63). This holistic orientation to support translates into varied culturally sensitive approaches, ranging from developing (or redeveloping) more inclusive documentation to gaining an awareness of each person's cultural orientation and needs (UPCCI 2007). Strategies and policies should also consider the complex, interconnected nature of some mental health issues, which may take time for individuals to share with their support person and, subsequently, to unpack (Department of Health and Social Care, UK 2015).

HEIs have a particular need and social responsibility to engage in culturally competent policymaking and practice, given the increasingly international make-up of their workforces and their foundation in education and research. Universities' reliance on international staff (and students) is well-known and well-documented in many parts of the world (Scott 2000; *The Economist* 2015). For example, universities in the United Kingdom have been the largest volume users of the immigration system; in 2010, more than 10 percent of all academic staff were non-EU nationals (Dandridge 2010). Universities, in their organizational communication collateral, also regularly promote their disregard for nation-state borders in their recruitment and hiring processes. Larger, research-intensive universities, in particular, emphasize their desire to retain and attract the world's *best and brightest* academic staff. This desire is also driven by *best practice* staffing criteria embedded in national and international published performance indicators, such as the Research Assessment Exercise (REF) in the United Kingdom and the Performance Based Research Fund (PBRF) in Aotearoa New Zealand.

Alongside these changes, universities face growing criticisms for not meeting the needs of their increasingly diverse workforces. For example, a 2015 report examining the state of Massachusetts Institute of Technology's (MIT) diversity found that, worryingly, racial minorities at the institution were significantly under-represented; the percentages of these under-represented ethnic groups hired as postdoctoral fellows (2 percent) and research staff (4 percent) were singled out as particularly low (Zuckerman and Barabas 2015). Universities in other parts of the world have been criticized for manipulating the presentation of diversity statistics. As McKenna (in Jolin 2016) points out, a university may boast that 15 percent of its staff, for example, have Black and minority ethnic backgrounds, yet that percentage of staff is likely to be occupying entry-level roles or serving as domestic assistants, rather than holding full-time, permanent (research and/or teaching) positions. Universities without diverse workforces—especially teaching staff—have greater problems engaging with students from diverse backgrounds. Scholars (such as Biesta 2011; Roxå, Mårtensson, and Alveteg 2011) emphasize that a culturally sensitive approach to pedagogical strategies enhances learning for students of diverse backgrounds. Hence, higher education staff from minority ethnic groups may be doubly disadvantaged; without permanent roles, they are more likely to suffer from stress and anxiety, and lack easy access to crucial emotional support as well.

Universities thus have an imperative to provide culturally competent mental health support to their increasingly diverse staff. This support needs to be as dynamic as culture itself. Our knowledge of culture has deepened: The definition of *culture* is understood to be constantly changing because it is founded on our emotions and social relationships (Bantock 1967). Strong support is especially important given the fact that academics' mental health has received far less attention than that of students (see, for example, Stanley and Manthorpe 2001; Reavley and Jorm 2010; Conley, Durlak, and Kirsch 2015). Academic staff have far fewer options for receiving well-being support than students. Gorczynski (2018) points out that, "Most universities will offer their staff the chance to see an occupational health nurse or contact an employee assistance program by telephone—but information about both services is limited and often difficult to find." Gorczynski (2018) adds that institutions often direct staff to services outside the university campus. Mental health problems will not go away in the current university climate, though. In an increasingly competitive neoliberal higher education sector, staff workloads are growing, and support (for administration, service, research, and teaching) is shrinking. Burnout among university teachers is extensive, compromises productivity, impairs personal and professional competence, and leads to emotional exhaustion in particular (Watts and Robertson 2010). According to a study by Gorczynski, Hill, and Rathod (2017), 43 percent of academic staff indicate at least a mild mental disorder. When academic staff (especially teaching staff) are mentally unwell and face ongoing obstacles to discharging their duties, they cannot fulfill their central, time-honored obligations of serving others (particularly students) as servant-teacher-leaders (Nichols 2010).

This chapter contributes to our knowledge about mental health in academia. On a scholarly level, it responds to the issue that current research does not canvas culturally competent mental health support approaches in academia, particularly with respect to staff moving across borders. At the time of writing, the post-COVID-19 global workplace presents unknown and unprecedented challenges to everyone, including staff in academia. For instance, the complex pressures of physical distancing and online teaching could increase workload stress and anxiety (World Health Organization

2020; Cipriano and Brackett 2020). Travel restrictions not only separate staff from friends and family but also present job insecurity when overseas student enrolments are negatively impacted (McKie 2020). This makes our case for recommending more comprehensive and robust mental health support policies and procedures for staff working in academia even more crucial in the months and years ahead. Although Carter and Goldie (2018) have examined the enablers of mental health and wellness for teaching staff in HEIs, and although other scholars (see, for example, Luquis and Pérez 2003; Treadwell et al. 2009) have investigated the ways in which educators and university leaders can become culturally competent, or encourage cultural competence in their institutions, no critical scholarship addresses this chapter's research focus. The chapter also remedies the acknowledged lack of research into migrant experiences in higher education with regard to work–life and work–family balance (Pillay and Abhayawansa 2014). On a practical level, it responds to the fact that migration continues to grow around the world, and universities' increasingly diverse staff confront more and more challenging workloads. The chapter therefore contributes to improving mental health support for university staff by assembling timely and useful knowledge about the strengths and limitations of current HEI practice. This knowledge will be useful not just for universities (and their executive groups, senior, or otherwise), but also individual staff at all levels.

The chapter is divided into five sections. The first delves more deeply into culturally sensitive mental health and its importance for HEIs. The second section outlines the research method used to understand how universities are providing staff with culturally competent mental health support (if at all). The third discusses the findings of the research, presenting illustrative examples and, importantly, highlighting the current limitations of HEI practice in those examples. The fourth section outlines recommendations for improving culturally sensitive mental health support for university staff. A conclusion that suggests avenues for further research rounds out the chapter.

Culturally Sensitive Mental Health

The provision of culturally sensitive mental health support requires a commitment to cultural competence. In the most fundamental terms, this refers to sensitivity and responsiveness to people's diverse needs (Lustig and Koester 1999). On a more personal level, this type of competence refers to:

> [T]he ability to participate ethically and effectively in personal and professional intercultural settings. It requires being aware of one's own cultural values and world view and their implications for making respectful, reflective and reasoned

choices, including the capacity to imagine and collaborate across cultural boundaries. (NCCC n.d.)

In practicing cultural competence, both individuals and institutions must be attuned to the ever-changing nature of cultures. The need for this responsiveness stems from the constantly changing emotions and social relationships (Bantock 1967) that underpin culture, which can broadly be described as a way of life of a group of people: that is, a social context. Culture encompasses the learning of shared values, norms, and beliefs within that group. It shapes the multiple ways in which we interact with others, including in our virtual worlds. Unsurprisingly, culture also includes the negative interactions that can impact our mental health. International research confirms the fact that negative interactions—perhaps most significantly in the form of workplace bullying—contribute to poor mental health (Verkuil, Atasayi, and Molendijk 2015).

Culturally sensitive mental health support takes different forms, including broad approaches. Nardi, Waite, and Killian's (2012) model helpfully establishes a holistic set of standards for culturally competent mental health care. In this model, six broad elements must be taken into account: (1) the involvement of various disciplines and professions (ranging from psychiatrists to culture-specific healthcare workers, like doulas); (2) the delivery of different resources for patients (including education and information resources); (3) the incorporation of particular economic practices or systems (such as a council of elders, who may need to sanction particular services); (4) an understanding of the surrounding ecological environment (including factors such as geography, housing, and community structures); (5) respect for patient and family systems; and (6) a sensitivity toward prevailing political systems, which shape diagnoses and treatments that are available (and even legal) within a specific setting. If any of these elements is ignored, and if cultural sensitivity more broadly is not systematically built into the mental healthcare that is provided to individuals, then inequalities and poor mental health outcomes will be "perpetuated and exacerbated" (Nardi, Waite, and Killian 2012, 5).

More specific approaches in culturally sensitive mental health support integrate the elements in this set of standards into targeted actions and resources. They consider the fact that cultural differences influence both providers and clients or patients (UPCCI 2007). Established culturally competent practices include:

- surveying clients or patients (and providers), using open-ended questions, to understand each person's unique cultural outlook and understanding of cultural competence (as well as culturally competent practice);

- creating and implementing culturally sensitive treatment plans featuring community-based resources, where appropriate or necessary, to aid each individual's recovery;
- employing qualified mental health workers fluent in the language(s) of the clients or patients;
- providing cultural competence training for existing staff to address, among other things, any identified cultural biases;
- developing or redeveloping more culturally sensitive policies, programs, and procedures (such as intake and assessment documentation) after identifying their current cultural biases.

Implementing culturally sensitive approaches not only enormously benefits the treatment of episodes of mental illness, but also potentially prevents them (UPCCI 2007).

As higher education workforces become increasingly ethnically diverse, and mental health needs are widespread, HEIs need to be responsive and sensitive to the complex needs of their diverse staff. As mentioned in this chapter's introduction, this diversity is no coincidence: HEIs are increasingly recruiting staff from around the world. On the one hand, more and more competitive universities seek out the *best and brightest* staff. On the other hand, the institutions are responding to aging populations, increasing numbers of retiring workers, and skills shortages in many countries, all of which necessitate skilled labor from overseas (Pillay and Abhayawansa 2014). For both locally born and migrant higher education staff, work pressures are increasing. Reports (see, for example, Fazackerley 2019; Richardson 2019) discuss unmanageable workloads, the pressure of performance management, data-led cultures of surveillance, higher expectations from students, the increasing pressure to *publish or perish*, the insecurity of ongoing short-term contracts, a sense of isolation and lack of collegiality, a loss of autonomy, the pressure to measure and provide evidence of *excellence* across all indicators (especially service, teaching, administration, and research), and high levels of rejection for research.

This cocktail of growing pressures has, unsurprisingly, equally led to growing mental health problems for HEI staff. Often, these problems go unreported. At the same time, more cases are being reported. For example, between 2009 and 2016, the average increase in referrals—whether self-referred or otherwise—to counseling services in larger UK HEIs (those with 2,000 staff or more) was 77 percent. However, in many universities, the increase in referrals was much higher during this time period: 316 percent at the University of Warwick, 292 percent at the University of Kent, 177 percent at Brunel University, and 126 percent at Newcastle University (Richardson 2019).

In light of these mounting pressures, HEIs have a responsibility to provide effective culturally sensitive mental health support to their increasingly ethnically diverse staff. This support should be available, in some form, before staff start at their new workplace and after they leave. Pre-arrival and post-departure support takes into account the increasing international mobility of staff, recognizes the ongoing nature of mental health issues, and particularly helps staff on non-permanent contracts. These insecure contracts have been shown to damage the mental health of staff who have to work unpaid hours, cut corners in their responsibilities (including marking and teaching preparation), and even hold down multiple jobs due to lack of job security and lack of steady income (UCU 2019). Our original research furthers understanding of how HEIs are providing culturally competent mental health support (when they do so at all) to staff before, during, and after their employment at particular institutions. The chapter now turns to this research and its findings.

RESEARCH METHOD

The original research used to substantiate this chapter's argument was guided by this question: What evidence is there of culturally competent mental health support in HEIs' policies and other organizational communication collateral? To answer this question, we used qualitative content analysis. This method involves systematically and closely examining texts in order to identify themes, patterns, and (manifest or latent) meanings (Zhang and Wildemuth 2017). We analyzed publicly available HEI policy documents and other organizational communication collateral (such as webpages and their contents) at one point in time (specifically, June 2019). Some might argue that private—in other words, internal—documents and collateral should also have been investigated; we would counter-argue that information outlining mental health support approaches should be fully transparent, readable, and publicly available for all staff to access at any time. This information should be available to staff before arriving at an institution, between teaching periods (in the case of casual staff whose electronic institutional accounts often expire at the end of every semester or trimester), and after leaving the institution. If HEIs fail to make this information public, then they already fail stakeholders (especially students) and neglect their wider social responsibilities. It was particularly important to understand which forms of support (if any) were available for the full spectrum of employment—before arrival and after departure—at each HEI for the reasons mentioned in the previous section.

The data-universe for the research was the forty-nine government-funded universities in Australia and Aotearoa New Zealand. This set of institutions constituted a robust research universe from which to gather data, due to the universities' location in richly multicultural (and, in the case of Aotearoa New Zealand, bicultural) populations. Carnegie Mellon University (Australia Campus) was excluded from the research as it is not an Australian university proper. Using keywords related to mental health, materials were identified and examined by: (a) using each university's internal search engine and Google, and (b) browsing the university websites without search engines. Data were collated using the conventional qualitative content analysis procedure of allowing "categories and names for categories to flow from the data" (Hsieh and Shannon 2005, 1279). The forms of mental health support for staff found on the university websites were divided into internally accessible forms of support and externally accessible forms of support. The following section outlines the results of the research and discusses their implications.

RESULTS AND DISCUSSION

Our analysis found that the forms of mental health support for staff varied between the forty-nine universities in Aotearoa New Zealand and Australia. Nine broad categories emerged from the data, representing the nine forms of support that these HEIs provided overall. The internally accessible forms of support entailed the universities: (1) offering an employee assistance program (EAP); (2) offering other mental health support services for staff; (3) holding an annual mental health week, month, or day promoted to staff; (4) holding general mental health–related events; and (5) running more specific mental health–related training for staff. The externally accessible forms of support entailed the universities: (6) offering a university-developed (publicly accessible) mental health–related online course; (7) providing links to external mental health resources; (8) providing text-based mental health information and advice; and (9) having a specific or stand-alone institutional mental health strategy or plan. The Appendix at the end of this chapter provides a snapshot of the data.

The findings indicated that support was mainly available once staff had arrived at the given institution and was centered on externally-delivered employee assistance. At the time of research and writing, an EAP was offered by nearly all of the universities and was mentioned in their publicly available communication collateral. At most universities, the EAP was the main form of mental health support available for staff; it was also nearly always provided by an external organization (particularly Benestar). At a handful of universities (La Trobe, Queensland University of Technology, the University of New England, and the University of Sydney), the EAP was the only publicly mentioned form of mental health support for staff. Other forms of support were presumably available, but were locked within staff intranets (and thus restricted to staff employed at the institution). This is a particularly significant problem for staff coming from overseas and lacking access to university systems, employees who have recently left the university, and the growing numbers of casual staff who may not be able to afford other, privately funded forms of mental health support.

Besides the EAP, two other sets of internally accessible forms of support for staff were prevalent. The first set comprised other mental health support services. At times, these were unspecified or general mental health services, such as those offered by the Bond University Psychology Clinic. At other times, they were specific, such as Edith Cowan University's human resources-run staff health and wellness program called *Live Life, Longer* that contains face-to-face and online elements. The second set comprised more specific mental health–related training for staff. This training dealt with various topics; for instance, one of the University of Auckland's *CPC (Combining Parenting and a Career)* seminars covered good mental health and well-being, while the Australian National University offered a *Responding to Mental Ill-Health in the Workplace Training for Managers* workshop. A detailed list of examples for each category is not provided here as it is unnecessary. Selected examples suffice in providing a snapshot of the different forms of support in each category.

Two sets of externally accessible forms of support were prevalent. The first set featured links to external mental health resources provided on the universities' websites. For instance, Federation University Australia provided links on its "Wellness" page, in its Staff section, to: FutureLearn's online course *Mindfulness for Well-being and Peak Performance* (hosted by Monash University); the *My Digital Health* platform; the Work Life Balance section of the *Harvard Business Review*; the Health section of *ABC News*; *The Conversation: Health+Medicine* site; and health service details for external providers in Ballarat and Gippsland. The second set of externally accessible forms of support comprised text-based mental health information and advice. These usually took the form of PDFs and webpages. For example, the University of Queensland Current Staff Information and Services webpage provided three PDFs with text-based information about different aspects of workplace stress: *10 Ways to Build Resilience*, *Dealing with Challenging Working Relationships*, and *Recognising Signs of Distress in the Workplace*.

In direct answer to the research question (What evidence is there of culturally competent mental health support in HEIs' policies and other organizational communication collateral?), this chapter found that there was virtually no evidence of culturally sensitive, publicly available mental health support for staff. There was also little explicit acknowledgment of the widespread need for this form of support for diverse workforces. Most of the time, in the policies and organizational communication collateral, the term *culture* was used in terms of workplaces or *institutional culture*. This was evident in the Australian National University's *Mental Health Strategy*, the University of Western Australia's *University Policy on Mental Health* webpage, the University of Queensland's *Mental Health Strategy 2018–2020*, the University of South Australia's *Mental Health and Wellbeing Guidelines*, the University of Wollongong's *Workplace Mental Health Strategy 2020–2025*, and Western Sydney University's *Mental Health & Wellbeing Strategy* and webpage.

That said, there were two exceptions: Two HEIs did make an effort at recognizing the importance of diverse cultures or ethnic diversity in terms of mental health support for staff. The University of Canterbury's *Wellbeing Strategy* has bicultural models of well-being, the second of which incorporates different threads of Māori health promotion: namely, Mauriora (access to Te Ao Māori, the Maori World), Waiora (Environmental Protection), Toiora (Healthy Lifestyles), Te Oranga (Participation), Ngā Manukura (Leadership), and Te Mana Whakahaere (Autonomy) (University of Canterbury 2019). Western Sydney University's *Mental Health and Wellbeing Pack for staff* contains information specifically related to culture (although, inappropriately, some of the information is student-focused); it features a link to the Western Sydney University transcultural support page, a link to the New South Wales Transcultural Mental Health Centre, a telephone number for 20/10 Gay and Lesbian Youth Services, a link to the Western Sydney University Welfare Service, a telephone number for support for international students, and a link to Western Sydney University–provided information about Overseas Student Health Cover.

The findings also reveal a wide disparity in the forms of mental health support apparently offered by the universities. Some institutions offer extensive resources (including guides with information and advice, online courses, video-recordings from events, and links to further resources, among others). Monash University is a stand-out in this respect, having even developed its own (publicly accessible) mental health–related online course. Other institutions simply listed web links to external resources in addition to providing the EAP for current employees only.

Online mental health resources for students far exceeded the numbers and types of mental health resources offered for staff. This mirrors the fact, discussed previously, that most of the focus on mental health in academia is directed at undergraduates. This is a problem, too, as staff often have different mental health support needs. If institutions genuinely want to promote their organizations as safe, positive, and healthy environments, then they need to respect and address these needs. They also need to send a serious signal to staff that they are valued, especially given universities' longstanding focus on students, and given this chapter's discussion about the profession's ever-sharper tolls on academics. Richardson (2019) points out that:

Until recently, the mental health of students rather than academics has been in sharp focus.... But the deaths by suicide of two respected academics, Malcolm Anderson, at Cardiff University, and Prof Stefan Grimm, at Imperial College, have highlighted the excessive pressure that some academics feel.

These findings open up a range of recommendations for all HEIs, not just institutions in Australia and Aotearoa New Zealand.

RECOMMENDATIONS

The research in this chapter highlights a clear need for culturally sensitive mental health support for higher education staff. HEIs should take two solid steps in this direction. First, they should expand their publicly available mental health resources, ensure that those resources are more easily accessible to staff (before, during, and after employment at a particular institution) and, crucially, ascertain that those resources adhere to culturally sensitive approaches that are based on research evidence. Second, they must ensure that their broader, institution-wide mental health policies and guidelines are culturally sensitive and promote cultural competence. This would raise awareness of diverse mental health needs, promote equality and respect within the institutions (and society more broadly), and even potentially prevent risks of discrimination. Implementing these two steps together would represent the best possible outcome for HEIs and their staff. However, just meeting the first step—that is, making more mental health resources publicly available—would already be an enormous boon, given the significant differences in the levels and types of support currently provided by HEIs, as this chapter has found.

In developing more culturally sensitive forms of mental health support for staff, HEIs would do well to adopt some of the standards and practices outlined in this chapter. For instance, more culturally sensitive forms of publicly available support should take into account Nardi, Waite, and Killian's (2012) six elements. Those forms of support should acknowledge, and help staff to also acknowledge, the various key disciplines and professions relevant to their mental health support; they should also be provided in different ways (through different modes of media and communication). Additionally, in adopting some of the established standards (UPCCI 2007), the more culturally sensitive forms of support should help staff, for example, recognize their own cultural biases in the area of mental health, assist staff in understanding their own culturally suitable forms of mental health support, and be available in multiple languages.

HEIs can also take other measures to strengthen the publicly available, culturally sensitive forms of support for staff mental health. They can divide staff and student online resources, thus recognizing that the two diverse populations also have differing mental health support needs. With regard to migrants arriving in a new locale, they can provide cultural insights into that new locale (and HEI) in a way that will help those migrants adapt to life there more effectively. On that note, to minimize costs, they might do well to pool resources and provide a national website with a forum to share widely applicable culturally sensitive mental health resources for staff (in addition to providing their own institutionally specific information). This would address some of the financial tensions between smaller HEIs lacking the budgets to develop extensive mental health support and larger, strongly endowed HEIs able to develop such support.

CONCLUSION

As demands on staff in HEIs continually increase, and as employees continue to arrive at HEIs from around the world, the need for innovative strategies to provide more effective mental health support for staff will continue to grow. This chapter has argued that HEIs have an obligation to their increasingly international workforces to provide culturally sensitive, publicly available forms of mental health support. Without this type of support, staff are unable to thrive in HEIs and deliver quality teaching, research, and service to their respective institutions and wider communities. Original research has identified that culturally sensitive, publicly available forms of staff mental health support in universities in Aotearoa New Zealand and Australia are minimal. The chapter has made recommendations for addressing this situation, and for providing support that will better support staff who work increasingly hard to serve others.

At the same time, there is an underlying need for deeper understanding of the cultural diversity in HEIs in Australasia, the ways in which that diversity is changing over time, and the implications that those changes entail. For example, some universities do not keep adequate records about migrant staff: particularly their recruitment, retention, and progress (Edgington and Swiatek 2018). Without this data, it is impossible to predict the types of support that staff from diverse backgrounds will require. Preventing mental health issues from escalating is likely to require long-term measures to help staff to stay well. The benefits to HEIs of such long-term, culturally sensitive care are numerous, and include enhanced productivity, as well as lower costs arising from staff absences and poorly delivered or undelivered work.

Future studies could also help overcome some of the other inevitable limitations of the research undertaken here. An analysis of a broader sample of

HEIs, beyond those in Australia and Aotearoa New Zealand, would help paint a more detailed picture of the different forms of culturally sensitive, publicly available forms of mental health support available for staff in different parts of the world. Other research methods, such as action research, could help develop better forms of support. Resources within HEI intranets could also be analyzed. On that note, it could be argued that online, publicly available forms of mental health support for staff will be less effective than one-on-one, personalized services with healthcare professionals. However, publicly available support can go a very long way in improving staff mental health. In particular, it can greatly assist casual staff, migrant staff, and staff who have recently left an institution and can no longer access internally provided support. The limitations of mental health support for these groups of staff in academia were already evident before the Coronavirus outbreak. Inevitably, because of the additional pressures resulting from the post-COVID-19 workplace, it will be even more essential for institutions now to address these needs. As long as higher education is marked by significant casualization and growing pressures on internationally sourced staff, good quality forms of publicly available, culturally sensitive support for staff will be vital.

REFERENCES

Bantock, Geoffrey Herman. 1967. *Education, Culture and the Emotions*. London: Faber and Faber.

Bennett, Joanna. 2009. "Black and Minority Ethnic Issues." In *Mental Health: From Policy to Practice*, edited by Charlie Brooker and Julie Repper, 57–69. Edinburgh: Churchill Livingstone Elsevier.

Biesta, Gert. 2011. "From Learning Cultures to Educational Cultures: Values and Judgements in Educational Research and Educational Improvement." *International Journal of Early Childhood* 43: 199–210. https://doi.org/10.1007/s13158-011-0042-x.

Carter, Margaret-Anne, and Donna Goldie. 2018. "Potential Enablers of Mental Health and Wellness for Those Teaching in Tertiary Education." *International Journal of Innovation, Creativity and Change* 4, no. 3: 3–20. https://www.ijicc.net/images/vol4iss3/Margaret-Anne_Carter_and_Donna_Goldie.pdf.

Cipriano, Christina, and Marc Brackett. 2020. "Teachers Are Anxious and Overwhelmed. They Need SEL Now More Than Ever." *EdSurge*, 7 April 2020. https://www.edsurge.com/news/2020-04-07-teachers-are-anxious-and-overwhelmed-they-need-sel-now-more-than-ever.

Conley, Colleen S., Joseph A. Durlak, and Alexandra C. Kirsch. 2015. "A Meta-Analysis of Universal Mental Health Prevention Programs for Higher Education Students." *Prevention Science* 16, no. 4: 487–507. https://doi.org/10.1007/s11121-015-0543-1.

Constanti, Panikkos, and Paul Gibbs. 2004. "Higher Education Teachers and Emotional Labour." *International Journal of Educational Management* 18, no. 4: 243–249. https://doi.org/10.1108/09513540410538822.

Dandridge, Nicola. 2010. "Universities Rely on International Staff and Students." *The Guardian*, October 12, 2010. https://www.theguardian.com/education/2010/oct/12/universities-rely-on-international-staff.

Department of Health and Social Care, UK. 2015. *Improving Mental Health Services for Young People: Report of the Work of the Children and Young People's Mental Health Taskforce*. London: Department of Health and Social Care, UK. https://www.gov.uk/government/publications/improving-mental-health-services-for-young-people.

Dept of Health, UK, and Dept of Education, UK. 2017. *Transforming Children and Young People's Mental Health Provision: A Green Paper*. London: UK Government. https://www.gov.uk/government/uploads/system/uploads/attachment_data/file/664855/Transforming_children_and_young_people_s_mental_health_provision.pdf.

Edgington, Ursula, and Lukasz Swiatek. 2018. "An Investigation of Induction Policies for University Teachers: (Re)valuing Staff and Cultural Diversity." In *Research and Development in Higher Education: (Re)Valuing Higher Education*, edited by Dale Wache and Don Houston, 41, 81–91. Adelaide: Higher Education Research and Development Society of Australasia. http://www.herdsa.org.au/system/files/Edgington_et_al_HERDSA2018.pdf.

Fazackerley, Anna. 2019. "'It's Cut-throat': Half of UK Academics Stressed and 40% Thinking of Leaving." *The Guardian*, May 21, 2019. https://www.theguardian.com/education/2019/may/21/cut-throat-half-academics-stressed-thinking-leaving.

Gorczynski, Paul. 2018. "More Academics and Students Have Mental Health Problems Than Ever Before." *The Conversation*, February 22, 2018. http://theconversation.com/more-academics-and-students-have-mental-health-problemstha n-ever-before-90339.

Gorczynski, Paul, Denise Hill, and Shanaya Rathod. 2017. "Examining the Construct Validity of the Transtheoretical Model to Structure Workplace Physical Activity Interventions to Improve Mental Health in Academic Staff." *EMS Community Medicine Journal* 1, no. 1: 1–4. https://researchportal.port.ac.uk/portal/files/8438799/Examining_the_Construct_Validity.pdf

Hsieh, Hsiu-Fang, and Sarah E. Shannon. 2005. "Three Approaches to Qualitative Content Analysis." *Qualitative Health Research* 15, no. 9: 1277–1288. https://doi.org/10.1177/1049732305276687.

Jolin, Lucy. 2016. "Do Universities' Workforces Reflect the Diversity of their Students?" *The Guardian*, November 23, 2016. https://www.theguardian.com/diversity-matters/2016/nov/22/do-universities-workforces-reflect-the-diversity-of-their-students.

Long, Helen, Jane Pirkis, Cathrine Mihalopoulos, Lucio Naccarella, Michael Summers, and David Dunt. 1999. *Evaluating Mental Health Services for Non-English Speaking Background Communities*. Melbourne: Australian Transcultural Mental Health Network.

Luquis, Raffy R., and Miguel A. Pérez. 2003. "Achieving Cultural Competence: The Challenges for Health Educators." *American Journal of Health Education* 34, no. 3: 131–138. https://doi.org/10.1080/19325037.2003.10603544.

Lustig, Myron W., and Jolene Koester. 1999. *Intercultural Competence: Interpersonal Communication Across Cultures*. New York: Longman.

Mindframe. 2020. *Guidelines for Communicating about Mental Ill-Health*. https://mindframe.org.au/mental-health/communicating-about-mental-ill-health/mindframe-guidelines/communicating-about-mental-ill-health.

McKie, Anna. 2020. "Covid-19: Universities Treating Staff in 'Vastly Different Ways.'" *Times Higher Education Supplement*, 20 April 2020. https://www.timeshighereducation.com/news/covid-19-universities-treating-staff-vastly-different-ways.

Nardi, Deena, Roberta Waite, and Priscilla Killian. 2012. "Establishing Standards for Culturally Competent Mental Health Care." *Journal of Psychosocial Nursing and Mental Health Services* 50, no. 7: 3–5. https://doi.org/10.3928/02793695-20120608-01.

NCCC. n.d. "What is Cultural Competence?" Sydney: National Centre for Cultural Competence. http://sydney.edu.au/nccc/.

Nichols, Joe D. 2011. *Teachers as Servant Leaders*. Lanham: Rowman & Littlefield.

Pillay, Soma, and Subhash Abhayawansa. 2014. "Work–Family Balance: Perspectives from Higher Education." *Higher Education* 68, no. 5: 669–690. https://doi.org/10.1007/s10734-014-9738-9.

Reavley, Nicola, and Anthony F. Jorm. 2010. "Prevention and Early Intervention to Improve Mental Health in Higher Education Students: A Review." *Early Intervention in Psychiatry* 4, no. 2: 132–142. https://doi.org/10.1111/j.1751-7893.2010.00167.x.

Richardson, Hannah. 2019. "University Counselling Services 'Inundated by Stressed Academics.'" *BBC News*, May 23, 2019. https://www.bbc.com/news/education-48353331.

Rickwood, Debra. 2006. *Pathways of Recovery: Preventing Further Episodes of Mental Illness*. Canberra: Commonwealth of Australia Department of Health. http://www.health.gov.au/internet/publications/publishing.nsf/Content/mental-pubs-p-mono-toc~mental-pubs-p-mono-pop~mental-pubs-p-mono-pop-cul.

Roxå, Torgny, Katarina Mårtensson, and Mattias Alveteg. 2011. "Understanding and Influencing Teaching and Learning Cultures at University: A Network Approach." *Higher Education* 62, no. 1: 99–111. https://doi.org/10.1007/s10734-010-9368-9.

Scott, Peter. 2000. "Globalisation and Higher Education: Challenges for the 21st Century." *Journal of Studies in International Education* 4, no. 1: 3–10. https://doi.org/10.1177/102831530000400102.

Stanley, Nicky, and Jill Manthorpe. 2001. "Responding to Students' Mental Health Needs: Impermeable Systems and Diverse Users." *Journal of Mental Health* 10, no. 1: 41–52. https://doi.org/10.1080/2-09638230020023606.

The Economist. 2015. "The World is Going to University." *The Economist*, March 28, 2015. http://www.economist.com/news/leaders/21647285-more-andmore-money-being-spent-higher-education-too-little-known-about-whether-it.

Treadwell, Henrie M., Ronald L. Braithwaite, Kisha Braithwaite, Desiree Oliver, and Rhonda Holliday. 2009. "Leadership Development for Health Researchers at Historically Black Colleges and Universities." *American Journal of Public Health* 99, no. S1: S53-S57. https://doi.org/10.2105/AJPH.2008.136069.

UCU. 2019. *71% of University Staff Say Insecure Contracts Have Damaged their Mental Health*. London: UCU [University and College Union]. https://www.ucu.org.uk/article/10194/71-of-university-staff-say-insecure-contracts-have-damaged-their-mental-health.

University of Canterbury. 2019. *University of Canterbury Wellbeing Strategy*. Christchurch: University of Canterbury. https://www.canterbury.ac.nz/media/Wellbeing_Strategy_doc.pdf.

UPCCI. 2007. *Cultural Competence in Mental Health*. Pennsylvania: UPenn Collaborative on Community Integration. http://tucollaborative.org/wp-content/uploads/2017/01/Cultural-Competence-in-Mental-Health.pdf.

Verkuil, Bart, Serpil Atasayi, and Marc L. Molendijk. 2015. "Workplace Bullying and Mental Health: A Meta-Analysis on Cross-Sectional and Longitudinal Data." *PLoS One* 10, no. 8: 1–16. https://doi.org/doi:10.1371/journal.pone.0135225.

Watts, Jenny, and Noelle Robertson. 2010. "Burnout in University Teaching Staff: A Systematic Literature Review." *Educational Research* 53, no. 1: 33–50. https://doi.org/10.1080/00131881.2011.552235.

World Health Organization. 2020. "Mental Health and Psychosocial Considerations during the COVID-19 Outbreak." WHO/2019-nCoV/MentalHealth/2020.1. WHO. https://www.who.int/docs/default-source/coronaviruse/mental-health-considerations.pdf.

Zhang, Yan, and Barbara M. Wildemuth. 2017. "Qualitative Analysis of Content." In *Applications of Social Research Methods to Questions in Information and Library Science*, edited by Barbara M. Wildemuth, 318–329. Santa Barbara: Libraries Unlimited.

Zuckerman, Ethan, and Chelsea Barabas. 2015. "Diversity Challenging Not Just Tech Companies But Universities Too." *The Conversation*, February 27, 2015. http://theconversation.com/diversity-challenging-not-just-tech-companies-but-universities-too-38108.

APPENDIX

The chart below captures the results of the original research into the evidence of the culturally competent mental health support in the forty-nine universities' policies and other organizational communication collateral. The key to the chart is as follows.

A: Offers an employee assistance program (EAP)
B: Offers other mental health support services for staff

C: Holds an annual mental health week, month, or day that is promoted to staff
D: Holds general mental health-related events
E: Runs more specific mental health-related training for staff
F: Offers its own (publicly accessible) mental health-related online course
G: Provides links to external mental health resources
H: Provides text-based mental health information and advice
I: Has a specific or stand-alone mental health strategy or plan

Table 9.1 A Summary of the Different Forms of Online, Publicly Accessible Mental Health Support for Staff Provided by Universities in Aotearoa New Zealand and Australia (Featuring Original Research by the Authors)

Universities (Beginning with Aotearoa New Zealand, followed by Australia)	Internally accessible forms of support					Externally accessible forms of support			
	A	B	C	D	E	F	G	H	I
AUT	✓								
Lincoln University			✓	✓					
Massey University	✓						✓		
University of Auckland	✓			✓		✓	✓		
University of Canterbury	✓			✓		✓	✓		✓
University of Otago	✓			✓		✓	✓		
University of Waikato	✓		✓	✓					
Victoria University of Wellington	✓			✓					
Australian Catholic University	✓					✓	✓		
Australian National University	✓			✓		✓	✓	✓	
Bond University		✓							
Central Queensland University	✓						✓		
Charles Darwin University	✓			✓		✓	✓		
Charles Sturt University	✓	✓				✓	✓		
Curtin University	✓	✓			✓				
Deakin University	✓	✓		✓		✓	✓		
Edith Cowan University	✓	✓			✓	✓			
Federation University Australia	✓				✓	✓	✓		
Flinders University	✓			✓	✓	✓	✓	✓	
Griffith University	✓	✓	✓	✓			✓		
James Cook University	✓						✓		
La Trobe University	✓								
Macquarie University	✓	✓			✓		✓	✓	
Monash University	✓	✓	✓			✓	✓	✓	✓
Murdoch University	✓					✓			
Queensland University of Technology	✓								

206 Lukasz Swiatek and Ursula Edgington

Universities (Beginning with Aotearoa New Zealand, followed by Australia)	Internally accessible forms of support					Externally accessible forms of support			
	A	B	C	D	E	F	G	H	I
Royal Melbourne Institute of Technology (RMIT)	✓	✓							
Southern Cross University	✓	✓					✓		
Swinburne University of Technology	✓		✓						
The University of Canberra	✓								
The University of Divinity									
The University of Newcastle	✓	✓	✓		✓		✓	✓	
The University of Notre Dame Australia	✓								
The University of Western Australia	✓	✓			✓		✓	✓	✓
Torrens University Australia									
University of Adelaide	✓	✓	✓		✓		✓	✓	
University of Melbourne	✓				✓		✓	✓	
University of New England	✓								
University of New South Wales	✓		✓		✓		✓	✓	
University of Queensland	✓	✓		✓	✓		✓	✓	✓
University of South Australia	✓	✓		✓	✓		✓	✓	
University of Southern Queensland	✓	✓		✓					
University of Sydney	✓								
University of Tasmania	✓	✓	✓	✓			✓		
University of Technology Sydney	✓	✓			✓		✓	✓	
University of the Sunshine Coast	✓	✓		✓					
University of Wollongong	✓		✓		✓		✓	✓	✓
Victoria University	✓		✓				✓	✓	
Western Sydney University	✓		✓	✓	✓		✓	✓	✓
	45	19	12	11	23	1	30	22	8

Chapter 10

Having Emotional Support Animals at College

Susan Hafen

INTRODUCTION

More students entering college today seek mental health services as soon as they arrive because of the psychiatric medications they are taking (Watkins, Hunt, and Eisenberg 2012) and because their mental health issues are more severe and long-term (Lipson et al. 2018). In addition, students who are military veterans are increasingly entering college with psychological disorders stemming from post-traumatic stress, brain injuries, depression, and substance abuse (Fortney et al. 2015). Although service dogs are understood and accepted in the public sphere for helping people with disabilities (blindness, deafness, loss of mobility, epileptic seizures, and other conditions), the need for emotional support animals (ESAs) for people with mental health issues is less well understood.

Existing research examines the therapeutic benefits of animal-assisted interventions (AAIs) on physical and psychological challenges and disorders (LaFrance, Garcia, and Labreche 2007; Maujean, Pepping, and Kendall 2015); reductions in anger, anxiety, depression, and general distress; beneficial effects on socialization (DeCourcey, Russell, and Keister 2010; Rosetti and King 2010); and employee job stress and satisfaction (Barker et al. 2012). Visiting therapy dogs decreased student stress (Barker et al. 2016; Binfet et al. 2018; Charles and Wolkowitz 2019; Crump and Derting 2015; Daltry and Mehr 2015; House, Neal, and Backels 2018) and increased classroom learning (Brelsford et al. 2017). No wonder that university counseling centers (UCCs) and disability student services (DSSs) are increasingly managing students' requests for accommodations for their ESAs to help them cope with psychological disorders and the stresses of school life (Kogan et al. 2016; Taylor 2016).

Von Bergen (2015) makes a case for why college administrators must prepare for increasing requests to accommodate students' companion animals. This case is validated by a survey of UCCs, which indicated that most administrators rarely write support letters to permit students to have ESAs in their classrooms or accommodation (Kogan et al. 2016). Most surveyed administrators said they needed guidelines for how to communicate official policies on ESAs (Kogan et al. 2016). However, understanding the legal issues around animals in their workplaces and developing appropriate policies is only the first step for college administrators, faculty, and staff: institutions must also create and implement campus support programs.

To examine how two institutions have responded to this need for clear policies around ESAs, I conducted in-depth interviews with administrators, faculty, staff, and students at a private college and a public university. The private college has a longstanding ESA policy because of its anthrozoology (ANZ) program, which was established in 2007 and trains dogs. I interviewed UCC and DSS staff at a public university with a newly implemented policy. I used McPhee's (2015) organizational model of four-flows: membership negotiation, self-structuring, activity coordination, and institutional positioning to compare the respondents' stories, advice, and guidelines for accommodating people and their non-service-animal relationships.

LEGAL STATUS OF ESAS

Any discussion of ESAs—also variously called companion, comfort, visitation, therapy, social/therapy, assistive, assistance, and psychiatric service animals (Von Bergen and Bressler 2015)—must begin by distinguishing them from service animals. Titles II and III of the 2008 Americans with Disabilities Act Amendments Act (ADAAA) defines a *service animal* as "any dog that is individually trained to do work or perform tasks for the benefit of an individual with a disability, including a physical, sensory, psychiatric, intellectual, or other mental disability" (Foreman et al. 2017, 2). The revised ADA regulations later provided for miniature horses that have been trained for service. The "service" distinction is essential: The dog (or horse) must perform a specific task related to the disability, which can be a psychiatric service, such as a dog trained to remind someone to take their medication or to stop someone from self-mutilation (Clay 2016).

Simply being present as a dog to give comfort does not qualify the animal as a service dog. Therefore, this animal is not legally protected in public places such as restaurants, public transit, and public buildings such as college or university campuses. However, under the Fair Housing Act of 1988, a housing provider must permit an ESA as a "reasonable accommodation" for a person with a disability, including mental or psychiatric impairments. Restrictions normally applied to "pets" cannot be applied to any animal certified as an ESA, nor can housing providers charge a "pet deposit" if the individuals rely on the assistance animals (Wisch 2019). The U.S. Department of Housing and Urban Development (HUD) investigates claims of housing discrimination. HUD outlines the only two questions that a housing provider is allowed to ask when someone requests accommodation for their ESA: (1) Does the person have a mental impairment that limits major life activities? (2) Does the animal provide emotional support that alleviates one or more of the identified symptoms or effects of the disability? Housing providers are also not legally allowed to ask what the impairment is or how the animal provides support.

Von Bergen (2015, 24) outlines ten lessons "for administrators regarding accommodations for mentally disabled students and 'no-pets' policies": First, institutions must prepare for growing student requests for ESAs, which result from online industries that qualify pets for a fee, as well as from educational institutions' increased service orientation toward students as consumers. Second, administrators must know the legal distinctions between service animals and ESAs. Third, institutions should have only one university office respond to questions about animals on campus, to eliminate contradictory responses. Fourth, administrators should avoid asking for "any overly intrusive, burdensome, confidential, unnecessary documentation for a student" (Von Bergen 2015, 26) to avoid lawsuits such as the 2011 case at the University of Nebraska at Kearney, which resulted in a $140,000 settlement for affected students (Brinn 2018). Fifth, institutions should determine whether the student has a disability and focus on reasonable accommodation, and clearly state that "exemptions from no-pet rules will be decided on a case-by-case basis" (Von Bergen 2015, 26). Sixth, campus policies should focus on housing, facilities, and other sites that employ students, remembering that housing requires ESA compliance. Seventh, institutional policies should mirror municipal and state language, which may vary from federal language regarding ESAs. Eighth, institutions should consider other students' objections to animals on campus because of allergies, phobias, and other conditions. However, these are not legally valid reasons for denying access to ESAs or service dogs. Ninth, institutions must recognize that accommodation requests will increase partly because "the definition of mental illness has broadened, creating a bigger tent with more people under it" (Rosenberg 2013, in Von Bergen 2015, 28). For example, a severely shy person might now be diagnosed with an "avoidant personality disorder" (Von Bergen and Bressler 2017). In the most recent 2016 *Diagnostic and Statistical Manual of Mental Disorders*, two new childhood mental disorders were added: social communication disorder and disruptive mood dysregulation disorder (Substance Abuse and Mental Health Services Administration 2016). Another way of extending the tent is by lowering the diagnostic criteria, such as having persistent symptoms of anxiety for three months instead of six months (Von Bergen and Bressler 2017). Finally, Von Bergen's (2015) tenth recommendation is that institutions must clearly address the responsibilities of ESA owners, including animal vaccination and license tags, leashes, cleanliness and cleanup, and disruptive behavior.

METHOD: INTERVIEWS AT A PRIVATE COLLEGE AND A PUBLIC UNIVERSITY

This chapter began as a case study at Carroll College in Montana (herein referred to as CC), which offers the only undergraduate ANZ major in the United States. Students from across the United States apply to CC's program to learn how to train service and therapy dogs. Dogs are highly visible on the college's campus. For example, students walk their canine trainees to and from their canine neuroscience and advanced canine training classes. With my overarching research question of how dogs on campus affect the campus culture, I attended classes where students sat with their service dogs-in-training under their desks. I conducted twenty-two interviews with students and faculty who taught in the ANZ program, communication faculty, administrators, and staff. I asked the respondents open-ended questions about their experiences with animals on campus. Administrators, faculty, and staff are not identified by name or specific position, and students are given pseudonyms.

The interviews had recurring themes. For instance, many respondents described the surge in applications for ESAs and the need to clarify, distinguish, and mediate difficulties among owners of program dogs, service dogs, ESAs, and student pets. Because of CC's increasingly popular ANZ program, the institution had a head start in collaborating with different departments to determine what policies or guidelines were needed and how to communicate them across campus.

I returned to my own campus, Weber State University in Utah (WSU), where a dog is only occasionally seen accompanying a student in a wheelchair or on a leash guiding a blind student. More often, dogs trot on-leash beside their owners. I interviewed a staff member from both Disability Services and Counseling and Psychological Services about policies and attitudes toward ESAs on campus. The open-ended questions focused on the staff members' experiences and personal philosophies about requests for ESAs from students, faculty, and staff. Through the theoretical lens of the communicative constitution of organizations (CCO), I contrasted the two campuses as case studies of how communication about organizational practices, policies, and potential problems can (re)structure the educational institution and (re)shape its identity.

THE FOUR-FLOWS MODEL OF CCO

CCO's roots are found in Giddens's *The Constitution of Society* (1984), which describes how human agents, acting alone or together, can transform or maintain social structures in a process called the *duality of structuration*. This structuration refers to the process of relying on individual and institutional resources and constraints to both produce and reproduce social systems. CCO rearticulated this theory into an organizational setting to explain how organizational cultures, practices, and decisions result from "communication that is at once both human and organizational," and includes the four flows of membership negotiation, reflexive self-structuring, activity coordination, and institutional positioning (McPhee, Poole, and Iverson 2014, 80).

The first flow, membership negotiation, focuses on members' relationship to the organization. Putnam, Nicotera, and McPhee (2009, 10) clarify that this relationship involves not merely recruiting and assimilating to the organization, but takes many forms, such as partial inclusion, commitment, identification, and leadership, and "focuses on the ways membership becomes a relationship formation." This flow asks the researcher to search for both authoritative and unauthorized voices.

The second flow, organizational self-structuring, "refers to any interactions that steer the organization in a particular direction" and includes "formal organizational charts and policies as informal processes of influence" (Putnam, Nicotera, and McPhee 2009, 10). Finding those informal processes is necessary to understand the everyday, unwritten realities of organizational structures.

The third flow, activity coordination, focuses on communication involving joint work processes, where organizational members must solve problems without pre-established norms "to creatively augment or even contravene organizational practices" (Nordbäck, Myers, and McPhee 2016, 400). To identify these flows, the researcher must learn how cooperative or beneficial these activities are perceived to be to the organization.

The fourth flow, institutional positioning, involves "societal interactions at the macro level with suppliers, customers, competitors, government regulators, and partners" (Putnam, Nicotera, and McPhee 2009, 11). This flow is particularly important from a legalistic or public relations perspective and has a top-down influence on the first three flows.

As universities and colleges grapple with competing demands of various constituencies arguing for and against animals on campus, they have been drawn into membership negotiation, reflexive self-structuring, activity coordination, and institutional positioning. Interviews with personnel at CC and WSU most invested with ESAs on campus reflect interconnections between the four flows in organizational communication and their structuring process in one aspect of campus culture and organizational practices. In addition, the interviews suggest that students' and employees' mental health and the well-being of the animals they love are at stake in communication about resources and constraints, public image, policies, precedents, and legalities around ESAs.

First Flow: Members Negotiating Animals in Public

The first flow of membership negotiation can be applied to examine how students, faculty, and staff encounter questions, issues, and opportunities about how having animals in public spaces might simultaneously enable one person and encroach upon another person or animal. A 2017 online survey indicates the public's mixed perceptions and acceptance of service, emotional support, and therapy dogs in school dorms and classrooms, with 46 percent agreeing with allowing ESAs in dorms and 34 percent agreeing with permitting ESAs in classrooms (Schoenfeld-Tacher et al. 2017). WSU and CC both have had increasing ESA requests for both dorms and classrooms in recent years. Therefore, this chapter's research anticipated that the respondents might similarly reflect mixed perceptions toward ESAs.

At CC, the ANZ major has attracted more students requesting ESAs in recent years. These students then have to be told by ANZ faculty that becoming an ANZ major does not allow them to train their own dog in their classes. The surge in ESA requests has included a bearded dragon (approved), a guinea pig (denied), and numerous dogs and cats. The uptick in kitten requests as ESAs has received skeptical responses because, as one staff member asked, is there really a long-term emotional support relationship there? The accessibility coordinator's job is to ask the applicant why they think they need the animal. For example, the officer might ask: Is this animal the best remedy for a mental health disability? In the case of one student's betta fish ESA, it was her best remedy, and that student is now working toward her doctorate in aquatic management.

Students requesting an ESA must have documentation from a legitimate provider who has known the student over a period of time and can explain why the need exists. Confirming "legitimacy" is part of the process, due to the proliferation of websites that provide letters verifying ESA requirements, for a fee, without any therapeutic consultation. CC's accessibility coordinator then reviews the rules on living accommodation with the students. Dogs must be taken out and exercised regularly; they must also be at least nine months old, and be potty and leash trained. Cats' litter areas must be kept clean.

Students living with ESAs in student housing comprise just one aspect of animals on CC's campus. The ANZ major has resulted in dogs present all over campus, including classrooms. Montana and Utah state laws specify that service dogs-in-training have the same rights and privileges as a service dog to being in public; for example, dogs can learn how to be in an elevator only by being in an elevator. Dogs being trained by ANZ majors are necessarily in the ANZ classrooms, but this situation has led to students requesting other faculty to allow dogs in non-ANZ classrooms. ANZ students are coached on how to politely ask faculty for permission and to graciously accept any response. According to students, most faculty say yes, but some say no, especially for laboratory-based classrooms. One student stated in an interview, "Professors only say no if there has been a problem. You have to talk to the professor before class. You also have to ask the class members themselves if anyone has an allergy or phobia and give them your email if they want to tell you no, but privately."

At WSU, questions about animals on campus predated ESAs. For many years, students and staff fed feral cats living outside an academic building. Geese also migrate from the campus pond across lawns and roads, and deer frequently trespass onto campus. Students, employees, and community members use the campus as a place to walk and exercise their dogs, usually on leash. The Disability Office gets requests for ESAs several times a month from students who want their rescued animals to live with them in student housing, and from faculty and staff who want to have their ESAs in their offices.

WSU's Disability Office has had to negotiate issues with a student club bringing birds on campus; students bringing animals into class (e.g., surreptitiously in a backpack or under clothing); pet dogs interacting inappropriately with service dogs; and service dogs that are disruptive and not well trained. One interviewed staff member said that, "Animals don't have the same coping mechanisms as humans . . . . WSU is an animal friendly campus, but we need to be able to say here is a list of behaviors that aren't accepted and where animals are restricted." Having that list and those policies leads to the next flow in CCO theory, reflexive self-structuring, which includes "authoritative acts" or "chains of decisions that absorb uncertainty in the organization system" (McPhee 2015, 489).

Second Flow: Reflexively Structuring ESA Policies/Guidelines

CC's Animals on Campus policy is four pages long in the school's Student Handbook. The policy includes an application to have an animal on campus.

The application requires the signature of Student Life Office for students, or Human Resources for faculty requests. The applicant must check the five boxes below:

- My animal is being used for instructional purposes from my enrollment in an anthrozoology canine course.
- As a professional staff member who resides in Carroll housing, my pet meets all of the requirements of the Animal on Campus policy.
- A one-time exception has been granted for a Carroll event involving animals.
- I am requesting to have an Emotional Support Animal as an accommodation and have provided additional documentation outlining my request.
- I am a licensed Therapist and request to use my Therapy Animal as part of the scope of my job duties at Carroll (Animals on Campus Policy 2018–2019)

The application then lists nine rules that the owner must agree to if bringing an animal on campus: (1) a health certificate of animal showing vaccinations; (2) animal is on a wellness program with a veterinarian; (3) registration of animal and notification of HR/Student Life if any changes; (4) a leash, collar, etc., with visible identification; (5) animal is housebroken, well-groomed, odor free, with no external parasites; (6) when outside, animal must not be in estrus and must be on leash and controlled by verbal commands; (7) owner must be responsible for sanitary disposal of animal's waste; (8) animal cannot be where food is being prepared, in research labs, or other restricted areas; and (9) owner is liable for animal's behavior, including any property damage or injuries (Animals on Campus Policy 2018-2019). Their application is a shorter version of a seventeen-point "Emotional Support Animal Memo of Understanding" used at Kutztown University in Pennsylvania. (Adams, Sharkin, and Bottinelli 2017)

Questions about animals as ESAs or service dogs are forwarded to CC's Campus Housing office, and a "triage" meeting then discusses all accommodations needed and the policies to be followed. Service dogs must be with their owners at all times. ESA dogs must be crated (placed in a cage) in their owner's absence. It should be noted that the student conduct process regarding animals was co-written with ANZ students. Although ESAs require no housing deposits, damage fees may be assessed, including for the odors from the animals. When there are policy violations, the student conduct process requires that the student repair damages to those impacted. The students' grades are affected by any complaints about their responsibilities to their dogs. Students are also often required to write apology letters or deliver door-to-door apologies.

CC's policies regarding ESAs certainly have gray areas. For example, students with dogs have specific housing with fenced yards and a $400/semester refundable cleaning fee. Because dogs are allowed on campus, the Dean of Students Office sends out annual emails about the animals and their colored bandanas. After each stage of testing behaviors, dogs graduate from yellow to green to the purple vests establishing them as AKC Canine Good Citizens. The emails explain that other students are welcome to meet the dogs, but they first need to ask permission from the dogs' handlers.

No working policy exists about animals in CC's faculty or staff offices, but "a common sense rule applies," explained one staff member respondent. Faculty may permit students to have ESAs in the classroom because they have full control of their own classroom, as long as the animal is not disruptive and the students obtain prior permission. The staff member quoted above acknowledged that a power imbalance could make a student afraid to challenge faculty permission and complain about an animal's potential disruption in the classroom. In general, the respondent said that CC could create guidelines for more possible situations, such as when a faculty member could not bring her dog to the office after it bit someone.

At WSU, the Faculty Senate approved the relatively new ESA policy when it became apparent that regulation was needed beyond state or federal statutes (Animals on Campus, PPM 5-50, 2018). The policy defines what is university property and differentiates between service and ESA animals, pets, and research/teaching animals. The policy also covers reasonable accommodations, prohibits animals on university-controlled property, animals used for institutional programs or services, control of the animal by the owner, and addresses policy violations.

Adhering to federal guidelines, WSU's policy section on ESAs limits these cases to those with disabilities who have requested reasonable accommodation and can provide requested documentation. ESAs are strictly limited to university housing, and their owners "must comply with all applicable laws and regulations . . . as well as University's rules in lease provisions regarding vaccination, licensure, leash control, cleanup rules, animal health, and community relationships" (Animals on Campus, PPM 5–50, 2018). Pets are not permitted to enter campus buildings, although they may walk on campus grounds if secured by a leash that is a maximum length of 6 feet. Pets can be left in a personal vehicle as long as they do not pose a threat to passersby and are not in danger of distress.

WSU's section on policy violations states that anyone observing unauthorized and/or unrestrained animals may contact Facilities Management or the university's Police Department. These animals may be immediately removed, and employees violating the policy may face disciplinary action. The Animals on Campus policy's overall tone is legalistic, similar to the rest of the Policies and Procedures Manual. As one staff member respondent said, in practice the policies are treated more as guidelines than policy. When

WSU first created the step-by-step policy, it was rejected because it creates a legal obligation, and the university "didn't want to get into the weeds in terms of enforcement," stated the staff member, adding that the university instead needed a "policy that's breathable but protects from disruptions."

When a problem on campus is reported to WSU's facilities management or campus police, it is typically a problem of eminent harm. The question of whom to call often arises for someone who wishes to report a complaint. For instance, if a service dog exhibits threatening behavior, what action should the observer take? Who decides what is a problem and its remedy? Giving these examples, a disabilities staff respondent stated that, "We need a concrete, intentional, and purposeful decision-making process for each individual." Another respondent, who was a counseling staff member, added that processes must be individually based: "Right person, right animal, right place, right time."

This lack of specificity in applying policies around animals on campus is not uncommon across different institutions. After Britain's national "Take Your Dog to Work Day" campaign, a British online survey from 2012 found that, of 776 respondents working in an office environment, 12 percent were permitted to bring their dogs to work and 64 percent respondents said no specific policy allowed it (Hall et al. 2017). Although guidelines give the flexibility needed to individualize organizations' responses to people's differing needs, the policies require CCO's third flow of activity coordination, which "emerges when members have to negotiate new cooperative patterns to get work done" (McPhee 2015, 489).

Third Flow: Addressing ESA Activities and Issues

When CC faculty, staff, and students are asked about the animals' general impact on campus (disregarding if the animals are ANZ dogs, ESAs, or just pets), their responses were overwhelmingly positive:

- "People stop to pet a dog and talk—it is an educational moment to be a neighbor."
- "The majority of students really connect and appreciate the dogs on campus."
- "Dogs have been integrated on campus. Lots of people keep dog treats in their office. I plan to bring my own puppy to work when it is potty trained."
- "Dogs have a calming effect on me and make me happy."

CC faculty and staff shared stories about the co-worker who keeps her little dog in her office; the colleague who often brings his dog to class; and the priest who brought his "200-pound-dog" for a staff member to mind while he was in a meeting because it was too cold in the car. One administrative member stated that she didn't know if there was a policy about bringing dogs to the office, but she had never heard a complaint or noticed dogs off-leash or dog excrement anywhere.

Not everyone shared this staff member's opinion about issues with animals on campus. For example, other CC staff shared complaints about grounds cleanup, which they described as one of the biggest issues, such as when students take dogs to the softball field and don't clean up after them. The question of having doggie bag dispenser stations on campus was raised, but, according to one respondent, was rejected by facilities management because it might be perceived as inviting the public to view the campus lawns as a dog park. Facilities management feared that it would only increase dog traffic and dog excrement on campus. They also complained that students needed to take their dogs to urinate in one area to reduce grass burn everywhere.

When asked about animal safety issues, the CC respondents shared many stories about unruly animals. Once, during an outdoor ANZ dog agility training class, one dog ran through the tunnel and bit a woman passing by on a bike. Fortunately, the woman decided not to litigate. A positive outcome was that CC realized it needed a training center for dogs. After renting a warehouse off campus for several years, CC raised several million dollars for a new training center, now being built.

Interviewees who were ANZ students at CC also shared complaints. Particularly, they complained about non-ANZ students' ESA dogs that bothered their service dogs-in-training. In one case, the ESA's conflict with a service dog resulted in the non-ANZ student moving off campus. A campus housing staff member said that although she had never removed an ESA from campus, she came close to doing so because of people's multiple accounts of ESAs being over-reactive.

ANZ students are also the first to point fingers at their ANZ peers: "Some students aren't adequate at socializing their dogs so the dogs don't learn to cope with their fears. [It's] important to know whether the dogs themselves are comfortable in public places and be sensitive to their discomfort or anxiety." Socializing their dogs is an essential prerequisite for bringing them into classrooms. One ANZ student admitted that dogs can definitely distract people in non-ANZ classrooms. When she takes her dog to her non-ANZ classes, she places him under her desk and tells students they can socialize with him before or after class, but not during class. Dogs must be vest-tested to stay on their mat and not wander. However, if a student objects, as did one student fearful of a professor's dog in the classroom, then the dog must leave.

When asked about dogs in CC student accommodation, a staff member stated that, though rare, there have been a few complaints. One dog chewed through walls and doors, while another barked incessantly. "Grace periods" are permitted for new arrivals with their animals (both ANZ and ESA dogs) on campus, and after that "issues are resolved quietly." Allergies have never been a problem because the dogs are only on the first floor of student housing, so the few (primarily foreign exchange) students who express concerns are placed on floors without dogs.

Housing has a roommate pairing system for CC students with ESAs. One problem recently arose when a student turned in paperwork for an ESA after being assigned a roommate, but the college resolved that situation. An ongoing, unresolved issue includes students who dog-sit for ANZ service dogs-in-training and take the dogs back to their own residences, which are not checked monthly, unlike ANZ rooms. A second issue arises when student halls are used for summer conferences. The two-week turnaround between the end of the school year and the summer conference season makes it difficult when carpets need to be replaced.

At WSU, the only animals in classrooms are service dogs, although Disability Services has been contacted about "fake service animals" on campus or "fake ESAs" in student housing. The school's Disability Services office has made it clear that they are not an enforcement agency. They try to educate students and employees that, for a dog to be considered a service animal, it must act like a service animal by being trained to perform a specific task. The WSU staff interviewee provided this example: "If the dog is not a service animal, but the person has an obvious disability, such as being in a wheelchair with a chihuahua, people will let it go. But if the person has a hidden disability, they think someone is trying to get away with something, even though the dog may be trained to predict an epileptic seizure." However, in general, she said that "most faculty have zero problems if the animal is not disruptive, only when it acts like an animal."

Animals acting like animals have occasionally created problems at WSU. For example, these incidents have included the service dog that gets sick in the office; pets or ESAs interacting with service dogs (in one instance, attacking a service dog); and the veteran's service dog that alerted people about possible danger, but barked when he saw a person in a dinosaur costume. WSU's Disability Services has tried to be flexible in instances when students have needed their ESAs on campus, but that flexibility can also backfire. In one case, a student who was going through an emotional crisis without a support network was permitted to keep her ESA cat in her backpack, but was then reported for animal endangerment. If students need to take a test for a course, they can use a private office testing room, but the room must be immediately vacuumed for future student users with allergies.

Because WSU's Counseling and Psychological Services does not give documentation for ESAs, this information must be provided by a licensed mental health practitioner who can diagnose the disorder following treatment with data justifying an ESA. Sometimes the disorder has not had years or even months to be established. For example, a sexual assault victim may need emergency housing and would feel more secure with a dog, so a temporary permit for an ESA will be issued. WSU's Counseling and Psychological Services and Disability Services work together to try to find solutions whenever possible. ESAs need to also be annually certified with campus housing so students must engage in the process.

Staff from both campus services mentioned that students' favorite campus event is during final exam week, when volunteers from Intermountain Therapy Animals bring dogs to the student union for students to pet and hold. A survey of sixty-eight American colleges and universities found that 62 percent had a stress relief program with animals on campus, most commonly in the school library or student union center (Haggerty and Mueller 2017). Although some schools reported negative responses, the positive feedback was overwhelming, and none of the schools terminated the program. However, someone observing these dogs on campus—without understanding the people, policies, or activities involved—might misinterpret the institution's position on animals. Indeed, one surveyed institution reported that the program "'encouraged' some students to bring their own pets to campus" (Haggerty and Mueller 2017, 384). As a result, institutions must be aware of public perceptions and proactively position themselves for ramifications of the organizational "flows" from members, policies, and activities.

Fourth Flow: Institutional Positioning and Ramifications of ESAs

At CC, the initial prospect of funding an undergraduate ANZ major encountered many naysayers: If you build it, will they come? Will the major attract too many ESAs, which could become a liability (such as the student on a suicide watch who had to be hospitalized)? Initial perception problems from some academic programs were that, as one respondent was told, "Too many students just want to play with dogs."

The ANZ program has since countered that perception with examples of student research studies on human–animal relationships. Students (referred to here with pseudonyms) interviewed proudly explained their research studies: Mary investigated the effect of human anxiety/anger on dogs using videotapes and a coding system to correlate with visual signs of stress. Amy refined a method to train a dog to alert for migraines using cotton balls with her saliva when she had migraines. Lily studied the effects of human introversion-extroversion on their interactions with horses. Xander, a psychology minor, studied subjects' responses to pictures of white versus Black men with a dog, to see if the presence of the dog mitigated responses based on race.

Since then, as one CC administrator interviewee pointed out, "The human-animal bond has become increasingly vogue." The consensus from all administrators, faculty, and staff interviewed is that the ANZ program, with its increase of dogs on campus, has strengthened enrollment and retention for students who need a sense of home. Having dogs on campus sets their school apart; as one staff member stated, the dogs give the campus a more "lively flavor visually with the colorful scarfs dogs wear based on their training level." Dogs on campus are now ingrained in the cloth of the campus and accepted as normal because they are present at sports games and campus events, and in the student union. As another staff member said, dogs are "Saints" by extension at this Catholic college, fitting in with its mission. For example, a campus "blessings for the animals" ceremony is held each year. People bring their pets, even their horses. The entire community is invited to the ANZ dog graduation ceremony held outside every spring. Students tell what each dog has achieved, so it is "graduation day" for both ANZ dogs and students, making the students doubly proud.

The ANZ program is now a college priority because of its draw for applicants and donors. Many donors are dog lovers. Among their donations is the $1.25 million gift for a canine center and canine director. One staff member stated that almost every potential donor wanted to help, especially when they hear stories about vets with PTSD or students with autism and what dogs can be trained to do. As for the future, CC has talked about having pet-friendly housing areas, but it has not happened yet. As one CC administrator pointed out, because CC's reputation as a very animal-friendly campus has impacted the types of students who enroll, including more students with ESAs, the college has also had to go "along with the national movement, close the floodgates to take control of any animal counting as an ESA." The administrator continued, "We are always asking ourselves, 'How can we make this the most successful and positive experience for everyone.'"

Without an ANZ program to advocate for ESAs and animals on campus generally, WSU has had a much shorter timeline to consider institutional positioning and ramifications. The disabilities coordinator interviewee said she believes that more education is needed about the benefits versus the liabilities of having a culture shift around animals on campus. A culture shift toward a more animal-friendly campus instead of policy ESAs is not an impossibility. The disabilities coordinator asked why the college could not have animal friendly apartments on campus without requiring ESA certification, or a kind of "affinity housing" with animals (like majors). She stated that not strictly separating one's work and personal life is part of having a whole life. However, she added that others who prefer keeping work effective and efficient might begrudge those combining work and personal life.

Disabilities Services raised important questions during the interviews. Primarily, if people are more productive when they are comfortable and happy, whose comfort and happiness is being prioritized? Do animals always help or can they prevent someone from engaging with others? A larger ESA issue is which animals have the most value and should therefore be protected? A more thorny issue for ESA advocates might be the therapists' liability if they recommend an animal and there's a problem. From one counseling staff member's perspective, many questions still need to be answered before WSU campus could become more animal friendly. A policy must have a process to address problems and remedies, while still allowing for the individual circumstances of "right person, right animal, right place, right time."

An article in *The Chronicle of Higher Education* about animals on campus reported that "the single biggest concern on the part of institutions [regarding animals] would be setting a precedent. They worry that if they say yes to this one, they won't be able to say no to the next one" (Field 2006, 15). Field's (2006) article was based on an interview with Jane Jarrow, president of Disability Access Information and Support (DAIS), who provides workshops, manuals, and webinars to help colleges and universities meet disability standards. In the area of ESAs, she has more recently focused on helping colleges reject illegitimate ESAs without violating Federal Housing Authority (FHA) rules with her course entitled, "Who Let the Dogs Out... IN!?!?" (Jarrow 2015) Jarrow explains that disability service providers represent a variety of philosophies. They may appear as social justice or civil rights advocates, grounding their approaches as legal eagles, universal design enthusiasts, or "weary warriors who just want to Make-It-Work" (Jarrow 2015). That is why the programs at different institutions vary so much, and yet can be equally successful in promoting equal access. The statutes and laws tell institutions to not discriminate on the basis of disability, but leave the interpretation of what that means to the institution.

CONCLUSIONS AND IMPLICATIONS

Using federal guidelines stipulated in Titles II and III of the 2008 Americans with Disabilities Act Amendments Act (ADAAA) and the Fair Housing Act of 1988, colleges and universities have differentiated service animals and ESAs to create clear, restrictive, and legal boundaries based on the potential and real conflicts with human-animal and animal-animal interactions. UCCs and DSSs struggle with accusations of "fake service animals" or "fake therapy animals," as well as with demands that they must become enforcement agencies so that campus does not become a "zoo." The institutions must create rules to address legitimate concerns from constituencies with allergies or fear/discomfort around animals; facility management with responsibilities of building and ground cleanliness; and animal welfare advocates who question the well-being of animals kept in crates and backpacks all day.

Common themes arising from the interviews included: the need for legal guidance; conflicts involving categorizing service dogs, ESAs, and pets; the value of flexible versus strict prescriptive policies; the use of therapy dogs on campus during final exams; the need for housing that permits student pets; the importance of staff and faculty support; and the well-being of all stakeholders, including animals. Institutional positioning ultimately becomes a primary determinant in an "animal friendly" campus cultural shift to support student mental health versus policing ESAs to minimize educational disruption and professional/personal life boundaries. Administrators and staff involved in managing ESAs on campus should consider not only the legalities in drafting policies, but also how those policies are communicated through stories that facilitate understanding of complex, situated relationships. Those interpretations flow, over time, from communication about membership, activities, policies, and institutional positioning, which likely varies considerably from a large public university to a small private religious college.

This chapter, which is based on in-depth interviews at two very different institutions, is only a temporal snapshot of a limited range of perceptions about how to balance student and employee mental health needs with the well-being and comfort of all stakeholders. To gain a more comprehensive understanding of stakeholders' perceptions, campus-wide surveys are needed. Any hesitancy about conducting such surveys may be due to the implicit understanding of how that action would constitute the flow of activity coordination and trigger the flows of membership negotiation and reflexive self-structuring, ultimately impacting institutional positioning. Indeed, just distributing a survey could signal possible institutional (re)positioning and result in reconstituting the organization itself. Ultimately, my hope is that educational institutions will continually prioritize students' mental health and well-being.

REFERENCES

Adams, Aimee C., Bruce S. Sharkin, and Jennifer J. Bottinelli. 2017. "The Role of Pets in the Lives of College Students: Implications for College Counselors." Appendix A. *Journal of College Student Psychotherapy* 31, no. 4: 306–324. https://doi.org/10.1080/87568225.2017.1299601.

"Animals on Campus." 2018–2019. Carroll College. Copy provided by administrative staff.

"Animals on Campus." 2018. Policies and Procedures Manual 5-50. Weber State University.
"Anthrozoology Major or Minor." Carroll College. Accessed October 23, 2020. https ://www.carroll.edu/academic-programs/anthrozoology.
Barker, Randolph T., Janet S. Knisely, Sandra B. Barker, Rachel K. Cobb, and Christine M. Schubert. 2012. "Preliminary Investigation of Employee's Dog Presence on Stress and Organizational Perceptions." *International Journal of Workplace Health Management* 5, no. 1: 15–30.
Barker, Sandra B., Randoph T. Barker, Nancy L. McCain, and Christine M Schubert. 2016. "A
Randomized Cross-Over Exploratory Study of the Effect of Visiting Therapy Dogs on College Student Stress Before Final Exams." *Anthrozoös* 29, no. 1: 35–46. https ://doi.org/10.1080/08927936.2015.1069988.
Binfet, John-Tyler, Holli-Anne Passmore, Alex Cebry, Kathryn Struik, and Carson McKay. 2018. "Reducing University Students' Stress Through a Drop-in Canine Therapy Program." *Journal of Mental Health* 27, no. 3: 197–2004. https://doi.org /10.1080/09638237.2017.1417551.
Brelsford, Victoria, Kersin Meints, Nanch R. Gee, and Karen Pfeffer. 2017. "Animal-Assisted
Interventions in the Classroom—A Systematic Review." *International Journal of Environmental Research and Public Health* 14, no. 7: 197–204. https://doi.org/10 .3390/ijerph14070669.
Brinn, Hope. 2018. "Case Profile, United States v. University of Nebraska at Kearney" (No. ED-NE-0001), Civil Rights Litigation Clearinghouse. https://www .clearinghouse.net/detail.php?id=15045.
Charles, Nickie, and Carol Wolkowitz. 2019. "Bringing Bodies on Campus: Inclusions and Exclusions of Animal Bodies in Organizations." *Gender, Work, and Organization* 26, no. 3: 303–321. https://doi.org/10.1111/gwao.12254.
Clay, Rebecca A. 2016. "Is That a Pet or Therapeutic Aid?" *Monitor on Psychology* 47, no. 8 (September 9, 2016): 38. https://www.apa.org/monitor/20 16/09/pet-aid.
Crump, Chesika, and Terry L. Derting. 2015. "Effects of Pet Therapy on the Psychological and Physiological Stress Levels of First-Year Female Undergraduates." *North American Journal of Psychology* 17, no. 3. https://link -gale-com.hal.weber.edu/apps/doc/A435796037/AONE?u=ogde72764&sid=AON E&xid=e22d7215.
Daltry, Rachel M., and Kristin E. Mehr. 2015. "Therapy Dogs on Campus: Recommendations for Counseling Center Outreach." *Journal of College Student Psychotherapy* 29, no. 1: 72–78. https://doi.org/10.1080/87568225.2015.976100.
DeCourcey, Mary, Anne C. Russell, and Kathy J. Keister. 2010. "Animal-Assisted Therapy: Evaluation and Implementation of a Complementary Therapy to Improve the Psychological and Physiological Health of Critically Ill Patients." *Dimensions of Critical Care Nursing* 29, no. 5: 211–214. https://doi.org/10.1097/DCC.0b013e3 181e6c71a.

Field, Kelly. 2006. "These Student Requests Are a Different Animal." *The Chronicle of Higher Education* 53, no. 8 (October 13, 2006). https://www.chronicle.com/article/these-student-requests-are-a-different-animal/.

Foreman, Anne M., Margaret K. Glenn, Barbara J. Meade, and Oliver Wirth. 2017. "Dogs in the Workplace: A Review of the Benefits and Potential Challenges." *International Journal of Environmental Research and Public Health* 14, no. 5: 498. https://doi.org/10.3390/ijerph14050498.

Fortney, John C., Geoffrey M. Curran, Justin B. Hunt, Ann M. Cheney, Liya Lu, Marcia Valenstein, and Daniel Eisenberg. 2015. "Prevalence of Probably Mental Disorders and Help-Seeking Behaviors among Veteran and Non-Veteran Community College Students." *General Hospital Psychiatry* 38: 99–104. https://doi.org/10.1016/j.genhosppsych.2015.09.007.

Giddens, Anthony. 1984. *The Constitution of Society*. Oakland, CA: University of California Press.

Haggerty, Julie M., and Megan Kiely Mueller. 2017. "Animal-Assisted Stress Reduction Programs in Higher Education." *Innovative Higher Education* 42: 379–389. https://doi.org/10.1007/s10755-017-9392-0.

Hall, Sophie, Hannah Wright, Sandra McCune, Helen Zulch, and Daniel Mills. 2017. "Perceptions of Dogs in the Workplace: Pros and Cons." *Anthrozoös* 30, no. 2: 291–305. https://doi.org/10.1080/08927936.2017.1311053.

House, Lisa A., Chelsea Neal, and Kelsey Backels. 2018. "A Doggone Way to Reduce Stress: An Animal Assisted Intervention with College Students." *College Student Journal* 52, no. 2: 199–204. https://eric.ed.gov/?id=EJ1180325.

Jarrow, Jane E. 2018. "Online Professional Development from DAIS." Course Catalog for Disability Access Information and Support, Fall 2018. http://www.daisclasses.com/?upf=dl&id=193.

Kogan, Lori R., Karen Schaefer, Phyllis Erdman, and Regina Schoenfeld-Tacher. 2016. "University Counseling Centers' Perceptions and Experiences Pertaining to Emotional Support Animals." *Journal of College Student Psychotherapy* 30, no. 4: 268–283. https://doi.org/10.1080/87568225.2016.1219612.

LaFrance, Caroline, Linda J. Garcia, and Julianne Labreche. 2007. "The Effect of a Therapy Dog on the Communication Skills of an Adult with Aphasia." *Journal of Communication Disorders* 40, no. 3: 215–224. https://doi.org/10.1016/j.jcomdis.2006.06.010.

Lipson, Sarah Ketchen, Emily G. Lattie, and Daniel Eisenberg. 2018. "Increased Rates of Mental Health Service Utilization by U.S. College Students: 10-Year Population-Level Trends (2007-2017)." *Psychiatric Services*, November 5, 2018. https://doi.org/10.1176/appi.ps.201800332.

Maujean, Annick, Christopher A. Pepping, and Elizabeth Kendall, E. 2015. "A Systematic Review of Randomized Controlled Trials of Animal-Assisted Therapy on Psychosocial Outcomes." *Anthrozoös* 28, no. 1: 23–36. https://doi.org/10.2752/089279315X14129350721812.

McPhee, Robert D., and Pamela Zaug. 2009. "The Communicative Constitution of Organizations: A Framework for Explanation." In *Building Theories of*

Organization: The Constitutive Role of Communication, edited by Linda L. Putnam and Anne M. Nicotera, 21–45. New York: Routledge.

McPhee, Robert D., Marshall Scott Poole, and Joel Iverson, J. 2014. "Structuration Theory." In *The Sage Handbook of Organizational Communication*, edited by Linda L Putnam and Dennis K., 75–100. Thousand Oaks, CA: Sage.

McPhee, Robert D. 2015. "Agency and the Four Flows." *Management Communication Quarterly* 29, no. 3: 487–492. https://doi.org/10.1177/0893318915584826.

Nordbäck, Emma S., Karen K. Myers, and Robert D. McPhee. 2017. "Workplace Flexibility and Communication Flows: A Structurational View." *Journal of Applied Communication Research* 45, no. 4: 397–412. https://doi.org/10.1080/00909882.2017.1355560.

Putnam, Linda. L., Anne Maydan Nicotera, and Robert D. McPhee. 2009. "Introduction: Communication Constitutes Organization." In *Building Theories of Organization: The Constitutive Role of Communication*, edited by Linda L. Putnam and Anne Maydan Nicotera, 1–20. New York: Routledge.

Rosenberg, Robin S. 2013. "Abnormal is the New Normal: Why Will Half of the U.S. Population Have a Diagnosable Mental Disorder?" *Slate*, April 12, 2013. https://slate.com/technology/2013/04/diagnostic-and-statistical-manual-fifth-edition-why-will-half-the-u-s-population-have-a-mental-illness.html.

Rossetti, Jeanette, and Camille King. 2010. "Use of Animal-Assisted Therapy with Psychiatric

Patients." *Journal of Psychosocial Nursing and Mental Health Services* 48, no. 11: 44–48. https://doi.org/10.3928/02793695-20100831-05.

Schoenfeld-Tacher, Regina, Peter Hellyer, Louanna Cheung, L., and Lori Kogan. 2017. "Public Perceptions of Service Dogs, Emotional Support Dogs, and Therapy Dogs." *International Journal of Environmental Research and Public Health* 14, no. 6. https://doi.org/10.3390/ijerph14060642.

Substance Abuse and Mental Health Administration. 2016. "DSM-5 Changes: Implications for Child Serious Emotional Disturbance." *Center for Behavioral Health Statistics and Quality Report.* https://www.ncbi.nlm.nih.gov/books/NBK519708/.

Taylor, Judy Sutton. 2016. "Colleges See an Uptick in Requests for Emotional Support Animals on Campus." *American Bar Association Journal* 102, no. 7. https://www.abajournal.com/magazine/article/colleges_see_an_uptick_in_requests_for_emotional_support_animals_on_campus.

Von Bergen, C. W. 2015. "Emotional Support Animals, Service animals, and Pets on Campus." *Administrative Issues Journal: Connecting Education, Practice, and Research* 5, no. 1: 15–34. https://doi.org/10.5929/2015.5.1.3.

Von Bergen, C. W., and Martin S. Bressler. 2017. "Animals in the Workplace: Employer Rights and Responsibilities." *Global Journal of Business Disciplines* 1, no. 1 (Summer): 87. *Gale Academic OneFile* (accessed February 21, 2020). https://link-gale-com.hal.weber.edu/apps/doc/A540211364/AONE?u=ogde72764&sid=AONE&xid=c8a4f83e.

Von Bergen, C. W., and Martin S. Bressler. 2015. "Employees' Best Friends and Other Animals in the Workplace." *Employee Relations Law Journal* 14, no. 1:

4–34. http://homepages.se.edu/cvonbergen/files/2015/03/Employees-Best-Friends-and-Other-Animals-in-the-Workplace.pdf.

Watkins, Daphne C., Justin B. Hunt, and Daniel Eisenberg. 2011. "Increased Demand for Mental Health Services on College Campuses: Perspectives from Administrators." *Qualitative Social Work*, Aug. 9, 2011. https://doi.org/10.1177/1473325011401468.

Wisch, Rebecca F. 2019. "FAQs on Emotional Support Animals." Animal & Legal Historical Center, Michigan State University College of Law. Accessed February 21, 2020. https://www.animallaw.info/article/faqs-emotional-support-animals.

Chapter 11

Navigating Boundaries while Creating Safe Spaces for Faculty and Students

Sandra Smeltzer, David M. Walton, Nicole Campbell

SETTING THE STAGE

It is a Tuesday afternoon in the Winter academic semester. Western University's Teaching Fellows have gathered for our monthly meeting to discuss our respective teaching innovation projects and educational experiences with colleagues from across campus. The Teaching Fellows Program, which is housed in Western's Centre for Teaching and Learning (CTL), supports teaching excellence and innovation "by bringing together a cohort of outstanding faculty members to provide educational leadership in their respective Faculties and the wider campus community" (Western University 2019). The program has been a productive venue for full-time tenured and untenured academic staff to discuss projects about the scholarship of teaching and learning, collaborate on professional development activities, and solicit advice from peers about how to most effectively fulfill their Fellow mandates. The program thus speaks to the value of interdisciplinary connections and the importance of fostering a "third space" in academia outside one's home discipline, especially in research-focused universities that can physically and intellectually silo scholars (Sharif et al. 2019). The Teaching Fellows Program is also an invaluable safe space for members to share their personal and professional struggles as university educators and mentors.

At this regular meeting, something unexpected transpired. One colleague[1] disclosed their emotional struggles after the tragic loss of one of their students. Although this faculty member knew professional support was available on campus, talking with their peers in a safe environment was vital to their nascent healing process. The meeting's agenda was set aside as we focused on our friend and colleague. This personal disclosure, combined with the supportive discussion afterward, inspired this chapter's co-authors to share our own mental health challenges associated with our academic lives.

We contextualize these personal narratives against the backdrop of growing mental health crises within (and beyond) the academy. These crises are compounded by the historical reticence of scholars to appear less than perfect in the eyes of peers and students. By sharing our stories of vulnerability, we contest the image of the stoic, dispassionate professor as the only path to success in higher education and instead imagine a world where professors embrace their human-ness through caring and compassion. By unpacking our experiences and beliefs about the potential for improved workplaces and teaching outcomes, we seek to create space(s) in the academy to share fears, vulnerabilities, and anxieties. As part of our call to action, we emphasize the Teaching Fellows Program's important role in our personal and professional lives as we navigate "the effects of changing academic environments on faculty well-being" (Mudrak et al. 2018, 325).

Intersections of Student and Faculty Mental Health

The neoliberalization of the Canadian university system reflects similar trends in post-secondary education worldwide. Problematically, the academy's increasing corporatization translates into greater emphasis on metrics-based evidence of scholarly output. Namely, well-positioned, peer-reviewed articles, single-authored monographs, and large-scale grants are prioritized at the expense of other forms of academic productivity, including teaching, service, and alternative venues for scholarly dissemination (Berg, Huijbens, and Larsen 2016; Mudrak et al. 2018; Peake and Mullings 2016; Tuck 2018). From our experiences, the academy's individualized and competitive nature undermines the collegial collaboration and support that would help build community within and across disciplinary lines (despite the increasing lip-service in support of interdisciplinary collaboration). To help counteract this antagonistic environment, Austin and Trice (2016) describe five factors essential to faculty members' emotional and mental well-being: academic freedom, flexibility, collegiality, professional development, and equity. The Teaching Fellows Program has played a vital role in helping this chapter's co-authors champion these factors—especially collegiality and professional development—in both their respective departments and across campus.

Yet, mental health issues continue to increase in both academic staff and student populations in an environment of chronic and cumulative stress (Kwan et al. 2016). Post-secondary institutions are thus under pressure to provide expanded support services for student mental health, a growing demand that mirrors trends in wider society. In North America, for example, current estimates place the prevalence of mood disorders and other psychopathologies at between 20–40 percent (Canadian Mental Health Association 2019) of the adult population.[2] Statistics for university and college students appear to be even higher. The National College Health Assessment (American College Health Association 2018), referred to as the "benchmarking climate survey conducted at postsecondary institutions across North America" (Western University 2018, 8), found a steady increase in the number of Canadian postsecondary students reporting psychiatric conditions. In 2016, 42 percent of all Canadian university students indicated that stress or anxiety negatively impacted their academic performance, up from 33 percent three years earlier (American College Health Association 2018). It is therefore not surprising that community and institutional supports are strained by the increasing demand. Reflecting these trends, the number of students seeking help from Western's Accessible Education Services tripled from 2007–2008 to 2017–2018, and students requesting psychiatric/mental health support more than quadrupled between 2010–2018 (Western University 2018, 5).

The university's upper administration has proactively tried to address the mental well-being of the large student population by developing a robust campus-wide strategy, "Western's Student Mental Health and Wellness Strategic Plan" (Western University 2018). The plan enacts the institution's financial and political commitment to give students, staff, and faculty members the mental health resources they need. However, the mental health of faculty members is only mentioned once in the thirty-page document under a recommendation that the institution "[d]evelop a mental health and wellness strategic plan for faculty and staff" (Western University 2018, 8). Further, faculty are encouraged to "be engaged," "talk to the students," and "trust [their] instincts" (Western University 2018, 8), especially if they are concerned about a student's mental health and well-being. Although we fully support the plan's proactive approach to mitigating crises, these requests of faculty members do not manifest easily in practice for reasons we discuss in this chapter.

We expect that the perspectives we share below will be familiar to most readers. However, our experience is that faculty members seldom publicly address or disclose personal struggles about mental health in academia. Indeed, we "rarely ever have discussions with each other about mental and emotional distress, even though its prevalence among students may be recognized" (Peake and Mullings 2016, 270). Yet, there is no reason to believe that faculty members, no matter where they are positioned in the tiered university system, are immune to the pressures facing other members of society. Despite occupying a position of relative privilege in many societal structures, university faculty members face at least as many, or more, chronic daily stressors than other work sectors. These include pressures to (often independently) produce high-quality publications in volume, secure grant dollars, attain promotion and tenure, manage lab budgets and resources, mentor highly qualified personnel, obtain strong teaching scores, and engage in myriad institutional- and community-level service activities. The expectation that we succeed in these multivariate categories, especially in the context of sociopolitical shifts in contemporary society (including trends toward anti-intellectualism and fiscal constraint), can manifest in considerable and chronic allostatic load[3] on the person. Further, academic pursuits often demand labor outside normal working hours, such as early/late meetings, community or institutional events, fieldwork, conference travel, and sitting in front of a computer for long periods of time to meet increasingly tight deadlines. These responsibilities often demand time and attention away from one's personal health and wellness, and from family members (e.g., children, aging parents) who themselves may be dealing with mental and physical health issues that require caregiver support.

Concomitantly, as student mental well-being becomes increasingly recognized on university campuses, faculty members often assume counseling roles beyond the scope of their traditional teaching responsibilities. These pastoral duties are one of the most emotionally taxing aspects of our academic positions, yet they are almost exclusively performed beyond normal workload expectations. That is, other than the very rare faculty appointment that explicitly includes student support and wellness (and therefore provides workload credit for such activities), most faculty members engage with students in distress out of an altruistic compulsion to help. These experiences often require significant physical and emotional energy, but there is no line on the annual performance evaluation for *number of crises averted*. The toll of providing this support is compounded at a time when universities' budgetary restrictions mean that faculty members are often asked to take on added workload to ensure institutional viability with fewer resources.

Further, in Canada (as in many other countries), we are witnessing significant growth in precariously employed academic staff and a decline in tenure-track appointments (Canadian Association of University Teachers 2018; Council of Ontario Universities 2018). Problematically, individuals in part-time and/or contract-based appointments experience "instability and uncertainty in relation to their own, their units', and/or their universities' absolute and relative position" (Polster 2016, 95). Contingent faculty members are often expected to carry a higher teaching load and thus, in another example of cumulative stress, can be particularly affected by students' adverse mental health challenges.

Having briefly summarized some key shifts occurring in the academic landscape, we now explore how institutions can prioritize faculty members' mental well-being. We particularly emphasize the importance of having safe spaces for faculty members to share their struggles and vulnerabilities, and to seek peer support. To this end, we offer our personal stories about mental health in the academy.

PERSONAL EXPERIENCES AND REFLECTIONS: THREE VIGNETTES

This chapter's co-authors are faculty members in three different academic units at Western University, a large research-intensive institution in London, Ontario, Canada. We have varied disciplinary backgrounds and come from different academic cultures; yet, we share a commitment to teaching and are members of Western's Teaching Fellows Program.

Our primary objective for the following discussion is to give readers permission to engage with their own mental health, particularly about their experiences working in higher education. However, we want to avoid perpetuating the stigma that mental health disorders are directly and causally linked to stress or the (in)ability to cope with it. Many people experience stress, but not all develop a diagnosable mental health disorder (El Hage, Powell, and Surguladze 2009). Evidence also indicates that mental ill-health is multifactorial and cannot be reduced to a single cause (Heim and Binder 2012; Sharma et al. 2016). As well, we are sensitive to possibly over-pathologizing normal experiences of transient sadness, worry, emotional or mental fatigue, and of contributing to an academic culture that stigmatizes and marginalizes people with mental health disorders. Emotional or mental fatigue, while possibly a sign of a mood disorder like depression (American Psychiatric Association 2013), can also be a perfectly rational result of managing stress in one's self or others. Peake and Mullings (2016) remind us that, "The stigma attached to mental and emotional distress encourages the assumption that it is a sign of weakness or of not being cut out to be an academic, an indication of unfitness to be in the academy" (270). Therefore, although we encourage readers to engage in personal exploration and to share their mental health challenges, we also advocate deep reflection on their biases, assumptions, and experiences in this regard.

The personal vignettes below represent threads from our lived experiences of mental health in the academy. With our vision of destigmatization, we hope that these stories will motivate readers to think about their own boundaries when engaging with students and colleagues, so that they can practice self-care within and outside work.

NICOLE'S STORY

Nicole is an Assistant Professor in Western University's Interdisciplinary Medical Sciences program. She is an emerging[4] faculty member in a teaching-focused, full-time contract position and serves as the department's academic counselor for students. She also coordinates and instructs her department's capstone courses and meets frequently with students to discuss their academic lives and postgraduation aspirations. When she was hired, Nicole's administration gave her explicit instructions to raise the capstone courses' rigor so that they aligned with the outcomes of the department's thesis programs. To successfully do this, Nicole recognized that students needed access to adequate support during their studies. As she modified her curriculum each year, Nicole emphasized building professional relationships with students, but noticed they were frustrated, anxious, and experiencing significant stress throughout the term. After attending an optional mental health first-aid workshop, and not hearing any concrete ideas about how faculty members could proactively support students, Nicole introduced greater awareness of mental health issues in her courses.

To this end, Nicole began having conversations with her students about mental health, provided them with institutional resources, and introduced strategies to help them manage their mental health and well-being. As an example of the latter, she introduced a *no questions asked* 24-hour coupon that students can *cash in* when they need another day to complete an assignment. Students can use the coupon once during the term for an individual task as long as they identify strategies to manage their time in the future.

Within a year of introducing these initiatives, Nicole noticed that students increasingly sought support from her about non-course–related issues. The extent and personal nature of these requests could be attributed to various determinants, including that Nicole is a relatively young, female professor who demonstrates care and compassion for her students. To manage these requests, Nicole completed additional training such as suicide intervention skills and how to respond to sexual assault disclosures. Nicole eventually recognized the negative impact that these experiences were having on her own mental health. She was distracted and having trouble sleeping due to emotional exhaustion from the vicarious trauma. At this point, she sought support from colleagues in the Teaching Fellows Program. Nicole found that she was not alone in feeling overwhelmed by trying to handle escalating student requests while also maintaining work–life balance.

From these experiences, Nicole realized that she needed to embrace self-care, and even make choices that she sometimes felt were even selfish. The next time she taught, she openly described her commitment to mental health with her students, but recognized that she needed boundaries to protect her own well-being. She remains committed to supporting her students, but is finding creative ways to build a community where students can support one another and access campus resources before they reach a crisis point. Additionally, in 2019, Nicole organized a well-attended, in-depth session on campus for faculty from across the university to discuss compassion fatigue and share self-care strategies.

DAVE'S STORY

Dave is a tenured Associate Professor in the School of Physical Therapy at Western University. Like many in a standard tenured or tenure-track position, Dave is expected to be successful in each of his appointment's teaching, research, and service components. He effectively fills these roles, earning recognition for his accomplishments. As a Caucasian, cisgender, upper-middle-class male, he is also a member of what is, by most standards, one of the most privileged demographic groups in North America. Despite this position, Dave is not immune to the effects of mental health disorders impacting his students, his family, or himself. Indeed, his success as a researcher and teacher has come at no small personal cost, including problems with anxiety, insomnia, and self-doubt. Whether from the pressures to be successful in large national and international funding competitions (with success rates in the 10–15 percent range); supervising a large interdisciplinary group of graduate students; providing an exceptional learning experience for students; or contributing to the university and academic communities more broadly (e.g., through manuscript and grant reviews, community volunteerism, editorial roles, board memberships), his dedicated energies are often disproportional to the time and resources available for success in every role. Even Dave's participation in the Teaching Fellows Program has been viewed as a *lesser than* pursuit by some colleagues who do not equate academic success with teaching innovation.

Academic martyr culture arises once again in Dave's story, as it is expected that if one is truly dedicated to their academic pursuits, then one will do work beyond what most would consider standard working hours. The tensions, worry, and self-doubt come to the fore when these traditional values of the academy conflict with one's personal values. In this case, Dave prioritizes his family; yet, they, too, are not immune to mental ill-health. Dave's increasing awareness of his burnout and fatigue, despite believing himself to be resilient, combined with mental health crises of family members (including those of a child), led him to focus on family care and self-care that sometimes conflicted with the highly meritocratic expectations of academic life. However, in an unexpected twist, by de-prioritizing his former publish or perish mindset, reducing his *quantity* of scholarly outputs increased Dave's sense of satisfaction with his work. Dave now creates a culture of wellness and satisfaction for his thesis-based graduate students, though he admits that it is easy to slip back into the overwork mindset without frequent self check-ups.

In the Teaching Fellows Program, Dave has received advice and encouragement from colleagues who are often dealing with similar life challenges and professional expectations. Like Dave, they are trying to successfully manage professional expectations while being partners and parents in life beyond the university's walls.

SANDRA'S STORY

Sandra is a tenured Associate Professor and Assistant Dean (Research) in Western's Faculty of Information and Media Studies. She recently lost her father and has struggled to find meaning in her academic life in the aftermath. Her father was her champion and cheerleader, the one individual who expressed unadulterated pride in her scholarly accomplishments. Sandra's initial grief was compounded by the sleeplessness that accompanies having a new infant at home and the fear that her long-standing eating disorder, which she had managed to keep at bay in her late thirties and early forties, would resurface. Moreover, she found that an increasing number of undergraduate and graduate students were requesting time to talk with her about their *big life* decisions. They wanted to divulge their personal struggles, which she often felt ill-equipped to address. Sandra continues to worry about their well-being long after they have completed their program of study.

Sandra adopted three strategies to move forward in a productive and healthy manner. First, she shifted some of her research to be more community-focused so that her job's 40 percent research component would be more meaningful for others and, by extension, for herself. By more consciously engaging in public-facing research, Sandra renewed her desire to produce scholarly material. Second, she chose to talk more openly about mental health issues in the academy to counter the stigma around mental health that persists among faculty. Third, Sandra relies on the Teaching Fellows Program as a safe space to share her challenges and decisions.

Despite these proactive steps to address her mental health concerns, Sandra struggles to accept that she cannot achieve perfection in every, or even any, aspect of her academic life. Her home life suffers when she overcommits to on- and off-campus events, extra committee memberships, and additional mentorship of undergraduate and graduate students. Further, by creating spaces for conversations about mental health within and beyond the classroom, Sandra has found that more students (quite understandably) want to talk with her about their personal adversities. This has, somewhat paradoxically, heightened her pastoral care stress. Increasingly, Sandra has also felt unprepared to appropriately respond to her students' various mental health concerns. Worryingly, during one semester in 2019, six students who were in full crisis and needed immediate professional attention contacted her before seeking support elsewhere. Sandra's Teaching Fellows colleagues have helped her to accept that personal boundaries are necessary, and that she must actively steer students to professional support personnel *before* they reach a crisis point.

Four Themes Emerging from Vignettes

Below, we briefly examine consistent themes in our three vignettes. Though the following discussion is not intended to be a rigorous discursive analysis, the themes distilled from our experiences can be used as conversation prompts for readers interested in developing their own communities of practice or versions of a Teaching Fellows Program at their institutions.

Theme #1: Navigating Boundaries

Faculty members often serve as parental or avuncular/materteral figures and emotionally engage with students beyond their programs' official curriculum. Because we care about our students' mental health and well-being, we sometimes find it difficult to determine where the lines should be drawn in these relationships. In their provocative article, "'Your Professor Will Know You as a Person': Evaluating and Rethinking the Relational Boundaries Between Faculty and Students," Chory and Offstein (2017) critically examine the expectations of students and/or institutional administrations that faculty members will develop ostensibly familial relationships with their students. Similar to Butler's (2017) response to the Chory and Offstein (2017) article, we are concerned that knowing our students on this more intimate level has "become embedded as a psychological contract 'obligation' complete with blurry boundaries and high-stakes outcomes" (Butler 2017, 46). Indeed, this *in loco parentis* has impacted our mental health. Although the traditional academic's role is to ignore one's "human-ness" and to be seen as unbiased and objective, we have experienced how strictly adhering to this role would have potentially risked a student's well-being. In these instances, we have stepped outside our roles as objective and dispassionate professors and into familial support roles that are not universally endorsed or even supported by institutional leadership. The stress of feeling responsible for our students' well-being, while second-guessing our actions and reactions in crisis situations, has affected us on a personal level. The Teaching Fellows Program helps us to talk through our past, current, and future decisions without fear of judgment.

On different occasions during our fellowship tenure, we have asked our peers: At what point should emotionally supporting students and ensuring their welfare take priority over academic protocols? Do you have red lines for what constitutes appropriate engagement with students regarding their mental health and well-being? If you do engage with a student in a personally supportive way, will institutional administration support those decisions? When students need certain types of help, who should we contact? Where can faculty members go for additional support that fits their individual needs? We contend that answers to these questions should be known to all part- and full-time faculty members *prior* to crises arising in order to avoid fear-based decision making.

Theme #2: Care Work

Different intersectional factors, including gender, race, ethnicity, sexual orientation, class, indigeneity, and labor precarity, can impact faculty members' capacity for, and commitment to, care work in the academy (Misra, Lundquist, and Templer 2012; Moore et al. 2010; Victorino, Nylund-Gibson, and Conley 2018). Faculty members educate potentially thousands of students. Many of us worry that we simply cannot *know* even a fraction of these individuals at the level that would allow us to support them beyond a traditional banking model of education. Nevertheless, many of us feel a strong sense of responsibility for student safety and well-being. Care work is thus intimately intertwined with emotional labor, which, as Lawless (2018) describes, includes "demonstrations of sympathy and empathy, one-on-one attention, supportive communication, counseling, general development of personal relationships, and making a person 'feel good'" ([86]; see also Berry and Cassidy 2013; Constanti and Gibbs 2004). These expectations are tremendously time-consuming, emotionally draining, and often require specific training to which few faculty members have been exposed (Lawless 2018).

For this chapter's three authors, the sense of responsibility to engage in emotional labor hits close to home because we each have two children, ranging from four to seventeen years of age. At our Teaching Fellows meetings, we have expressed our hope that when our children are of university age, an authority figure would help look out for their welfare as we have done for others' children. Collectively, we also acknowledge that this care work can cause us emotional distress (Toffoletti and Starr 2016).

Problematically, the angst faculty members can experience is often compounded for those who are precariously employed. For our peers who are first-time teachers in unstable employment situations, who are struggling with mental health, and/or who are members of one or more marginalized demographic, the issues we raise in this chapter can be even more detrimental to their welfare (Berg, Huijbens, and Larsen 2016; Ivancheva, Lynch, and Keating 2019; Watts and Robertson 2011). Further, part-time faculty members may have neither an office space nor a sense of community in their program/school/department. When combined with the common need to teach at more than one institution for financial stability, the lack of an institutional home base interferes with their ability to support themselves and their students. Female faculty particularly tend to be over-represented in precarious academic labor positions (O'Keefe and Courtois 2019). They also usually experience greater student expectations to do emotional labor than their male counterparts and are often not rewarded in promotion and tenure for this outlay of time and energy (El-Alayli et al. 2018; Gonçalves 2019; Henry 2018; Winslow and Davis 2016).

The situation for graduate Teaching Assistants (TAs) is equally fraught, especially given that many TAs are new instructors and often for large first- or second-year undergraduate courses. As graduate students, they may struggle with their own mental health issues (Wedemeyer-Strombel 2019). They are also usually in a vulnerable position as both students and employees of the institution, likely live without financial security, and are often (though not always) relatively young with a dearth of life experience from which to draw. As the first contact for many undergraduates, TAs can witness mental health crises and must navigate how to handle them, where to refer students for assistance in the institution, and how to manage their own self-care as the result of the experience (Broeckelman-Post and Ruiz-Mesa 2018; Evans et al. 2017). The compounding impact on faculty members in this case occurs when undergraduates in these situations contact their TAs, who in turn may have their own mental health challenges and contact their faculty supervisors for assistance.

Theme #3: Lack of Formal Training

Identifying and responding to signs of mental ill-health in students or colleagues is not a regular component of training for graduate students, postdoctoral fellows, or new faculty members. Consequently, individuals who are first points of contact are rarely prepared to respond effectively when crises arise. Even the most effective campus resources for supporting students are only useful inasmuch as faculty members are aware of and know how to access them. Moreover, instructors often do not get a warning that a student is about to disclose a sensitive subject, which adds a layer of complexity for how to appropriately direct a student, especially when those resources remain unknown. Additionally, we cannot require students to take advantage of these supports; we merely provide what we hope is useful information without usually knowing (for privacy reasons) whether they seek professional assistance.

As our vignettes demonstrate, not knowing this information also causes stress for faculty members. Adding to the challenge, many institutions prioritize greater diversity and internationalization of their student body, pursuits we fully endorse. However, the unique needs of an increasingly diverse student population requires appropriate intercultural training, especially about mental health as well as an equally diverse faculty and support staff complement.

Our biggest concern is that, with the increasing population-level prevalence and burden of mental ill-health, coupled with governmental constraints to healthcare and post-secondary funding, the situation on campuses will get worse before it gets better. Although many campuses espouse student wellness, their expectation of faculty members to know what to do, especially in crisis situations, places us in a precarious position if we make the "wrong" decision. As Broeckelman-Post and Ruiz-Mesa (2018) suggest, faculty members should be "trained to watch for symptoms that students might be struggling as well as to gently refer students to campus mental health resources when needed" (97). We encourage taking this one step further by providing opportunities for faculty to develop their competencies in recognizing and responding to signs of mental ill-health in not only their students, but also in their part- and full-time faculty and staff colleagues.

Theme #4: Going against the Grain

This chapter's co-authors have each felt that the more we counsel a student, the less time we have to read, write, apply for grants, prepare lectures, and other compulsory aspects of our jobs. Although we cannot morally turn our backs on any student in need, we are also somewhat sensitive to being labeled as *professors who care*. Our sensitivity stems, in part, from the mixed messaging we receive: On the one hand, we must meet expectations of scholarly productivity, especially in a neoliberal institution that rewards quantifiable research-oriented achievements (i.e., external exigencies). On the other hand, we must support and counsel increasing numbers of students, which we feel is our moral obligation as educators and as individuals (i.e., internal pressures).

Importantly, we know that many of our peers who feel similarly torn between competing external and internal demands experience negative reactions from some colleagues who view care work as pandering to students for better teaching evaluations and/or helping to undermine students' resiliency. Not only are these critiques difficult to accept, if colleagues eschew caring for students' mental health and well-being, then an even greater burden is placed on those of us who take on this work.

Conclusion: Valuing Community and Developing an Action Plan

As this chapter highlights, we see tremendous value in our institution's Teaching Fellows Program as an interdisciplinary and supportive community.

When institutions place greater emphasis on metrics-oriented publishing outputs and grant funding accumulation, teaching seems to be relegated further down the ladder of importance. The program affords us an opportunity to connect with other faculty who value teaching and mentorship, but also an even broader view of wellness and success in the entire academic and lay community.

Much academic literature quite understandably focuses on how established faculty members can mentor emerging colleagues (Ambler, Harvey, and Cahir 2016; Johnson 2015). Arguably, this paternal arrangement presupposes that the former have it *all figured out,* even though faculty burnout is common at all career levels. It is our experience from participating in the Teaching Fellows Program that emerging scholars, and especially those in teaching-intensive streams at the university, bring perspectives and experiences to bear that benefit more established colleagues. Self-reflexively, this chapter's co-authors recognize that we are all in relatively secure academic positions. For obvious reasons, contingent and pre-tenured faculty members may be reluctant to share mental health challenges. However, those in privileged positions may also be hesitant to reveal struggles for fear of appearing as though they are complaining about their jobs, which further stigmatizes voicing mental health concerns or seeking support.

As our primary call to action, we propose that institutions take a proactive approach to ensuring all faculty and staff are equipped to identify and appropriately respond to subtle signs, or outright disclosures, of mental ill-health in their students *and* colleagues. We believe much could be achieved through creating accessible policies and procedures, by offering dedicated training sessions geared toward supporting faculty, and in ensuring that access to the information needed to respond to such disclosures becomes a routine part of new faculty on-boarding. The nature of this information depends on the context of the academic unit. However, *at minimum,* leadership should facilitate discussions with faculty and staff about how to build a culture in which every member of the unit is aware of expectations and feels prepared to be called upon to respond to a student mental health crisis.

Lastly, through the process of writing this chapter, we have shared with one another our respective stories and distilled the themes that emerged from our disparate experiences. This process was valuable in and of itself for our well-being by giving us further permission to talk openly about our mental health. Given this experience, and capitalizing on our Teaching Fellowship Program, we are collectively developing workshops and opportunities for our colleagues to share their struggles with the issues described in this chapter. Our goal is to not only provide additional resources, but to also help destigmatize talking about our mental health and the impact that our students' mental health issues have had on our own well-being.

The environment of Canadian academia is in transition because of shifts in student demographics; expectations of job-oriented experiential learning opportunities; changes to funding models for post-secondary institutions; government expectations of quantitative, corporatized performance metrics; and wide-ranging impacts of the global pandemic. Indeed, it seems clear that the higher education terrain in our country, like elsewhere around the world, will look very different in the next five toten years. We close this chapter by encouraging readers to give themselves permission not to be perfect in this ever-shifting milieu. We must all respect our physical and emotional health by engaging in activities that destigmatize mental ill-health on our campuses.

NOTES

1. This account is presented with permission of the faculty member who shared it.
2. The recent trend in mental health demand is perhaps best exemplified by the *opioid epidemic* that has gripped North America for nearly ten years. As a diagnosable condition, opioid use disorder reached such a crescendo in the latter half of the 2010's that deaths from opioid overdose have been blamed for reducing the average life expectancy of United States citizens (Kochanek, Murphy, Xu, and Arias 2017).
3. *Allostatic load* refers to the cumulative stress on an organism that is simultaneously a driver of adaptation or evolution and also a burden on emotional and physical coping resources to maintain relative *normality*.
4. In this chapter, we adopt the terms *emerging* and *established* rather than *junior* or *senior*, respectively.

REFERENCES

Ambler, Trudy, Marina Harvey, and Jayde Cahir. 2016. "University Academics' Experiences of Learning Through Mentoring." *The Australian Educational Researcher* 43, no. 5: 609–627. https://doi.org/10.1007/s13384-016-0214-7.
American College Health Association. 2018. National College Health Assessment II: Canadian Consortium Executive Summary Spring 2019. Silver Spring, MD: American College Health Association. Accessed November 20, 2019. https://www.acha.org/documents/ncha/NCHA-II_SPRING_2019_CANADIAN_REFERENCE_GROUP_EXECUTIVE_SUMMARY.pdf.
American Psychiatric Association (APA). 2013." Diagnostic and Statistical Manual of Mental Disorders." *BMC Med* 17: 133–137.
Austin, Ann E., and Andrea G. Trice. 2016. "Core Principles for Faculty Models and the Importance of Community." In *Envisioning the Faculty for the Twenty-first Century*, edited by Adrianna Kezar and Daniel Maxey, 58–80. New Brunswick, NJ: Rutgers University Press.

Berg, Lawrence D., Edward H. Huijbens, and Henrik G. Larsen. 2016. "Producing Anxiety in the Neoliberal University." *The Canadian Geographer/Le Géographe Canadien* 60, no. 2: 168–180. https://doi.org/10.1111/cag.12261.

Berry, Karen E., and Simon F. Cassidy. 2013. "Emotional Labour in University Lecturers: Considerations for Higher Education Institutions." *Journal of Curriculum and Teaching* 2, no. 2: 22–36. http://dx.doi.org/10.5430/jct.v2n2p22.

Broeckelman-Post, Melissa A., and Kristina Ruiz-Mesa. 2018. "Best Practices for Training New Communication Graduate Teaching Assistants." *Journal of Communication Pedagogy* 1, no.1: 93–100. https://doi.org/10.31446/JCP.2018.16.

Butler, Deborah. 2017. "On Professional Calling: Rejoinder to 'Your Professor Will Know You as a Person': Evaluating and Rethinking the Relational Boundaries Between Faculty and Students." *Journal of Management Education* 41, no. 1: 46–51. https://doi.org/10.1177/1052562916673864.

Canadian Association of University Teachers (CAUT). 2018. "Shattering Myths about Contract Academic Staff." September 2018. https://www.caut.ca/bulletin/2018/09/shattering-myths-about-contract-academic-staff.

Chory, Rebecca M., and Evan H. Offstein. 2017. "'Your Professor Will Know You as a Person' Evaluating and Rethinking the Relational Boundaries Between Faculty and Students." *Journal of Management Education* 41, no. 1: 9–38. https://doi.org/10.1177/1052562916647986.

Constanti, Panikkos, and Paul Gibbs. 2004. "Higher Education Teachers and Emotional Labour." *International Journal of Educational Management* 18, no. 4: 243–249.

Council of Ontario Universities (COU). 2018. "Faculty at Work: The Composition and Activities of Ontario Universities' Academic Workforce." January 22, 2018. https://cou.on.ca/reports/2018-faculty-at-work/.

El-Alayli, Amani, Ashley A. Hansen-Brown, and Michelle Ceynar. 2018. "Dancing Backwards in High Heels: Female Professors Experience More Work Demands and Special Favor Requests, Particularly from Academically Entitled Students." *Sex Roles* 79, no. 3–4: 136–150. https://doi.org/10.1007/s11199-017-0872-6.

El Hage, Wissam, J. F. Powell, and Simon A. Surguladze. 2009. "Vulnerability to Depression: What is the Role of Stress Genes in Gene × Environment Interaction?" *Psychological Medicine* 39, no. 9: 1407–1411. https://doi.org/10.1017/S0033291709005236.

Evans, Teresa M., Lindsay Bira, Jazmin Beltran Gastelum, L. Todd Weiss, and Nathan L. Vanderford. 2018. "Evidence for a Mental Health Crisis in Graduate Education." *Nature Biotechnology* 36, no. 3: 282–284. https://doi.org/10.1038/nbt.4089.

"Fast Facts about Mental Illness." N.d. Canadian Mental Health Association (CMHA). Accessed December 1, 2019. https://cmha.ca/fast-facts-about-mental-illness.

Gonçalves, Kellie. 2019. "'What Are You Doing Here, I Thought You Had a Kid Now?' The Stigmatisation of Working Mothers in Academia—A Critical Self-Reflective Essay on Gender, Motherhood and the Neoliberal Academy." *Gender & Language* 13, no. 4: 469–487. https://doi.org/10.1558/genl.37573.

Heim, Christine, and Elisabeth B. Binder. 2012. "Current Research Trends in Early Life Stress and Depression: Review of Human Studies on Sensitive Periods, Gene–Environment Interactions, and Epigenetics." *Experimental Neurology* 233, no. 1: 102–111. https://doi.org/10.1016/j.expneurol.2011.10.032.

Ivancheva, Mariya, Kathleen Lynch, and Kathryn Keating. 2019. "Precarity, Gender and Care in the Neoliberal Academy." *Gender, Work & Organization* 26, no. 4 (May): 448–462. https://doi.org/10.1111/gwao.12350.

Johnson, W. Brad. 2015. *On Being a Mentor: A Guide for Higher Education Faculty*. London: Routledge.

Kochanek, Kenneth D., Sherry L. Murphy, Jiaquan Xu, & Elizabeth Arias. "Mortality in the United States, 2016." NCHS Data Brief, no. 293 (2017): 1–8.

Kwan, Matthew Y. W., Kelly P. Arbour-Nicitopoulos, Eric Duku, and Guy Faulkner. 2016. "Patterns of Multiple Health Risk–Behaviours in University Students and Their Association with Mental Health: Application of Latent Class Analysis." *Health Promotion and Chronic Disease Prevention in Canada: Research, Policy and Practice* 36, no. 8: 163–170. https://doi.org/10.24095/hpcdp.36.8.03.

Lawless, Brandi. 2018. "Documenting a Labor of Love: Emotional Labor as Academic Labor." *Review of Communication* 18, no. 2: 85–97. https://doi.org/10.1 080/15358593.2018.1438644.

Misra, Joya, Jennifer H. Lundquist, and Abby I. Temple. 2012. "Gender, Work Time, and Care Responsibilities Among Faculty." *Sociological Forum* 27, no. 2: 300–323. Oxford, UK: Blackwell Publishing Ltd. https://doi.org/10.1111/j.1573-7861.2012.01319.x.

Moore, Helen A., Katherine Acosta, Gary Perry, and Crystal Edwards. 2010. "Splitting the Academy: The Emotions of Intersectionality at Work." *The Sociological Quarterly* 51, no. 2: 179–204. https://doi.org/10.1111/j.1533-8525.2010.01168.x.

Mudrak, Jiri, Katerina Zabrodska, Petr Kveton, Martin Jelinek, Marek Blatny, Iva Solcova, and Katerina Machovcova. 2018. "Occupational Well-Being Among University Faculty: A Job Demands-Resources Model." *Research in Higher Education* 59, no. 3: 325–348. https://doi.org/10.1007/s11162-017-9467-x.

O'Keefe, Theresa, and Aline Courtois. 2019. "'Not One of the Family': Gender and Precarious Work in the Neoliberal University." *Gender, Work & Organization* 26, no. 4: 463–479. https://doi.org/10.1111/gwao.12346.

Peake, Linda J., and Beverley Mullings. 2016. "Critical Reflections on Mental and Emotional Distress in the Academy." *ACME: An International Journal for Critical Geographies* 15, no. 2: 253–284. https://www.acme-journal.org/index.php/acme/article/view/1123.

Polster, Claire. 2016. "Vicious Circle: Academic Insecurity and Privatization in Western Universities." In *Routledge Handbook of the Sociology of Higher Education*, edited by James Coté and Andy Furlong, 94–105. London: Routledge.

Sharif, Afsaneh, Ashley Welsh, Jason Myers, Brian Wilson, Judy Chan, Sunah Cho, and Jeff Miller. 2019. "Faculty Liaisons: An Embedded Approach for Enriching Teaching and Learning in Higher Education." *International Journal for Academic*

Development 24, no. 3: 260–271. https://doi.org/10.1080/1360144X.2019.1584898 .
Sharma, Sumeet, Abigail Powers, Bekh Bradley, and Kerry J. Ressler. 2016. "Gene× Environment Determinants of Stress- and Anxiety-related Disorders." *Annual Review of Psychology* 67: 239–261. https://doi.org/ 10.1146/ annurev-psych-122414-033408.
Surguladze, Simon A. 2009. "Vulnerability to Depression: What Is the Role of Stress Genes in Gene x Environment Interaction?" *Psychological Medicine* 39, no. 9 (2009): 1407–1411. https://doi.org/10.1017/S0033291709005236.
"Teaching Fellows Program." 2019. *Western University*. December 30, 2020. https://teaching.uwo.ca/programs/allprograms/teaching-fellows.html.
Toffoletti, Kim, and Karen Starr. 2016. "Women Academics and Work–Life Balance: Gendered Discourses of Work and Care." *Gender, Work & Organization* 23, no. 5: 489–504. https://doi.org/10.1111/gwao.12133.
Tuck, Eve. 2018. "Biting the University That Feeds Us." In *Dissident Knowledge in Higher Education*, edited by Marc Spooner and James McNinch, 149–167. Regina: University of Regina Press.
Victorino, Christine, Karen Nylund-Gibson, and Sharon Conley. "Prosocial Behavior in the Professoriate: A Multi-level Analysis of Pretenured Faculty Collegiality and Job Satisfaction." *International Journal of Educational Management* 32, no. 5 (2018): 783–798.
Watts, Jessica, and Noelle Robertson. 2011. "Burnout in University Teaching Staff: A Systematic Literature Review." *Educational Research* 53, no. 1: 33–50. https://doi.org/10.1080/00131881.2011.552235.
Wedemeyer-Strombel, Kathryn R. 2019. "Why We Need to Talk More About Mental Health in Graduate School." *The Chronicle of Higher Education*, August 27, 2019. https://www.chronicle.com/article/Why-We-Need-to-Talk-More-About/247002.
Western University. 2018. "Western's Student Mental Health and Wellness Strategic Plan." *Western University*. March 8, 2018. http://studentexperience.uwo.ca/student_experience/strategic_planning/mental_health_strategic_plan/MH_Stratplan_DRAFT.pdf.
Winslow, Sarah, and Shannon N. Davis. 2016. "Gender Inequality across the Academic Life Course." *Sociology Compass* 10, no. 5: 404–416. https://doi.org/10.1111/soc4.12372.

Chapter 12

The Mental Health Impacts of Making a Workers' Compensation Claim for a Mental Injury

Philip Dearman and Beth Edmondson

PART 1—INTRODUCTION

Although universities in Australia and New Zealand promote attention to staff well-being and acknowledge their government-mandated responsibilities for providing safe working environments, many academics still experience workplace mental injuries. Those injuries have been linked to numerous psychosocial work factors, including manageable workloads, sociable work hours, confidence in leadership and management, and satisfaction in work tasks (Richards and McTernan 2014). On these and other potential measures, academics in Australia and New Zealand have been identified as experiencing considerable workplace mental injury risks (NTEU 2018; Sedgwick and Proctor-Thomson 2019). Some academics lodge workers' compensation claims, but many choose not to, or are simply overwhelmed by the prospect of having to prove the specific work-related causes of their injury.

Broadly framed by critical interpretivist approaches to health communication, this chapter considers the relationships between individual academic workers and the organizations that employ them, and the implications of the mandated workers' compensation schemes in Australia and New Zealand (Martin and Nakayama 1999; Zoller and Kline 2008). Adopting a critical perspective, it examines the management and delineation of individual/employee and organizational/employer rights and responsibilities in these workers' compensation governance systems. This takes into account the "human-made systems" of power that underpin universities, models of public and employment health, and the broader roles of governmental regulation of employer–employee relations (Zoller and Kline 2008, 94). The ethnographic elements of our work provide a focus, which would otherwise be lost, for Australian academic workers' personal experiences and observations in navigating their way through complex organizational and policy settings. While the ethnographic dimension of the chapter extends only to Australian academic workers, similarities in workers' compensation legislation in Australia and New Zealand suggest that academics in both countries experience similar obstacles in successfully claiming compensation for workplace mental injuries. In these ways, this chapter reflects upon "connections between local practices and larger systems of power" as structural determinants of workers' compensation claims outcomes for academic workers in Australia and New Zealand (Zoller and Kline 2008, 96).

We consider various workers' compensation systems in Australia and New Zealand in order to explore key factors that shape academic workers' decisions and actions when they experience workplace mental injuries. In these countries, most universities are publicly funded institutions, and in both countries universities are subject to legislation that specify their responsibilities to provide safe working environments for employees. We note the formal aspects of that legislation, and we pay particular attention to the roles of compensation systems as instruments that simultaneously prescribe and proscribe academic workers' rights to protections from mental injuries. We add a focus on the personal circumstances of university workers by including autoethnographic narratives to provide a "thick description" of individual experiences in navigating workers' compensation claims (Geertz 1973, 56). In doing so, this chapter considers the experiences of individuals as situated outcomes of organizational and regulatory contexts.

Academic Workforces in Australia and New Zealand

In 2017, almost a quarter of Australian academics surveyed by the National State of the University Survey (undertaken by National Tertiary Education Union) reported that they worked an average of more than sixty hours per week during a typical teaching week. Less than one-third believed themselves to be treated respectfully by university management (NTEU 2017). Similarly, Sedgwick and Proctor-Thomson's (2019) report on the *2018 State of the Public Tertiary Education Sector Survey* in New Zealand painted a grim picture of academic satisfaction levels. Notably, they reported considerable staff dissatisfaction with reduced autonomy in their work roles, increased workloads, and anxieties regarding "unrealistic expectations from management" (Sedgwick and Proctor-Thomson 2019, 2). Across both countries, academic workers report increasing (and often excessive) workloads and many also identify bullying and discrimination as common experiences in their workplaces. Additionally, Sedgwick and Proctor-Thomson (2020) report that qualitative comments from more than 10 percent of respondents reflected that a "bullying and discriminatory environment is embedded in the tertiary education sector" (2). On average, full-time academic workers in this survey reported working for approximately forty-nine hours per week, and more than half said they felt excluded or ignored in their workplaces (Sedgwick and Proctor-Thomson 2019).

In both Australia and New Zealand, academic workers have in recent years increasingly been held to account for quantified reporting of their work activities. Such measures include, but are not limited to: annual outcomes-focused goals for their teaching, research, scholarship and/or service activities; research productivity measures, whereby past production/output rates determine access to work sanctioned hours available for current or future research activities; and, demands to demonstrate higher than average student evaluations of teaching and curriculum as criteria whereby promotions applications are assessed. Similarly, many universities (or relevant management centers within them) have adopted customized measures of academic work activities, using either numbers of hours per week (or year), or points-based systems of various kinds, whereby tasks such as writing journal articles, supervising PhD students, and conducting lectures or tutorials are equated to specified volumes within their overall workload. Hence, across Australia and New Zealand, academics increasingly demonstrate their knowledge production according to measured outcomes. For many, their eligibility for certain academic roles and opportunities is determined by such performance measurement systems.

Legislated Health Conditions

The Australian Council of Trade Unions (ACTU), Australia's peak trade union body, recently reported that the "most common form of injury at work is a mental health issue caused by the conditions of a person's employment" (ACTU 2019). A number of other studies have reported increased rates of injury compensation claims in Australia for mental health conditions (Brijnath et al. 2014). Despite these claim incidences, relevant scholarly literature, applied research, and governmental data all confirm that workers' compensation claims for mental injuries in Australia and New Zealand have notoriously low rates of success. The rhetoric of "no-fault" insurance that has accompanied the revised versions of workers' compensation since the 1990s has not led to better outcomes for these workers. For example, LaMontagne et al. (2008) found that claims for workers' compensation for mental injuries "were four times more likely to be rejected than other kinds of claims" in workforce groups that included academic workers (190).

We argue that legislation and organizational practices across Australian and New Zealand universities create very real obstacles for many academic workers seeking recognition of their workplace mental injuries and compensation for them. The following sections present a comparative analysis of different legislative contexts in Australia and New Zealand that particularly considers their accessibility and implications for academic mental injury claims, and a set of case studies in the form of snapshots of recent personal observations and experiences. From this data, we draw conclusions regarding the circumstances of injured academic workers. These employees are typically caught up in the details of their injuries, concerned about their recoveries, and trying hard to access medical support and treatment.

Our case studies highlight how, in the midst of juggling immediate demands on their cognitive and emotional skills, as well as organizational and administrative capacities, academic workers are also trying hard to understand the workplace practices and psychosocial/environmental workplace factors that have led to their mental injuries. Their injuries, return to work (RTW) planning, and decisions regarding whether and how to claim workers' compensation inevitably embroil them in new challenging circumstances. As mentally injured workers, when they claim workers' compensation for workplace injuries, they are thrown into complex adversarial processes of documentary investigation, which are set by a variety of legal institutional processes. We argue that these processes can—and often do— present to injured workers as unpredictable and are skewed in favor of their employers. Additionally, these case studies affirm how mentally injured academics who claim worker's compensation experience new imperatives to navigate the entrenched contemporary culture and practices of academic labor. The culture and practices consist of individualized work patterns, a tendency to social isolation, and a sense of taboo and secrecy about the details of their personal lives, especially around mental health.

Organizational Health Communication

Academic workers' experiences reflect other findings of the dosuble-edged impacts of managerial and mandated workplace health promotion programs in emphasizing individual health responsibilities (Zoller 2003). In recent years, universities in Australia and New Zealand (and elsewhere) have implemented numerous policies and programs to promote the health (and well-being) of their workforces (Taylor, Saheb, and Howse 2018; Australian Health Promoting Universities Network 2016; Dooris et al. 2010). Health promotion is not the only form of health communication influencing the psychosocial work contexts experienced by academics, whose professional roles are characterized by mixed experiences of complex interpersonal relationships, implicit and explicit hierarchies, and individual self-reliance for achieving key performance goals/criteria. However, health communication is a key feature of the dialectics of worker-organizational relationships and judgments made regarding performance, productivity satisfaction, and commitment to achieving university goals (O'Brien and Guiney 2018; Zoller 2003; Taylor, Saheb, and Howse 2018).

Indeed, health communication and health promotion within universities remind academic workers that university management has power to intervene in their private decision making and their workplace conduct. Sherry (2013) has astutely observed that academics "cannot truly separate our personal lives from our work" (283). In various ways, academic workers are reminded that they are individually accountable and morally responsible for cultivating and maintaining both physical and mental health. Some university health promotion undertakings (and workplace policies and procedures that embed these as elements of psychosocial work conditions) also serve to remind academics of their social positions as leaders or intellectuals whose work carries moral responsibilities and social obligations for improving the societies in which they live and work (Zoller 2003; Hanawa et al. 2015; Taylor, Saheb, and Howse 2018; Watts and Robertson 2011; O'Brien and Guiney 2018).

In examining academic workers' experiences of workplace mental injuries, we draw on Gill's (2009) argument that mental injuries—and workers' compensation claims arising from them—are both highly personal (and often secret) experiences for academics, as well as being emblematic of broader organizational, sectoral, and governmental policies, procedures, and regulations. In setting out the limits of action specified by legislation, and through the detail of our ethnographic snapshots, we consider the broad structural possibilities established by legal/policy frameworks, as well as the local personal circumstances that we and our colleagues confront in our workplaces. In doing so, we seek to provide new insights into the emotionality of the stresses and strains involved in mental injury claims, and the compounding impact these can have on the outcome of a claims process.

PART 2—CONTEXT

In this chapter, we bring perspectives from our combined work experiences (more than fifty years) in seven universities across three Australian states. In our respective workplaces and academic roles, we have witnessed significant changes in academic workforces and in the broader economic and social contexts of Australian universities. We have felt first-hand the force of the expectation that academic workers diversify their skills and intensify their demonstrated performances. We have seen how this has unfolded through a flood of positive incitements about, for example, collaboration and innovation in both teaching and research, and through a collection of increasingly parsimonious criteria used to measure "outcomes" and "outputs."

Although the following list is far from exhaustive, some key changes we have witnessed (and of which we have experienced the impact) include:

- Increased casualization and reduced employment security among ongoing academic workers (Sedgwick and Proctor-Thomson 2019; NTEU 2018)
- Massification of university education, pressures to teach increased numbers of students, and increased pressures to attract/successfully teach fee-paying (international) students (Watts and Robertson 2011; Gill 2009)
- Corporatisation of university management, and management practices, and marketization of student recruitment and reputation management (Kenny 2018; Gill 2009)
- Increased quantification of research productivity and performance measures (Kenny 2018; Sedgwick and Proctor-Thomson 2019; NTEU 2018)
- An intensification of work routines, including through the development of mixed-mode "delivery systems," and increased average working hours among ongoing academics (Kenny 2018; Sedgwick and Proctor-Thomson 2019; NTEU 2018; Gill 2009; Watts and Robertson 2011).

These changes are not the sole contributors to increased workplace stress felt by academics, but they have been identified as influential contributors to increasing levels of workplace dysfunction (see Kenny 2018, 366). They have also been the objects of innumerable conversations in tea rooms, office doorways, and corridors, as we and our colleagues navigate the changing expectations. In these conversations and in meetings of various kinds outlining the next new policy, procedure, guideline, organizational change, strategic direction, or workload realignment, we have often reflected on the various institutional responses to the widely circulating stories about problems in the mental health of working populations. We have noted, too, research indicating that when universities engage in staff health promotion endeavors, they often do so to preserve productivity or limit flow on impacts for students (Watts and Robertson 2011; Taylor, Saheb, and Howse 2019). Even as Australian and New Zealand universities have acknowledged their roles as leaders in health communication and health promotion, their policies and practices have not always reflected such leadership. As noted by Taylor, Saheb, and Howse (2019), "staff health" is not generally approached using "whole-of setting or system" models (287).

Media and Health Communication

The news media has increasingly covered mental health as a public health issue, reporting on— for example—government commissions of inquiry and publishing stories about high-profile public figures (including politicians, actors, and athletes) outing themselves as suffering mental injuries (Roberts 2017; Smith 2010; Caldwell 2018; Pickstar Blog 2018). Additionally, in 2019, New Zealand's government "attracted widespread praise" for introducing what was described as "a 'world first' wellbeing budget" (Roy 2019). In both Australia and New Zealand, governments and employers have responded through different programs, such as by updating legislation on workplace bullying, formulating policies and procedures for notifying hazards, and responding to the country's national suicide crisis. Between July 2018 and June 2019, 685 suicide deaths were recorded in New Zealand, becoming the "highest since recording began" (Henry 2019). The Australian Black Dog Institute has reported that "more than 3000 Australians died by suicide in 2017" and "65000 Australians make a suicide attempt" (Black Dog Institute 2020). In New Zealand, WorkSafe/Mahi Haumaru Aotorea (2020) reported a workplace bullying incidence rate of between one in five and one in three workers and also provides mechanisms whereby workers can directly report their experiences. Notably, other researchers have found that 65.3 percent of academic staff in New Zealand experience workplace bullying at their current university (Raskauskas and Skrabec 2011).

Experiential Challenges

Our experiences, and the perspective we have derived through witnessing many other people's experiences, suggest that the best intentions behind the increased apparent mental health protections are often derailed by the substantive workplace activities required of academic workers by their employers, and by the performance/productivity expectations associated with them. We have known many academics who have experienced mental health challenges (and mental injuries) in their workplaces. Indeed, we have experienced our own workplace mental injuries. Some of the injuries experienced by our colleagues have been recognized as having been caused directly by the workplaces in which they occurred. Sometimes, our colleagues have reported their injuries, and their reports have led to successful workers' compensation claims for insured periods of sick leave and some paid medical treatment. Sometimes, our colleagues have chosen not to report their injuries. Sometimes, we have made the same choices. Sometimes, we, and colleagues we have known, have been "in denial" about the symptoms of injury, and have been so unwell that we were unable to process a clear path through the available options. Sometimes, claims have been made, but our employers have refused them, or they have failed the necessary proof tests demanded by workers' compensation schemes, with considerable consequences for some claimants.

The situations we and our colleagues have found ourselves in have been partly determined by wider legal and contextual frameworks, including the legislative and regulatory settings and structures associated with workers' compensation in Australia and New Zealand. The following section examines these settings and structures in detail. Along with emergent university-focused health communication models and workplace health promotion practices, these settings and structures influence "intersections between professional and personal roles and identities" such that academic workers have become subject to "new relational fluidities between the public and private spheres that we inhabit" (Edmondson 2020, 332).

PART 3—LEGISLATIVE FRAMEWORKS

Across Australia's federated systems of government, ten key workers' compensation acts regulate insurance provisions for workers. Academic workers are covered by eight state- and territory-based workers' compensation acts and insurance frameworks. New Zealand has a unified national workers' compensation approach. In all jurisdictions in Australia and New Zealand, the legislation provides a framework for establishing eligibility to receive compensation for a work-related injury.

Across Australia and New Zealand, different jurisdictions recognize, in slightly different ways, that psychological or mental injuries arising from the "significant, material, substantial" or "major contributing factor" of employment are "compensable" injuries (SafeWork Australia 2019; WorkSafe/Mahi Haumaru Aotorea 2020). Possible compensation for injury is one aspect of the legislation and employment policies applied in these jurisdictions. Alongside these are broadly common goals of ensuring "the safe, timely and durable return to work," which provides a dominant cultural frame that structures the limits of agency (and control over individual psychosocial factors) that workers with mental injuries can have as they navigate claims processes *and at the same time* seek to recover from their injuries (Wyatt, Cotton, and Lane 2017).

Those legislative frameworks, and the policies and procedures used to enact them, can create onerous thresholds that obfuscate the realities of mental injuries arising from workplace relations and work practices. Problematically, the compensation approaches used in Australia privilege critical incidents as injurious moments. In doing so, they underscore historical models that recognized workplace health and safety responsibilities for physical health and well-being, but did not appropriately consider mental health and mental injuries. In the context of Australian universities, these settings exacerbate the effects of workplace policies, procedures, and practices that cause mental injuries for significant numbers of staff.

In theory, by at least recognizing workplace mental injuries as compensable, workers' compensation legislation establishes the grounds for ascribing equal importance to mental and physical health. However, across Australian jurisdictions, their reliance on specific critical incidents or identified time-specified injurious moments effectively ignores the fact that many mental injuries occur over time through accumulated experiences, including through work-related stress, and through multiple changes in work practices, organizational structures, and systems for managing workloads.

In such reliance, they fail to recognize that universities routinely engage in practices that adversely affect the health of many staff—even as they apparently promote new health and well-being policies, procedures, and practices. Although outside the central focus of this chapter, it is nevertheless worth noting that, in some instances, the very policies and procedures that universities develop and implement mirror broader tendencies to make individual workers responsible for their own mental health (see Richards and Bailey 2014). Arguably, the proliferation of short-term mental health support through employer funded counseling programs falls into this category. These institutional and sectoral practices might contribute to under-reporting of workplace mental injuries, especially because workers' compensation regulations in Australia and New Zealand require that claimants carry a burden of proof in providing firm evidence that their injuries occurred in their workplace.

As can be seen in Figure 12.1 below, the legislative frameworks used in Australia and New Zealand establish different parameters for compensating workers and supporting their recoveries following workplace mental injuries. As noted above, common across them is recognition that workplace injuries to mental health can and do occur. However, they use different injury reporting and evaluation processes, set different injury thresholds, and follow different prescribed claims processes. As shown in Figure 12.1, workers in New Zealand simultaneously report their mental injury and claim compensation for both their absence from work and their recommended treatment plan when they first seek medical treatment. Their treating doctor completes and submits the relevant documentation to initiate a workers' compensation claim. The documents become the basis of the relevant insurance claim. Across Australia, more complex claims processes pertain, with more onerous obligations and intrusive process for injured workers to prove the validity of their claims.

Across Australia and New Zealand, workers' compensation legislative frameworks also restrict the types of injuries that are permissible for mental injury claims. These restrictions arise from the regulatory definitions regarding mental injuries: the limits and thresholds that are set, and the approvals and investigations processes associated with them. Many

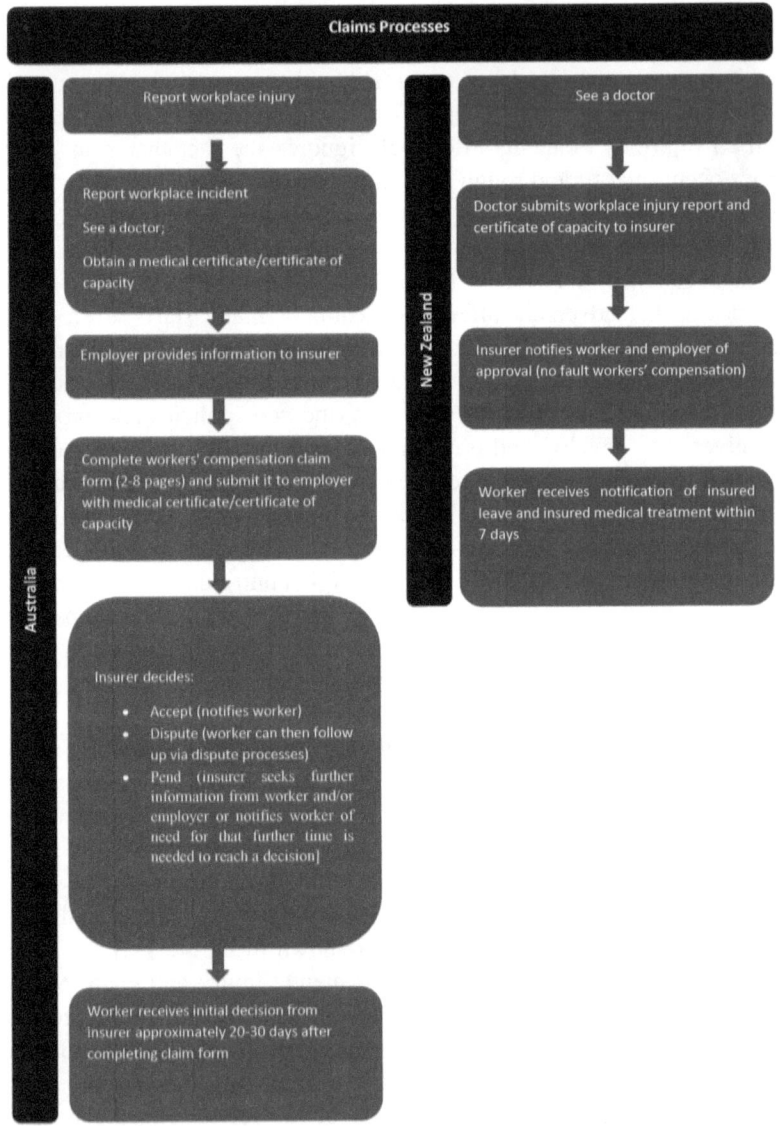

Figure 12.1 Navigating Workplace Mental Injury Claims in Australia and New Zealand.

injury-causing behaviors and practices that are expressly precluded by workers' compensation legislation across Australia and New Zealand have previously been identified as key sources of workplace stress among academics. For instance, management decisions requiring staff relocation, organizational restructuring, performance management practices, and unsuccessful applications for promotion or leadership opportunities are all identified exclusions under current workers' compensation regulations. However, these have also been identified as key causes of academic workplace stress, and some have also been identified as factors in workplace experiences of bullying among academic workers (Watts and Robertson 2011; Raskauskas and Skrabec 2011). As shown in Table 12.1 below, several exclusions in workers' compensation legislation across Australian and New Zealand jurisdictions pertain to management practices and changes in work roles/functions that pose foreseeable, potential mental health risks among academic workforces.

Across Australian and New Zealand jurisdictions, the possibility that mental injuries arise from accumulated workplace stress is universally precluded. Specifically, this means that the possibility of making a successful claim in respect of a mental injury arising from accumulated workplace stress is limited by a range of disallowances that constitute "get out of jail free" clauses embedded in legislation (as outlined in Table 12.1). In each jurisdiction, legislation limits workplace mental injuries to those arising from specific identified events, and some restrict these to traumatic incidents. This is most explicit in New Zealand's requirement that workers reporting a workplace mental injury must have been directly involved or have closely witnessed a traumatic event. Australian jurisdictions also distinguish between mental injuries caused by such events (in other words, defined as a time-bound incident) and those caused by working in workplaces where workloads, management decisions, or employer behaviors lead to mental injuries.

In each jurisdiction, workers face very real challenges in proving that their mental injuries have been directly caused by an event or events in their workplace. They must be able to directly link their mental injury with a workplace incident or traumatic event and be able to exclude other potential contributing factors from outside their workplace. These workers' compensation frameworks therefore create very real obstacles for many academic workers who experience workplace mental injuries, most especially when their injuries result from work-related stress. They face acute challenges in meeting the mandated requirements of proving direct workplace responsibilities for mental injuries. Workers' compensation settings for academic workers in Australia and New Zealand would be significantly improved by amending these regulatory requirements to better acknowledge the likelihood that many workplace mental injuries occur through ongoing work stresses, such as escalating workload or performance expectations, changed work settings, or ongoing bullying practices that do not culminate in a major reported incident. Some research has also suggested that the recent formation of university health promotion networks in Australia and New Zealand, through initiatives such as the Australian Health Promoting Universities Network (APHUN) and Tertiary Wellbeing Aotearoa New Zealand (TWANZ), might also increase

Table 12.1 Jurisdictional Mental Injury Disallowances

Victoria	*Workplace Injury Rehabilitation and Compensation Act 2013*	Disallowance of mental injuries caused by reasonable management actions
New South Wales	*Workplace Injury Management and Workers Compensation Act 1998*	Disallowance of mental injuries arising as a consequence of/secondary to physical injuries Focus on permanent impairment of at least 15 percent (lump sum compensation requires 20 percent or more of permanent impairment)
Queensland	*Workers' Compensation and Rehabilitation Act 2003*	Disallowance of mental injuries caused by reasonable management actions including transfer, demote, discipline, redeploy, retrench, or dismiss the worker or decision not to award promotion, reclassification, or leave of absence Employment as "the major significant contributing factor" for psychiatric or psychological disorders
Western Australia	*Workers' Compensation and Injury Management Act 1981*	Disallowance of mental injuries caused by reasonable management actions including transfer, demote, discipline, redeploy, retrench, or dismiss the worker or decision not to award promotion, reclassification, or leave of absence Recognizes that mental injuries can be associated with either sudden or gradual development, but does not include stress unless it arises from "unreasonable and harsh" actions by an employer
South Australia	*Return to Work Corporation of South Australia Act 1994 & Return to Work Act 1994*	Disallowance of mental injuries caused by reasonable management actions including transfer, demote, counsel, discipline, redeploy, retrench, or dismiss the worker or decision not to award promotion, reclassification, or leave of absence, decision not to renew or extend a contract Distinguishes between mental injuries and psychiatric injuries

Jurisdiction	Act	Disallowance/Recognition details	Further details
Tasmania	Workers Rehabilitation and Compensation Act 1988	Disallowance of mental injuries ("an illness or disorder of the mind") caused by reasonable management actions including transfer, demote, counsel, discipline, redeploy, retrench, or dismiss the worker or decision not to award promotion, reclassification, or leave of absence	Recognizes post-traumatic stress disorder when confirmed by medical diagnosis linking condition with workplace trauma
Northern Territory	Return to Work Act 1986	Disallowance of mental injuries caused by reasonable management actions including transfer, training, demote, discipline, redeploy, retrench, or dismiss the worker or decision not to award promotion, reclassification, or leave of absence or communication in connection with these matters	Recognizes mental stress as "anxiety, depression or other mental condition that affects a person's psychological, emotional or physical wellbeing"
Australian Capital Territory	Workers Compensation Act 1951	Disallowance of mental injury (including stress) caused by reasonable action taken or proposed to be taken by an employer in relation to transfer, demotion, promotion, performance appraisal, discipline, retrenchment or dismissal, or in relation to the provision of employment benefits	Recognizes stress as mental injury
New Zealand	Accident Compensation Act 2001	Disallows mental injuries caused by a gradual process	Recognizes work-related mental injuries caused by a single event that "could reasonably be expected to cause mental injury to people generally." Also recognizes mental injuries caused by physical injuries. Cover applies to all workers experiencing injuries in New Zealand and also to all New Zealand residents who experience injuries outside of New Zealand on or after October 1, 2008

sectoral recognition of inadequacies in current workplace mental injury protections (Taylor, Saheb, and Howse 2017).

Jurisdictional Disadvantages

Academic workers disadvantaged by current limits include: people who have previously reported a pre-existing mental injury or medical condition relating to their mental health; those who have previously taken periods of personal leave or told their employer of stressful or traumatic events occurring outside of their workplaces; and people who have previously experienced a workplace mental injury or workplace stress.

Although workers' compensation legislation across Australia and New Zealand recognize that workplace injuries might be caused by events or incidents that aggravate pre-existing medical conditions, they also simultaneously require proof that workplace events/incidents are the primary or sole aggravating factors. These conditions restrict the likelihood of achieving successful claims for academics who have previously provided their employers with knowledge of external factors, such as life events that foreseeably might have affected their mental health at key points in the past. For instance, as outlined in some of the following case studies, workers who take periods of personal leave while experiencing grief-related depression might later find this information used as evidence of a pre-existing non-work–related medical condition or injury. Further, in some jurisdictions, workers' compensation legislation restricts workers' capacities to claim compensation for mental injuries that are caused by physical injuries that occurred in the workplace.

When internal university procedures and policies have been successfully used to recognize employer responsibility—such as in recognizing bullying behavior in the workplace or a confirmed breach of a university procedure/policy—academics have successfully identified a "critical incident" of the kind required by workers' compensation frameworks. Both our and our colleagues' experiences suggest that having previously gained university recognition of workplace bullying can improve the prospects of success in subsequent workers' compensation claims. However, many academics report low levels of confidence in their universities' responses to workplace bullying reports, and some forms of bullying remain outside the scope of bullying policies and procedures (Raskauskas and Skrabec 2011). In Raskauska and Skrabec's (2011) illuminating study of university workplace bullying in New Zealand, 45.6 percent of participants "said that nothing happened as a result of reporting" (26). Other studies of academic work–related mental health and workplace experiences have identified links between bullying, occupational stress, and worker burnout (Watts and Robertson 2011).

Across Australia and New Zealand, workers' compensation legislation universally requires workers to prove their injuries occurred as a direct result of one or more specific incidents. This is problematic for university workers whose employment settings are likely to expose them to slow-burn mental injuries arising from "more subtle" workplace behaviors, such as feeling belittled by colleagues and supervisors, experiencing overwork, or shifting deadlines (Raskauskas and Skrabec 2011). Without a clear reportable incident (that has been duly recognized by the university as an event of such nature), academic workers are unlikely to successfully claim workers' compensation for mental injuries caused by workplace stress. The requirement to provide direct proof of a specific injury-causing incident as validity tests for workers' compensation claims creates "get out of jail free" clauses for universities. These workers' compensation frameworks significantly restrict the abilities of academic workers to claim compensation, especially paid medical leave and treatments, for the mental injuries that arise from shifting work roles, increasing performance expectations, repeated university organizational restructuring, increasing workloads, changed reporting lines, and increasing productivity and performance monitoring.

PART 4—LOCAL/PERSONAL EXPERIENCES: ILLUSTRATIVE SNAPSHOTS

How, then, can affected workers navigate these obstacles? What options do they have? What factors affect a reasonable outcome of making a claim for a mental injury? We attempt to answer these questions by briefly summarizing observations derived from local, personal experiences, and a series of snapshots of individual cases.

This combined ethnographic/autoethnographic approach engages with worker-agency-organizational dimensions of workplace mental injuries and the associated workers' compensation claims management processes. This enables an examination of how the stages of making workers' compensation claims—and the health communications approaches associated with their legislative settings—frame claimants' identities and influence the outcomes of their claims. Our observations indicate that these intersect with university policies of various kinds, including staff health and well-being, complex management, workload monitoring, and performance measuring practices. Collectively, these factors lead to under-reporting of workplace mental injuries, and even lower levels of claims for workers' compensation. As shown in Table X.2 below, among these academics, taking periods of personal leave was much more commonly chosen over submitting workers' compensation claims following workplace mental injuries.

Academic staff who experience workplace mental injuries are often reluctant to initiate a claim for worker's compensation. During periods of managing staff, we have often heard colleagues express concerns that they might later be perceived as weak, or alternatively as trouble-making, if they report their mental injuries or even the events/experiences that might contribute to them. Their concerns have also been reflected by other academics in other studies (O'Brien and Guiney 2018). The health promotion and health communication roles of universities, and the skilled professionalism of academic workforces, create complex intersectional dynamics for Australian and New Zealand academics (Taylor, Saheb, and Howse 2018). It seems that few staff are prepared to report workplace mental injuries and, instead, many choose to take periods of personal leave. Whether these injuries arise from work overload, bullying, or harassment by peers or supervisors, unpredictable work tasks, or job insecurity seems to make little difference. Indeed, as Table 12.2 shows, in approximately two-thirds of the mental injury cases we have observed, staff took periods of personal leave, although their cases might legitimately have led to workers' compensation claims. Similarly, staff who have experienced a physical injury (including those who successfully claim worker's compensation for such an injury) are often reluctant to include associated/correlated mental injuries in their reporting and/or claims.

Our experiences and observations suggest that, in many cases, medical practitioners play influential roles in determining whether or not academics report their mental injuries to their employers, submit claims for workers' compensation, take periods of sick leave (either as insured leave or as personal leave), and request RTW plans. In the cases we have followed, medical practitioners often encourage academic workers to avoid the stressful experiences of making such claims. As these practitioners point out, the use of personal leave averts the immediate challenges of navigating demanding claims

Table 12.2 Unreported Mental Injuries

Total number of individuals taking periods of personal leave for workplace mental injuries (instead of workers' compensation claims)	30*
Pre-existing physical conditions aggravated by workplace events (secondary mental injuries)	6
Pre-existing mental health conditions aggravated by workplace events	8
Changing work roles	16
Uninvestigated workplace bullying (by senior managers)	15
Uninvestigated breaches of formal workplace procedures as cause of mental injury	11
Uninvestigated breaches of normal workplace practices and processes as cause of mental injury	6
Increasing or unmanageable workloads as cause of mental injury	22

* Includes three staff members who also took a separate period of approved workers' compensation leave

lodgment processes. This course of action protects workers from ongoing repercussions in their workplaces following their return to work.

To Claim, or Not to Claim?

What reasons have our colleagues offered, in their thinking about why not to report or claim? At best, many believe their careers would experience short-term setbacks. At worst, others fear that reporting a workplace mental injury will mark the beginning of their career's end. In countless conversations with our colleagues and staff we have managed, and in meetings of various kinds in our workplaces, staff have often expressed low levels of confidence in the policies, procedures, and processes surrounding mental injury reporting, treatment, support, and RTW, both within their universities and in jurisdictional settings. This pattern of reluctance to report, and mistrust toward achieving a positive long-term outcome, was apparent even when the circumstances in which our colleagues had sustained their workplace mental injuries met workers' compensation claims criteria.

Our direct experiences of working with academics who have successfully sought workers' compensation for workplace mental injuries are limited to seven instances, all of them within Victoria (see Table 12.3 below). Six of these claims were lodged by staff who experienced harassment or bullying. In each instance of a successful claim, individual academic workers were provided with periods of paid absence, medical services, and tailored RTW plans. In an additional instance, the academic worker abandoned their application approximately one month after lodging it. Although their Employee Assistance Program (EAP) provided a psychologist who supported their claim, the staff member believed that their career trajectory might be set back by the ripples created by following through with investigating their injuries. In the seventh instance, an academic who had previously received

Table 12.3 Successful Workers' Compensation Claims by Colleagues

Total number of successful claims	7
Successful claims where pre-existing physical conditions had been aggravated	2
Mental injury/ies arising from critical incident	1
Physical workplace injury with secondary mental injury	1
Investigated confirmed workplace bullying identified as cause of mental injury	5
Investigated confirmed breach of formal workplace procedures as cause of mental injury	1
Investigated confirmed breach of normal workplace practices and processes as cause of mental injury	3
Mental injury circumstances being focus of internal workplace investigations (in addition to workers' compensation investigation)	6

workers' compensation for a workplace physical injury subsequently submitted a workplace mental injury during their approved period of paid absence.

In both Australia and New Zealand, it is common for university workers to be eligible for three to four paid sessions per year with an approved psychologist. Typically, these services are accessed by registering with the EAP provider nominated by their university. Workers can do so without reporting either the nature of their service need or the forms of support received. Both the identities of staff using these services and the details of their support requests remain confidential. Although limited, providing these opportunities for staff to access employer paid medical care is an important pillar in universities' health promotion status.

Our experiences also suggest that, even when academic workers successfully claim workers' compensation for workplace mental injuries, they do not always recover from their injuries within the insured time period. Even after an approved period of insured work absence, numerous colleagues required further personal leave absences to support their continued recoveries. Additionally, we have also observed that our colleagues have not always experienced supportive work settings upon their RTW, in spite of the raft of policies and procedures that might claim to ensure this occurs.

In reflecting on these experiences, we have realized how many of our colleagues have stopped working as academics after periods of insured sick leave for workplace mental injuries. In each of these cases, recovered/recovering workers have returned to their roles for periods of time (usually six months to two years) before resigning or taking early retirement. In each of these cases, they expressed disappointment that the structural factors, work practices, and shifting measures of work performance that contributed to their initial mental injury remained unresolved in their workplaces. In short, they each formed the view that their workplace had not learned from their injuries or modified their practices to ensure that they (and others) were now better protected from future mental injuries.

As case studies, these accounts provide snapshots of individuals' experiences, creating a composite narrative regarding broader sectoral patterns to provide insights into health communication practices and their consequences (Bosticco and Thompson 2008). We share the view of Crowe et al. (2011) that case studies are especially "useful to employ when there is a need to obtain an in-depth appreciation of an issue, event or phenomenon of interest, in its natural real-life context" (1). Numerous other studies validate the benefits of learning from the workplace and health experiences of individuals (Kidd et al. 2016; Moll 2014; Mental Health Commission of Canada 2017). Some studies also suggest that case studies highlight often neglected considerations of potential workplace mental injuries for academics (Sherry 2013).

Snapshots of Workers' Compensation Claims

In the following snapshots, names have been coded to protect identities, and gender is presented in the neutral form "they."

1. An injury arising out of bullying

WG was a junior academic who carried a heavy teaching and curriculum development load while on probation with a probationary condition of completing a PhD within three years. In brief, after two years of working with limited peer support and supervision, WG notified the university grievance office that they were being bullied by their disciplinary supervisor.

In their claim, they outlined a pattern of erratic work supervision, escalating and often unreasonable work demands, and multiple breaches of relevant university policies and procedures. This bullying claim was not fully investigated or resolved because the disciplinary supervisor departed the university before it was completed. By this time, however, WG's mental and physical health had deteriorated and progress toward PhD completion had stalled. With support from the head of department, WG took a three-month medical leave of absence from PhD candidature and accepted an extension to their initial employment probationary period.

Several months later, WG's physical and mental health further deteriorated, necessitating an extended period of leave. Following a diagnosis of chronic fatigue syndrome, the psychologist they had been consulting since the earlier period of workplace bullying supported WG's application submission for Workcover-funded medical leave. WG's PhD supervisor was called to meet with investigating team members on two occasions. They were asked to provide details of earlier meetings with WG, any notes they had taken or emails received in which WG had reported problematic work experiences, or in which they had noted concerns about WG's health or work conditions. Fortunately, they had plenty of information to share with the investigators.

WG's claim for funded medical leave was successful, and they were absent from work for approximately five months before commencing a staged RTW plan. Again, the PhD supervisor was asked to participate in these formally mandated RTW planning discussions. The university's RTW officer took care to ensure that WG's return-to-work commitments would provide intrinsic rewards, measurable outputs, and opportunities to re-engage with supportive colleagues. Following medical advice and supported by Workcover, WG initially returned to work for six hours per week, engaging in work activities for two hours per day, three days per week. After two to three months, these hours increased to ten hours per week.

Over several months during this period, WG's physical health issues became increasingly complex. Ultimately, medical practitioners could no longer directly connect their ongoing health problems with the initial workplace injury. After more than a year and a half of Workcover-supported medical leave, WG was not yet fit to return to full-time work. In the months that followed the cessation of Workcover-funded medical leave, WG's accumulated personal leave was expended. Their mental health also declined during this time. They were acutely aware of their precarious finances and protracted health recovery period. Some months later, WG committed suicide.

2. An injury arising out of breaches of policies and procedures

This successful claim arose from breaches of academic promotion policies and procedures that caused a senior academic, BG, to experience a mental injury. These events, together with an earlier unsuccessful application for a sabbatical, provided the basis of a staff grievance against senior university management.

BG was fully absent from the university on Workcover-funded medical leave for approximately seven months. At the end of that period, they returned to work at a reduced fraction (0.7) for a further two months, enabling resumption of research and postgraduate supervision activities (which accounted for 0.5 of their work allocation), and a progressive return to program coordination at a reduced level (0.2).

Three months after resuming full-time work, BG commenced an extended period (seven months) of long service leave. Subsequent to their return, conflicts arose between them and other members of their disciplinary team. Mediation did not improve these relationships and, within two weeks, BG commenced a period of sick leave. After an absence of approximately nine months, they departed the university.

3. An injury arising from a critical incident

AB was an early-career staff member who submitted a claim for workers' compensation medical leave following a series of experiences in which an aggrieved senior colleague expressed anger and displayed threatening behavior. The EAP psychologist who was consulted by staff members in the midst of this distressing situation supported this claim.

AB was able to show they had experienced a workplace mental injury arising from a series of emails, received over a two-day period, which showed escalating expressions of aggression by the colleague. In addition, they were also able to provide evidence of threatening text messages sent to their mobile phone from this same colleague.

4. A mental health injury arising from a physical injury

SG experienced multiple physical injuries in a workplace accident. At the time of writing, approximately fifteen months after the incident, SG continues to require modifications to their normal work role alongside physio and occupational therapies. The nature of SG's injuries, and the close presence of others who witnessed the incident, readily enabled them to submit a claim for workers' compensation-approved sick leave.

After being absent from work for about two months, SG's mental health began to be affected by a sense of isolation and the realization that recovery from the physical injuries would involve a protracted time period, and ongoing and time-consuming treatments. At a planned medical review, SG's general practitioner (GP) added a mental health plan to the overall treatment plan and supported the staff member in claiming workers' compensation funding for consultations with a psychologist. This claim was accompanied by the GP's request to add treatment/consultation with an occupational therapist to assist SG with adjustments and modifications to routine activities. SG's GP clearly outlined links between the physical injuries suffered, their long-term nature, and impacts upon SG's mobility and mental health. Funding for consultations with a psychologist was subsequently provided for the remaining period of SG's full absence from work and also for the first three months following their return to work.

SG's initial RTW plan involved working for two hours per day over two days per week, with monthly reviews to consider adjustments. After two months of working four hours per week, SG's RTW plan was amended to two hours per day for three days per week, before increasing to three hours per day for three days per week. In these early RTW plans, numerous activities were proscribed, which took into account SG's mental and physical health. Subsequent incremental adjustments have been made such that, after more than a year since the initial injuries, SG's RTW enables them to work for five hours per day for three days per week.

From our experiences, and on the basis of what we have witnessed among our colleagues, it seems clear that deciding to take a period of leave to recover from a workplace mental health injury involves a series of decisions that can be difficult to navigate. Some of these decision making demands tap into the personal emotional and interpersonal aspects of academic professional competencies. Our observations suggest that academics who take leave to recover and seek treatment for workplace mental injuries are likely to experience new stresses as they do so. In light of studies that examine some of the causal links and interplay between these factors in other workforces with high incidences of mental injuries (Varker et al. 2018), we suggest that academic workers have similar experiences.

We are persuaded that all workplace mental injuries bring new exposures to foreseeably stressful experiences, whether involving workers' compensation claims or not. Our experiences and observations of others also suggest that claiming workers' compensation for workplace mental injuries leads to increased stresses because of the processes involved in making these claims–processes, which are inquisitorial, invasive, and often adversarial. At a time of elevated mental and emotional stress, and distress, claimants are required to use high-level interpersonal communication, self-comportment, organizational, and administrative skills.

The following snapshot considers reasons why workers' compensation claims processes bring new experiences of stress for workers with mental injuries. This snapshot of a claim that was refused also outlines how investigations of a claim, and subsequent conciliation processes available to the worker after refusal of the claim, can continually affect individual workers, with potential emotional/psychosocial impacts, too, for their managers and colleagues.

5. A case of unrecognized burnout, compounded by "reasonable management action"

Following an unsuccessful application for promotion, DC sought medical attention for the workplace mental injuries they had experienced as a result of this surprising outcome, poor communication processes, and protracted timeframes. Their supervisor and colleagues had encouraged them to apply for promotion. In their views, DC had already been performing beyond the expected performance thresholds for their academic level, and their roles, responsibilities, and achievements as a manager of others also reflected this. Their referees underscored these views as well.

More than three months after submitting this application, DC received a brief email notifying them it had not been successful. They felt overwhelmed by anger, shame, and anxiety. In a state of distress, they packed up their half-eaten lunch and work bag and walked home. Some weeks later, they realized that their response was triggered not only by the email, but also by a gradual descent into depression caused by burnout. The email was described subsequently as the critical incident in workers' compensation documents. DC understood this was a consequence of the manner in which the legislation was enacted through the form they and their GP filled out, but this only added to their distress.

Early the following week, DC consulted their GP, explaining they were overcome with stress at work and needed a week of personal leave. The GP agreed and provided a medical certificate to support that leave period. During that week DC sought written feedback from the promotions committee. Ultimately, they learned that the committee had not prepared written notes or feedback, just some numeric scores, and the task of providing written feedback rested with the committee chair who was now overseas and unable to meet this request for approximately two months.

As DC puts it, they "steadied [themselves] and returned to work the following week." Over subsequent weeks, they could not resolve the dissonance they experienced as they tried to reconcile the harmful effects of this institutional process with the kindness and support of colleagues. At this point, they were still not clear that they were experiencing burnout and falling into depression. They again consulted with their GP, who urged them to take an extended period of leave and lodge a compensation claim because, in their view, "Everything you're telling me says your work is hurting you."

Subsequently, DC submitted a Workcover claim, with an accompanying certificate of capacity. Realizing they did not understand the claims process, DC sought advice from their union representative, who explained that an investigation would be undertaken to consider the circumstances of the injury, its nature, and its impact upon the worker's capacities. This investigation would include an examination by an independent psychiatrist and by a private investigator who would seek to establish the facts of the case. They learned also that their line managers and colleagues would be interviewed and that records of work (and personal leave) history would be investigated.

At the end of these processes, DC was informed the claim had been rejected. It was rejected on the basis that a decision about promotion constituted what the *Workplace Injury Rehabilitation and Compensation Act*, 2013 called "reasonable management action." At this point, DC could have chosen to simply accept this outcome but following advice from a support organization (without whom they might not have known there was an alternative option), DC applied for a conciliation hearing. This would involve a meeting with the insurer's legal representative and a representative from the employer, in a formal process chaired by a conciliator.

DC was taken aback to learn that the conciliation request triggered a delivery to them of all the documents collected by the investigator, amounting to several hundred pages. This included their entire medical record for the previous ten years, including references to intimate personal relationships, and accounts of interviews with line managers that included implied references to their "history and background" of a previous episode of depression (experienced after the death of their father).

While the investigation and conciliation processes were themselves deeply stressful, DC ultimately achieved some success. They persuaded the conciliator that their illness was a consequence of a series of work-related stresses and, in turn, the insurer and employer agreed to pay their medical costs for nine months. They then established a detailed return to work plan, with appropriate adjustments made to DC's roles and responsibilities.

Some seven–eight months later, DC remained on a RTW plan with adjusted responsibilities. They regularly experience a heightened emotional response to many of their university's internal communications, especially those pertaining to promotion, but also the various incitements about the need for workers to appropriate the language and tactics of self-promotion now so prized among their colleagues: In other words, the rhetorics of outperformance, such as "passion," "impact," and "excellence." At this time, DC began to actively consider alternative options to working in higher education. Almost exactly one year after the critical incident that triggered the submission of a workers' compensation claim, DC departed the university sector to work in a different field.

In summary, we can conclude from these snapshots that it is imperative we pay attention to the stresses associated with making a claim, as well as those leading up to and causing a mental injury. It is evident that an estimation of work stresses and distress do not begin or end with calculations of what the original cause/s of the injury was or might have been. It is apparent, too, that the investigation itself, and the subsequent negotiations around the conditions of returning to work, present a range of stresses that are perhaps not yet fully appreciated.

PART 5—CONCLUSION

Academics in Australia and New Zealand cannot easily access effective workers' compensation and legal recognition of the workplace factors that cause their mental injuries. Across these jurisdictions, many of the most common causes of mental injuries are excluded from workers' compensation provisions. Most notably, work stress associated with increasing workloads, workplace burnout, or the impacts of organizational cultures and policy contexts are not compensable causes of workplace mental injuries (Watts and Robertson 2011; Richards and McTernan 2014; O'Brien and Guiney 2018). Consequently, although mental health is included in Australia's and New Zealand's national work health and safety models, many academics experiencing workplace mental injuries are unable to claim workers' compensation to support their treatment and recovery (Potter et al. 2017).

Current workers' compensation approaches across Australia and New Zealand offer few opportunities for academic workers to have their mental injuries appropriately recognized as insured claimable workplace injuries. So many aspects of their work environments are associated with potential mental injury risks that they are unlikely to successfully prove that a specific event caused their mental injury. The likelihood that they have experienced many different moments of change, along with increasing uncertainty about their roles and work activities, directly undermines their already restricted capacities to claim workers' compensation for workplace mental injuries.

Our experiences, and those of our colleagues whose mental injury experiences we have witnessed, suggest that, when academics use formal university complaints procedures to report specific experiences such as bullying, they also increase the likelihood of gaining workers' compensation for the mental injuries that arise from those experiences.

Our observations presented here are broadly reflected in other studies, which have found that many academics experience demanding "culture[s] of performativity" alongside "bad management" (O'Brien and Guiney 2018, 12). The recent findings of national surveys of academic workforces in Australia and New Zealand concerning low levels of confidence in senior management, poor practices of consultation, long working hours, and low rates of job satisfaction suggest that many academics experience ongoing workplace mental injuries (NTEU 2018; Sedgwick and Proctor-Thomson 2019). These findings intersect with other research, which confirms that "how work is structured and organised" can "present persistent psychological and physical hazards which are just as dangerous to the physical and mental health of working people" (ACTU 2019). We therefore conclude that the current health and safety frameworks of universities and relevant workers' compensation legislation do not adequately protect academics from suffering workplace mental injuries. Neither do they protect injured workers from experiencing compounding adverse mental health impacts following the lodgment of a claim for workplace mental injuries.

For academics, identified sectoral and institutional mental injury risks include shifting work roles, increasing performance expectations, repeated university organizational restructuring, increasing workloads, changed reporting lines, increasing productivity, and performance monitoring. Both individually and collectively, these sit largely outside the scope of current workers' compensation provisions across Australia and New Zealand. Current workers' compensation legislation across these jurisdictions do not yet provide appropriate support for workplace injuries resulting from these circumstances However, both Safework Australia and WorkSafe/Mahi Haumaru Aotorea have implemented national public awareness and education campaigns to increase understanding of compensation claims processes and employer responsibilities for providing safe working environments.

Although workplace mental health frameworks in Australia and New Zealand now include increased recognition that workplace stress strongly contributes to poor mental health, the workers' compensation schemes that insure injured workers do not recognize workplace mental injuries resulting from workplace stress. Observable changes have occurred in governmental and university policy settings to increase access and equity assurances for workers with mental health conditions, injuries, or illnesses. For instance, some Australian and New Zealand universities have implemented workplace management and/or health communication guidelines and mandated policies that recognize job stressors as health risks (Memish et al. 2017). Alongside these, organizational and sectoral approaches to academic mental health, such as new university health promotion networks in Australia and New Zealand, might be indicators of more comprehensive awareness of mental health vulnerabilities among academic workforces. However, these initiatives do little to improve the circumstances of academic workers when they experience workplace mental injuries.

University networks, policies, and practices can and do affect the levels and forms of mental health risks among academic workers. However, they cannot provide Australian and New Zealand academics with publicly funded workers' compensation when such injuries occur. Improving the likelihood that academic workers might receive appropriate workers' compensation for their workplace mental injuries requires changes to relevant legislation. In turn, universities and their academic workers have a key role in contributing new insights into health communication debates and shifting current policies and practices.

As this chapter has pointed out, change is needed in the legal and policy parameters that shape employer responsibilities for safeguarding their employees' mental health. We have discussed how most academics who experience workplace mental injuries in Australia and New Zealand are unlikely to succeed in workers' compensation claims. As a result, many are unlikely to submit a claim following a workplace mental injury. Our observations of the mental injury experiences of many colleagues, and our own personal struggles to reconcile the challenges involved in overcoming mental injuries, suggest that, even when universities adopt policies and guidelines, their workplace cultures, management practices, and work role routines can detail their intended worker protections.

Overall, we confirm the findings of other studies of workers' compensation claims for workplace mental injuries. Namely, our study affirms the existing research's findings of low rates of claim submission and claim success, and high rates of added stress among claimants during claims processes and negotiations (see Brijnath et al. 2014). The sources of additional stresses experienced by workers in these cases include:

- The burden of definitive proof of a mental injury and proving that this injury arose from experiences at work
- The burden of conflicting opinions between medical practitioners
- Exclusions of some mental health medical interventions from workers' compensation and/or employer funded medical support
- The burden of project managing their claim/medical evidence while also seeking/accessing treatment for their mental injury

- Fears and anxieties concerning the possibility that their claim will not be regarded as legitimate
- Fears and anxieties that their privacy/confidentiality will be breached, leading to diminished professional status, eroded reputation, and constrained future opportunities
- Fears and anxieties that workplace (and other) relationships might be adversely affected by the mental injury and/or by their workers' compensation claim (Brijnath et al. 2014; O'Brien and Guiney 2018; Guthrie, Ciccarelli, and Babic 2010).

Existing research also indicates that managerialized approaches to mental health across universities pose additional barriers to reporting workplace mental injuries (O'Brien and Guiney 2018).

Ongoing Challenges

Related research also suggests that academic workers in Australia and New Zealand have low confidence that university health and safety policies protect them from workplace mental injuries (Taylor, Saheb, and Howse 2018; Raskauskas and Skrabec 2011). Alongside these findings sits additional research of university workforces in Australia and New Zealand that reveals low confidence in overall university management practices, and especially with regard to staff health and well-being (Sedgwick and Proctor-Thomson 2019; NTEU 2018). Our case studies outline the stories of some academic workers who have experienced shortcomings around health communication in their universities, with contingent mental injury impacts. By validating our colleagues' stories, and through expression of our own experiences as academic workers, we seek to mitigate the shortcomings around health communication and highlight key institutional factors that perpetuate them.

Intersecting organizational factors, institutional backdrops, and legislative frameworks contribute to the emotionality of workplace mental injuries. These intersecting factors and the emotionality of workplace mental injuries interweave with the conversations, and the stories embedded in them, and other evidence to validate the perspectives expressed in our case studies (Varker et al. 2018). By connecting broader health communication and workforce research with the experiences and stories of academic workers, we highlight opportunities for changed approaches to staff health communication and promotion across Australian and New Zealand universities. We locate these stories in the broader emergent health communication settings that underpin the recent formation of the Australian Health Promoting Universities Network and Tertiary Wellbeing Aotearoa New Zealand. These networks and other initiatives—such as Healthy Universities models (Dooris et al. 2010)—indicate the awareness that new health communication and promotion steps are needed to improve workplace mental health for university workers.

Seeking New Approaches

Broader institutional, sectoral, and governmental approaches are now also needed to better recognize that academic workers often experience workplace stressors and burnout risk factors. This recognition ensures that new health communication and promotion practices can reduce and eliminate the stressors and risk factors from university workplaces. These goals will not be fully achieved for academic workers in Australia and New Zealand without legislative changes that adequately recognize workplace mental injuries. We recommend that new health communication approaches inform workers' compensation legislation across Australian and New Zealand jurisdictions, as well as the workplace health and safety policies and procedures adopted by universities within them.

Our findings suggest that there are many explanations for why increasing numbers of academics at Australian and New Zealand universities experience mental injuries. At the same time, successful workers' compensation claims remain low because of sectoral and institutional factors. The structural and cultural dimensions of workers' compensation policies, procedures, and processes present additional contributing factors. Specifically, the so-called "no fault" workers' compensation claim processes in Australia and New Zealand privilege employers over employees. Employers are advantaged by the burden of proof placed on employees requiring them to confirm that their mental injuries result directly from workplace events. This results in low rates of workers' compensation claims for academic mental injuries. Without further changes to the regulatory frameworks, academics in Australia and New Zealand will continually be among the 70 percent of workers who report having "experienced work-related mental stress" but do not apply for workers' compensation (SafeWork Australia 2019).

REFERENCES

Australian Council of Trade Union. 2019. *Work Shouldn't Hurt: A Survey on the State of Work Health and Safety in Australia.* ACTU D No. 27. https://apo.org.au/node/253121.

Black Dog Institute. 2020. "Facts about Suicide in Australia." https://www.blackdoginstitute.org.au/clinical-resources/suicide-self-harm/facts-about-suicide-in-australia.

Bosticco, Cecilia, and Teresa L. Thompson. 2008. "Let Me Tell You a Story: Narratives in Health Communication Research." In *Emerging Perspectives in*

Health Communication, edited by Heather Zoller and Mohan J. Dutta, 39–62. New York and London: Routledge.
Brijnath, Bianca, Danielle Mazza, Nabita Singh, Agnieska Kosny, Rasa Ruseckaite, and Alex Collie. 2014. "Mental Health Claims Management and Return to Work: Qualitative Insights from Melbourne, Australia." *Journal of Occupational Rehabilitation* 24, no. 4: 766–776. https://doi.org/10.1007/s10926-014-9506-9.
Caldwell, Olivia. 2018. "Sport, Fame, Money and Pressure a Cocktail for Mental Illness." *Stuff*, May 20, 2018. https://www.stuff.co.nz/sport/other-sports/103564949/sport-fame-money-and-pressure-a-cocktail-for-mental-illness.
Crowe, Sarah, Kathrin Cresswell, Ann Robertson, Guro Huby, Anthony Avery, and Aziz Sheikh. 2011. "The Case Study Approach." *BMC Medical Research Methodology* 11, no. 100. https://doi.org/10.1186/1471-2288-11-100.
Chang, Su-Chao, and Ming-Shing Lee. 2008. "The Linkage between Knowledge Accumulation Capability and Organizational Innovation." *Journal of Knowledge Management* 12, no. 1: 3–20. https://doi.org/10.1108/13673270810852359.
Dollard, Maureen F., and Tessa S. Bailey, eds. 2014. *The Australian Workplace Barometer: Psychosocial Safety Climate and Working Conditions in Australia.* Samford Valley, Queensland: Australian Academic Press.
Dooris, Mark, Jennie Cawood, Sharon Doherty, and Sue Powell. 2010. *Healthy Universities: Concept, Model and Framework for Applying the Healthy Settings Approach within Higher Education in England: Final Project Report.* Manchester Metropolitan University, University of Central Lancashire, Royal Society for Public Health.
Edmondson, Beth. 2020. "Vulnerable Researchers: Opportunities, Challenges and Collaborative Co-Design in Regional Research." In *Located Research: Regional Places, Transitions and Challenges*, edited by Angela Campbell, Michelle Duffy, and Beth Edmondson, 319–334. Singapore: Palgrave Macmillan.
Geertz, Clifford. 1973. *The Interpretation of Cultures.* New York: Basic Books.
Gill, Rosalind. 2009. "Breaking the Silence: The Hidden Injuries of the Neo-Liberal University." In *Secrecy and Silence in the Research Process: Feminist Reflections*, edited by Róisín Ryan-Flood and Rosalind Gill, 228–244. London: Routledge.
Guthrie, Robert, Marina Ciccarelli, and Angela Babic. 2010. "Work-Related Stress in Australia: The Effects of Legislative Interventions and the Cost of Treatment." *International Journal of Law and Psychiatry* 33, no. 2: 101–115. https://doi.org/10.1016/j.ijlp.2009.12.003.
Hanawa, Annegret F., Leonarda García-Jiménez, Carey Candrian, Costanze Rossmann, and Peter J. Schulz. 2015. "Identifying the Field of Health Communication." *Journal of Health Communication* 20, no. 5: 521–530. https://doi.org/10.1080/10810730.2014.999891.
Henry, Dubby. 2019. "New Zealand Suicides Highest Since Records Began." *New Zealand Herald,* August 26, 2019. https://www.nzherald.co.nz/nz/news/article.cfm?c_id=1&objectid=12262081.
Kenny, John. 2018. "Re-Empowering Academics in a Corporate Culture: An Exploration of Workload and Performativity in a University." *Higher Education* 75: 365–380. https://doi.org/10.1007/s10734-017-0143-z.

Kidd, Sean A., Athena Madan, Susmitha Rallaband, Donald C. Cole, Elisha Muskat, Shoba Raja, David Wiljer, and Kwame McKenzie. 2016. "A Multiple Case Study of Mental Health Interventions in Middle Income Countries: Considering the Science of Delivery." *PLOS One* 11, no. 3. https://doi.org/10.1371/journal.pone.0152083.

LaMontagne, Anthony D., Tessa Keegel, Deborah Vallance, Aleck Ostry, and Rory Wolfe. 2008. "Job Strain – Attributable Depression in a Sample of Working Australians: Assessing the Contribution to Health Inequalities." *BMC Public Health* 8, no. 181: 1–9. https://doi.org/10.1186/1471-2458-8-181.

LaMontagne, Anthony. D., Angela Martin, Kathryn M. Page, Nicola J. Reavley, Andrew J. Noblet, Allison J. Milner, Tessa Keegel, and Peter M. Smith. 2014. "Workplace Mental Health: Developing an Integrated Intervention Approach." *BMC Psychiatry* 14, no. 131. https://doi.org/10.1186/1471-244X-14-131.

Martin, Judith N., and Thomas K. Nakayama. 1999. "Thinking Dialectically about Culture and Communication." *Communication Theory* 9, no. 1: 1–25. https://doi.org/10.1111/j.1468-2885.1999.tb00160.x.

Memish, Kate, Angela Martin, Larissa Bartlett, Sarah Dawkins, and Kristy Sanderson. 2017. "Workplace Mental Health: An International Review of Guidelines." *Preventive Medicine* 101: 213–222. https://doi.org/10.1016/j.ypmed.2017.03.017.

Moll, Sandra E. 2014. "The Web of Silence: A Qualitative Case Study of Early Intervention and Support for Healthcare Workers with Mental Ill-Health." *BMC Public Health* 14, no. 138. https://doi.org/10.1186/1471-2458-14-138.

National Tertiary Education Union. 2018. *State of the Uni Survey Report 1: Overview.* https://www.nteu.org.au/stateoftheuni/2017_results.

O'Brien, Tim, and Dennis Guiney. 2018. *Staff Wellbeing in Higher Education: A Research Study for Education Support Partnership.* London: Education Support Partnership.

Pickstar Blog. 2018. "Australian Sports Stars Put the Spotlight on Mental Health." March 28, 2018. https://www.blog.pickstar.com.au/post/sports-stars-mental-health.

Potter, Rachel E., Maureen F. Dollard, Mikaela S. Owen, Valerie O'Keeffe, Tessa Baily, and Stavroula Leka. 2017. "Assessing a National Work Health and Safety Policy Intervention Using the Psychosocial Safety Climate Framework." *Safety Science* 100, Part A: 91–102. https://doi.org/10.1016/j.ssci.2017.05.011.

Raskauskas, Juliana, and Chris Skrabec. 2011. "Bullying and Occupational Stress in Academia: Experiences of Victims of Workplace Bullying in New Zealand Universities." *Journal of Intergroup Relations* 35, no. 1: 18–36.

Richards, Penelope. A. M., and Tessa Bailey. 2014. "The Impact of the Psychosocial Work Environment on Worker Health and Wellbeing." In *The Australian Workplace Barometer: Psychosocial Safety Climate and Working Conditions in Australia*, edited by Maureen F. Dollard and Tessa S. Bailey. Samford Valley, Queensland: Australian Academic Press.

Richards, Penelope. A. M., and Wes P. McTernan. 2014. "Psychosocial and Health Risk by Industry in Australia." In *The Australian Workplace Barometer: Psychosocial Safety Climate and Working Conditions in Australia*, edited by

Maureen F. Dollard and Tessa S. Bailey. Samford Valley, Queensland: Australian Academic Press.
Roberts, Jane. 2017. *Losing Political Office*. Basingstoke: Palgrave Macmillan.
Roy, Eleanor. 2019. "New Zealand 'Wellbeing' Budget Promises Billions to Care for Most Vulnerable." *The Guardian*. May 30, 2019. https://www.theguardian.com/world/2019/may/30/new-zealand-wellbeing-budget-jacinda-ardern-unveils-billions-to-care-for-most-vulnerable.
Sherry, Emma. 2013. "The Vulnerable Researcher: Facing the Challenges of Sensitive Research." *Qualitative Research Journal* 13, no. 3: 278–288. https://doi.org/10.1108/QRJ-10-2012-0007.
Taylor, Patricia, Rowena Saheb, and Eloise Howse. 2018. "Creating Healthier Graduates, Campuses and Communities: Why Australia Needs to Invest in Health Promoting Universities." *Health Promotion Journal of Australia* 30, no. 2: 285–289. https://doi.org/10.1002/hpja.175.
SafeWork Australia. 2018. *Comparison of Workers' Compensation Arrangements in Australia and New Zealand*, 26th edition. https://www.safeworkaustralia.gov.au/system/files/documents/1812/comparison-workers-compensation-arrangements-australia-and-new-zealand-2018.pdf.
Sedgwick, Charles, and Sarah B. Proctor-Thomson. 2019. *The State of the Public Tertiary Education Sector Survey, 2018*. Wellington: Tertiary Education Union Te Hautū Kahurangi o Aotearoa.
Smith, Deborah. 2010. "Politicians Hailed for Facing Up to Depression." *Sydney Morning Herald*. July 16, 2010. https://www.smh.com.au/national/politicians-hailed-for-facing-up-to-depression-20100715-10crt.html.
Varker, Tracey, Mark Creamer, Juhi Khatri, Julia Fredrickson, and Meaghan O'Donnell. 2018. "Mental Health Impacts of Compensation Claim Assessment Process on Claimants and their Families: Final Report." Phoenix Australia – Centre for Posttraumatic Mental Health, The University of Melbourne.
Watts, Jenny, and Noelle Robertson. 2011. "Burnout in University Teaching Staff: A Systematic Literature Review." *Educational Research* 53, no. 1: 33–50. https://doi.org/10.1080/00131881.2011.552235.
Wyatt, Mary, Peter Cotton, and Tyler Lane. 2017. "Return to Work in Psychological Claims: Analysis of the Return to Work Survey Results." Safework Australia. https://www.safeworkaustralia.gov.au/system/files/documents/1711/return-to-work-in-psychological-injury-claims.pdf.
WorkSafe/Mahi Haumaru Aotorea. 2020. "A-Z Topics and Industry -- Bullying." WorkSafe/Mahi Haumaru Aotorea. https://worksafe.govt.nz/topic-and-industry/bullying/.
Zoller, Heather M. 2003. "Working Out: Managerialism in Workplace Health Promotion." *Management Communication Quarterly* 17, no. 2: 171–205. https://doi.org/10.1177%2F0893318903253003.
Zoller, Heather M., and Kimberly N. Kline. 2008. "Theoretical Contributions of Interpretive and Critical Research in Health Communication." *Annals of the International Communication Association* 32, no. 1: 89–135. https://doi.org/10.1080/23808985.2008.11679076.

Appendix
Mental Health–Related Resources for the Communication Classroom

Teresa Heinz Housel, Andrea L. Meluch, Vanessa R. Sperduti, Sandra Smeltzer, Rahul Mitra

Over the past few years, more institutions in the United States and other countries are offering general wellness programs and mental health services on their campuses. As Chapter 1 points out, most mental health programming targets undergraduate students but, increasingly, institutions are recognizing the importance of supporting the mental health of their graduate students, faculty, staff, and administrators.

As part of this support for the wider academic community, this volume's authors collectively share the goal of bringing mental health into classroom practice. Our students will be future faculty, staff, administrators, and graduate students. How we communicate about mental health in the classroom can have future implications for academic and other types of workplaces. To this end, this Appendix includes ideas from this book's contributors for suggested class assignments and class readings to connect mental health to the classroom.

As you read this book's chapters, you will notice that a number of this book's contributors regularly support their students' mental health through different strategies. In this Appendix, Rahul Mitra shares below how he has reached out to students experiencing mental distress during the COVID-19 pandemic, which has placed extraordinary stress on students and academic employees. I encourage you to note the other teaching strategies discussed in the chapters.

Website addresses can change or be removed from the internet with no notice. Therefore, you can find web-based resources from this volume's contributors in the Features tab on this book's webpage of the publisher's website: https://rowman.com/ISBN/9781793630247/Mental-Health-among-Higher-Education-Faculty-Administrators-and-Graduate-Students-A-Critical-Perspective.

I also point our readers to my website www.ourmindstogether.com, which I've written and curated. This website offers additional information about institutional best practices around mental health; academics' stories of how they care for their mental health and well-being; resources for mental health–related assignments, class readings, and other classroom activities; and a directory of campus programming around mental health support for students, faculty, staff, and administrators.

I also invite you, our readers, to share your contributions to www.ourmindstogether.com. I seek your ideas for classroom activities and assessments; programming that your campus is planning or currently doing (and is working well, or perhaps what your institution learned from the experience to improve future programming); your own stories about how you are supporting your own mental health and well-being as an academic; and other ideas that will build this website as a community of resources.

In October 2020, I invited this volume's contributors to share their resources and ideas for bringing mental health–related topics into the communication classroom. We invite you to use or modify the resources that contributors have shared below.

WRITING MENTAL HEALTH PERSONAL NARRATIVES: CLASS ACTIVITY

Andrea L. Meluch

Courses: Undergraduate and Graduate; Health Communication, Interpersonal Communication and Health, and Narrative Health, among others

Course Format: Can be used in both online and face-to-face courses

Objectives: To provide students with the opportunity to explore their personal stories related to mental health and how these experiences intersect with course theories and concepts.

Background: As mental health concerns increasingly become part of our everyday lived experiences, it is no longer possible for individuals to avoid confronting how these issues intersect in our everyday lives. Whether through personal experience living with a mental health condition, having a family member with a mental health condition, or navigating how mental health is discussed in the media and broader societal discourses, everyone has some level of experience with mental health issues. The stigmatized nature of mental health and how we provide social support to individuals managing mental health conditions are of particular concern to health communication scholarship (Kreps 2020, 14).

Telling our stories is an integral part of making sense of our experiences and showing their importance in regard to broader life concerns (Norman

2020, 3963). Narratives are especially important in health contexts where we make sense of our health experiences by telling our stories (Charon 2006, 4). Instructors are increasingly recognizing how narrative can be a powerful pedagogical tool, especially in the health communication classroom (Thompson 2019, 133). The following course assignment/activity provides students with the opportunity to explore and reflect on their personal stories related to mental health, and how these experiences intersect with health communication theories and concepts and reducing social stigma around mental health.

Activity: Instructors should assign this activity after they have discussed mental health issues and health narratives in their course. During class, instructors should provide assignment directions to students (see below). Specifically, instructors should highlight the guiding questions to help students reflect on their experiences related to mental health and write their mental health narratives. Students should write their mental health narratives outside class. These brief narratives will highlight the student's mental health story and how it relates to course concepts (e.g., stigma, identity). When discussing this assignment, instructors should discuss what campus resources (e.g., counseling) are available to students who are managing mental health issues, and emphasize that students should only include what they are comfortable discussing. Providing trigger warnings related to mental health issues (e.g., suicide, depression) alongside the assignment is strongly recommended.

After students have written their personal narratives, the instructor should lead a class discussion about their written narratives. In particular, this class discussion should cover how mental health has impacted students' lives, how stigma was present in their narratives, and what they can do to reduce mental health stigma on college campuses. This discussion should include how, through our interpersonal communication about mental health, we can reduce stigma related to mental health and create a more inclusive community. Further, the discussion should again emphasize how campus resources can be used by students.

Assignment Instructions: Write a short personal narrative (three–five pages) that tells *your story* of experiencing and/or considering mental health issues. Your personal narrative can be about your own experiences dealing with a mental health condition (if you are comfortable sharing), your experiences dealing with a family member's mental health condition (if you are comfortable sharing), and/or your experiences learning about mental health through the media and/or broader societal discourses. In particular, consider the following guiding questions as you write your narrative:

- What does mental health mean to you?
- When did you first encounter mental health issues either personally or through learning about them abstractly? What did this encounter look like?

- When you think about mental health, what comes to mind?
- How does mental health impact or intersect with your life?
- In what ways do you see health communication concepts and/or theories (e.g., stigma, identity) present in your story?

PERSPECTIVE-TAKING ASSIGNMENT: THE POWER OF SPEAKING "I"

Teresa Heinz Housel

I have used this Perspective-Taking Assignment many times in my undergraduate communication courses. The assessment could be easily adapted to focus on understanding the perspectives of people who have felt silenced in some way because of their experiences of mental illness and/or mental distress. The instructor could build the assignment into larger lessons that cover effective communication around mental health and mental distress. In addition, the Perspective-Taking Assignment could be adapted to graduate courses, such as courses in interpersonal communication, health communication, and teaching pedagogy courses. The assignment could also be used as a counterpoint to common media stereotypes around mental illness. Finally, the assessment could be used in staff development workshops, either as a whole or broken down into parts, depending on the time available.

As Andrea Meluch points out in her assignment shared earlier in this Appendix, the instructor should embed this assignment in relevant theory and strategies around communication competency in the course. I typically cover the power relationships involved in speaking through the first-person voice, and how speaking from someone else's perspective (and *for* someone else) can impact how we understand another person's experiences, though we must be ethical and sensitive when doing so.

Before introducing the assignment, the course should also cover different types of interview questions; how to conduct interviews on potentially sensitive topics; safety during interviews (hold the interview in a public place and other matters); and how to sensitively word interview questions. The instructor should also provide information about mental health resources at the institution when introducing this assignment. In addition, the instructor should give trigger warnings alongside this assignment. Because the material focuses on mental health and distress, I also recommend that the instructor discuss the assignment's topical matter with their supervisor (e.g., department chair) before building it into the course.

I have written the Perspective-Taking Assignment below from a general perspective.

PERSPECTIVE-TAKING ASSIGNMENT OVERVIEW

Identify a specific person who you think has a perspective that is not heard (or often heard) in our society because it has been silenced by the dominant culture. You can interview someone who has felt silenced in the past, someone who feels currently silenced, or someone whom others attempt to silence, but refuses to be silenced.

Conduct an interview of at least thirty minutes. The interviews can be in person, by phone, or online (e.g., video).

Before going to the interview, prepare and type at least fifteen to twenty open-ended and closed questions to ask this person. Take notes during the interview. Do not record the interview unless you have asked the interviewee for permission. Also, do not use the interviewee's real name unless with their permission. Ask yourself as you prepare for the interview: If this person were to visit our class, what would this person want to convey? What would this person want us to know in order to communicate more effectively with him or her?

ON THE DAY OF THE PRESENTATION

Here are the instructions that I provide to students: Prepare a detailed outline of your eight-to-nine-minute presentation. To the class, introduce yourself as the person you interviewed (use "I" as you speak from the person's perspective) and give voice to this person's experiences and perspectives. Make a compelling case that the person is silenced. Your presentation should somehow address these questions: Why has this person been silenced? If this person were to visit our class, what would this person want to convey to us? What would this person want us to know in order to communicate more effectively with him or her?

After the presentation, turn in a stapled packet to your instructor that includes:

- Blank grading rubric with name at top (you will receive a blank rubric in class)
- Typed and detailed outline of presentation that is free of typos
- Interview notes taken during the interview (you are not being asked to identify the person)
- List of questions asked during the interview

You will be graded on:

- Quality of presentation (organization, main thesis)
- Interview topic relevant to assignment
- Ability to convincingly portray another's perspective through your writing

- Ability to impact your peer audience
- Professional presentation of assignment materials (hand in all required materials, detailed and typo-free outline)

STAGES OF PERSPECTIVE-TAKING ASSIGNMENT

I explain these stages of the assignment to the students when I first introduce it in class:
Paragraph describing your proposed topic due in class. You do not need to list the person's real name; only use their real name with their permission. You should indicate why the person feels silenced now or in the past. *I advise that instructors provide students with a date by which they should have scheduled their Perspective-Taking Interview date and time with the instructor. Instructors can also schedule the presentations themselves. In addition, I set a due date for the topic proposal paragraph.*

Presentations given in class. Do Perspective-Taking Presentations in peer groups of two to three students. *There are several presentation options for this assignment. I have also asked students to deliver the presentations in front of the entire class. I have also split the class into small groups and asked students to deliver their presentation to small peer groups as above. Both methods work well. However, I've found that, for larger classes, the peer group method encourages discussion among the smaller groups.*

On the day of your presentation, you should turn in your typed presentation outline, notes taken during the interview, a list of questions asked during the interview, and a blank assignment grading rubric (stapled on top). *Provide students with a date when they should complete their follow-up reflection.*

PERSPECTIVE-TAKING FOLLOW-UP REFLECTION

I ask students to type a half to three-fourth single-spaced response that reflects on the experience of doing the Perspective-Taking Assignment. Set a due date. I've often set the due date for the next class session after the student's presentation.

Instructions to students: Now that you have completed your interview and delivered your presentation in class, thoughtfully reflect on the experience of presenting another person's perspective in their voice (using first person "I"). Respond to these two questions:

- What role did speaking in the first person have on your ability to take someone else's perspective? Now that you've completed this assignment, what do you think is the role of perspective-taking in the development of communication competency? *The instructor can modify these questions*

depending on their course needs. My past students have found this reflection process to be quite powerful. Many of them said that speaking in the person's voice as "I" helped them better understand why some people are marginalized and how others do not know how to communicate with them.
- *Finally, describe the experience of listening to your peer's presentation(s). How did listening to someone else's experience of being silenced impact you as the listener? In my experience, students often had thoughtful whole-class discussions as they listen to the presentations on each class day. In a class of around twenty-five students, the Perspective-Taking Assignment typically required two weeks of class time for a class that met two or three times a week. I often used the follow-up reflection questions, or variations of them, as discussion prompts in class.*

PERSPECTIVE-TAKING ASSIGNMENT: GRADING RUBRIC

I used this basic rubric (see Table A.1) to grade the Perspective-Taking Presentations. It can easily be adapted to your own needs.

SUPPORTING STUDENTS' MENTAL HEALTH DURING THE COVID-19 PANDEMIC

Rahul MitraDuring the COVID-19 pandemic, I am quite clear both in my syllabi and in my email/online course communication with my students that my goals are twofold: their enhanced learning and engagement with the course material, and encouraging them to do their best, ending the semester on a positive note. To these ends, I told students that, should they want an extension to any class assignment (quizzes, weekly response papers, etc.) for any personal or professional reason, then they should ask me (preferably in advance) and I will grant it to them, no proof required or questions asked. Deadlines are important but not crucial, and especially not at the cost of mental health and meaningful learning. I also converted all my online quizzes (for the undergrad class) into open-book quizzes.

RESOURCES FOR INCORPORATING MENTAL HEALTH RESOURCES INTO CURRICULA

Vanessa R. Sperduti, Sandra Smeltzer

The selected resources included below offer examples of how we proactively incorporate mental health resources into two curricular areas: critical media/

Table A.1

	Excellent	Good	Fair	Poor
In-depth Interview: Asked insightful questions, had follow-up probing questions, elicited stories and examples, took notes during interview				
Choice of Interviewee: Relevant choice, compelling case for silencing				
Outline: Very detailed and reflects good organization. Free of typos and grammatical errors.				
Presentation:				
Presents perspective of interviewee; perspective is important, and likely to have an impact on classmate peer audience; presented perspective that challenges our stereotypes and preconceptions				
Written presentation had a thesis (main point) and was well-organized. Presentation ran appropriate length of time (no less than 7:45 or more than 9:30 minutes)				
Professional Presentation of Materials: Handed in all required materials (blank grading rubric stapled to top, typed presentation outline, interview notes, typed follow-up reflection, and typed interview questions)				
Assignment Grade and Comments: Will be typed and attached to your graded presentation materials				
Presentation Outline, Follow-Up Reflection, Interview Questions, Interview Notes:				
In-Class Presentation:				
Note: The topic proposal will be graded separately				

communication studies; and community-engaged learning, a type of experiential learning geared toward the public good and designed to benefit both students and community partners. These materials are also relevant to, and the activities can be modified for, other disciplines.

On the Features tab of this book's webpage on the publisher's website (https://rowman.com/ISBN/9781793630247/Mental-Health-among-Higher-Education-Faculty-Administrators-and-Graduate-Students-A-Critical-Perspective), you can find information about websites and other resources that we use in our classrooms.

READINGS USED IN OUR CLASSROOMS

Cora Learning. 2020. "Employing Equity-Minded and Culturally-Affirming Teaching and Learning Practices in Virtual Learning Communities." https://www.niu.edu/keepteaching/workshops/equity-in-virtual-learning.shtml.

Evans, Teresa M., Lindsay Bira, Jazmin Beltran Gastelum, L. Todd Weiss, and Nathan L. Vandelford. 2018. "Evidence for a Mental Health Crisis in Graduate Education." *Nature Biotechnology* 36, no. 3: 282–284. http://dx.doi.org/10.1038/nbt.4089.

Flaherty, Colleen. 2019. "How Mindfulness Helps Grad Students." *Inside Higher Ed*, November 15. https://www.insidehighered.com/news/2019/11/15/mindfulness-significantly-benefits-graduate-students-says-first-study-its-kind.

Gardner, Paula, and Jill Grose. 2015. "Mindfulness in the Academy—Transforming Our Work and Ourselves 'One Moment at a Time'." *Collected Essays on Learning and Teaching* 8: 35–46. https://doi.org/10.22329/celt.v8i0.4252.

Gardner, Paula, and Kaitlyn Kerridge. 2019. "Everybody Present: Exploring the Use of an In-Class Meditation Intervention to Promote Positive Mental Health Among University Students." *Canadian Journal of Community Mental Health* 37, no. 4: 9–21. https://doi.org/10.7870/cjcmh-2018-022.

Kaler, Lisa S., and Michael J. Stebleton. n.d. "Graduate Student Mental Health: Examining an Overlooked Concern." *Journal of Student Affairs* 29: 101.

Massey, Kyle D. 2019. "Student Affairs and Services in Canadian Higher Education." In *Preparing Students for Life and Work*. Edited by Walter Archer and Hans G. Schuetze, 78–97. Brill Sense.

Mental Health Commission of Canada. 2019. "Catalyst - March 2019 - Getting Mental Health Up to Standard on Post-Secondary Campuses." https://mentalhealthcommission.ca/English/catalyst-march-2019-getting-mental-health-standard-post-secondary-campuses.

Mick, Connie Snyder, and James M. Frabutt. 2017. "Service-Learning in Higher Education: Teaching about Poverty and Mental Health." In *Service-Learning* 12: 215–240. Emerald Publishing Limited.

Provoe, Jill. "Equity, Diversity and Inclusion-Minded Practices in Virtual Learning Communities." Nova Scotia Community College. https://www.nscc.ca/docs/about-nscc/applied-research/equity-report-english.pdf.

Seppälä, Emma M., Christine Bradley, Julia Moeller, Leilah Harouni, Dhruv Nandamudi, and Marc A. Brackett. 2020. "Promoting Mental Health and Psychological Thriving in University Students: A Randomized Controlled Trial of Three Well-Being Interventions." *Frontiers in Psychiatry* 11: 590. https://doi.org/10.3389/fpsyt.2020.00590.

Wedemeyer-Strombel, Kathryn R. 2019. "Why We Need to Talk More About Mental Health in Graduate School." *Chronicle of Higher Education*. August 27, 2019. https://www.chronicle.com/article/Why-We-Need-to-Talk-More-About/247002.

ADDITIONAL CLASSROOM RESOURCES

In our interdisciplinary "Introduction to Doctoral-Level Scholarship" class in the Faculty of Information and Media Studies, students read Samira Shackle's "The Way Universities Are Run is Making Us Ill: Inside the Student Mental

Health Crisis," *The Guardian*, September 27, 2019. https://www.theguardian.com/society/2019/sep/27/anxiety-mental-breakdowns-depression-uk-students. Participants also write a 2,000-word reflective essay about their first year as doctoral students.

Our faculty offers a popular third-year undergraduate course, "Media and Mental Health," which explores the media's role in shaping our understanding(s) of mental health and mental illness. Students produce traditional, academic assignments as well as work aimed at non-academic audiences.

EMBODIED FORMS OF SUPPORT TO PROMOTE MENTAL HEALTH AND WELL-BEING

Providing students with clear, easy-to-understand information about how and where to access both on- and off-campus mental health resources is critically important. However, we have found that passive provision of URL links, phone numbers, and checklists is not enough for many students. These resources often fail to reach those students who may need them the most for a range of reasons (e.g., they may not feel comfortable seeking mental health support in-person, do not anticipate benefiting from the process, or may have had a negative experience with professional help in the past). Many students may not even realize that they need support or what kinds of resources would benefit them the most.

Moreover, on-campus mental health professionals often do not have the capacity or human resources to visit individual classrooms or to tailor their mental health support to specific courses or programs. Therefore, at the beginning of the term in our fourth-year "Media & the Public Interest" (MPI) community-engaged learning course, a support person from a local community-based organization that focuses on youth mental health and well-being comes into the classroom. This individual facilitates discussions within a safe space for students to articulate and proactively address emotions they may experience while working in the local community and with their host organization.

INTERACTIVE MENTAL HEALTH WORKSHOP

Part-way through the term in the MPI community-engaged learning course, students participate in an interactive mental health workshop. Drawing on applied theater tools, the objective of this workshop is for both students and instructors to proactively engage with mental health issues through embodied interactive exercises. Learning and thinking about mental health issues, situations, and responses through physical activities provide participants with insight into their own understanding of, and relationship with, mental health.

Discussing, imagining, and role-playing community engaged learning experiences—whether fictional or actual—can trigger myriad emotions that can positively and negatively impact students' mental health. Given the possibility of emotional upheaval from participating in an interactive workshop of this nature, a professional mental health support person is available during and after the workshop's activities to address students' needs.

A BUDDY SYSTEM OF SUPPORT

In our MPI community-engaged learning course, we created a buddy system whereby students entering into the course are given the contact information of (consenting) graduates who previously worked with the same community partner and can share their positive experiences and the challenges they encountered. Through this peer-to-peer mentoring process, incoming students receive first-hand insight into what the placement will entail, which helps to alleviate their anxiety and manage expectations regarding their placements.

REFERENCES

Charon, Rita. 2006. *Narrative Medicine: Honoring the Stories of Illness.* New York: Oxford University Press.

Kreps, Gary L. 2020. "The Chilling Influences of Social Stigma on Mental Health Communication: Implications for Promoting Health Equity." In *Communicating Mental Health: History, Contexts, and Perspectives*, edited by Lance R. Lippert, Robbie D. Hall, Aimee Miller-Ott, and Daniel Cochece Davis, 11–26. Lanham, MD: Lexington Books.

Norman, Taylor. 2020. "Methods of a Narrative Inquirist: Storying the Endured Teacher Identity." *The Qualitative Report* 25, no. 11: 3962–3975. https://nsuworks.nova.edu/tqr/vol25/iss11/10/.

Thompson, Marie. 2019. "Narrative Mapping: Listening with Health, Healing, and Illness Narratives in the Classroom." *Communication Teacher* 33, no. 2: 132–138. http://dx.doi.org/10.1080/17404622.2017.1400673.

Index

abuse, 86–87, 107, 174; alcohol, 9; environmental, 107; ongoing, 174; sexual, 7, 169, 174–75; substance, 85, 207, 209
academic: careers, xxiv, 15–16, 37, 44, 69, 71, 76, 78–79, 83; culture, 1, 5, 69, 74, 82, 84, 87, 116, 231; employees, 5, 7, 9–11, 14, 16–18, 75, 277; goals, 36, 45; institutions, 5, 14, 18–19, 85, 105, 116–17; labor, 178, 181, 248; life-long, 84; self-concept, low, 129; self-efficacy, 72, 130; staff, 190–91, 228, 251, 260; White environment, 106
accommodations, 19, 45, 153, 176, 179, 208, 214; requests for, 14, 207
ACEs. *See* Adverse Childhood Experiences
ACHA. *See* American College Health Association
actions: corrective, 112; disciplinary, 215; empowered, 54; legal, 151; reasonable, 257; symbolic, 171; unconscious, 108
activities: daily, 42; extracurricular, 13; leisurely, 140; physical, 286; routine, 265; social, 74

administrators, xxi, 6–8, 10, 13, 15–19, 64–65, 87–88, 90, 114–15, 179, 181, 208–10, 220, 222, 277–78
adolescents, 73
Adverse Childhood Experiences (ACEs), xxi, 181
African Americans, 13, 77, 108, 175
allergies, 5, 209, 213, 218, 222
allostatic load, 230, 240
American College Health Association (ACHA), 10–11, 38–39, 229
analysis: academic, 4; discursive, 235; feminist rhetorical, 170; textual, 145; thematic, 145
animals: on campus, 209–10, 212–17, 219–22; companion, 208; fake therapy, 221; rescued, 213; research/teaching, 215; unrestrained, 215
anxiety, xxi–xxiv, 6–7, 9, 11–12, 16–17, 35–48, 54, 85, 127–29, 191, 228–29, 271; severe, 45, 73
ANZ (anthrozoology) program, 208, 212–13, 218, 220
assessments, 18, 131, 141, 278, 280; multicultural, 132
attrition rates, 126–27, 129, 131
autism, 220
autoethnography, 36–37

289

290   Index

awareness: critical, 19; racial, 113

backgrounds: diverse, 189, 191, 200; ethnic, 190; multiethnic, 57; scholarly, 59; varied disciplinary, 231

barriers, 40, 46, 106, 111, 114, 122–23, 125, 131, 189; attitudinal, 177; cultural, 13; identified, 127

behaviors, 106, 108, 113–15, 117–18, 128, 148, 154, 180–81, 213, 215–16; employer, 255; erratic, 4; injury-causing, 254; positive, 84; toxic, 87; unexplained, 58; workaholic, 84

biases, 65, 117, 171, 231

boundaries, 112, 150, 154–55, 231–32; implicit, 149–50, 154

bullying, xxii–xxiii, 246–47, 255, 258, 260–61, 263, 269; academic, 174; culture, 5

burnout, xxiv, 38–39, 53, 69–71, 73–78, 109, 128, 191, 233; cause, 69; chronic, 85; expected, 77; graduate student, 69, 73, 82, 89–90; higher levels of, 71, 74; mentor, 81; romanticizing, 80; severe, 75; stigma, 70–71, 76, 83; tenure, 76; unrecognized, 266

campus: communities, 172, 227; culture, 210, 212; diversity, 18; policies, 181, 209, 213–15; programming, 11, 17, 278; resources, 44, 279; staff, 155; therapy dogs on, 222

Canadian Mental Health Association (CMHA), 229

careers, xxi, xxiv, 41, 43, 58–59, 69, 72, 76, 79, 81–82, 261; academic, 89; choice, 89; mobility, 122; norms, 53; opportunities, 64; professional, 12, 126, 176

cats, 212–13

Caucasian, 144, 233

challenges, 11, 16, 43, 45–46, 129, 132, 270, 284, 287; acute, 255;
psychological, 207; significant, 121, 125; unprecedented, 191

chronic mental health information (CMHI), 139–43, 145, 148–49, 151–52, 154–55, 157

classism, 126

classmates, 54, 56, 60, 62–63

classrooms, 149, 153, 173, 176, 208, 212–13, 215, 217–18, 277, 284, 286–87; non-ANZ, 213, 217

colleagues, xxii–xxiii, 3, 5, 8, 16–17, 40, 42, 113–15, 124, 227, 231–35, 237–39, 251–52, 258–62, 264–71; aggrieved senior, 264; emerging, 239; former, 4–5; scholarly, 144–45; silent, xxii; supportive, 263

college: instructors, 151, 153; liberal arts, 15; private, 208, 210; small private religious, 222; students, 5, 10, 157, 222

collegiality, 177, 194, 228

color: academics of, 106, 116, 118; people of, 46, 105, 107, 109, 111, 113, 115, 117, 179; students of, 57, 65, 178

combat fatigue, 169

communication: cultural, 59; effective, 19, 280; empathic, xxiii; intercultural, 59; mentor-mentée, 90; organizational, 18, 212; person-centered, 18–19; poor, 189; public, 171; unspoken, xxiii

community, 16, 19, 140, 220, 228–30, 232, 235–36, 238–40, 278; inclusive, 279; role-playing, 287; small, xxiii; supportive, 238

compensation claims, 247–48, 252–53, 259–62, 265, 268–70, 272

competence: emotional, 17; professional, 191

conferences, academic, 177

confidants, 140, 142, 143, 146–49, 153–54

control, xxii, 14–15, 41, 54, 130, 215, 220, 252; perceived, 180–81

counseling, 5, 9–10, 13, 42, 44, 46, 71, 210; roles, 230
courses: capstone, 232; undergraduate communication, 280
COVID-19 pandemic, xxiv, 12, 14, 16, 18, 65, 277, 283
crises: current, xxiii; emotional, 218; mitigating, 229; national suicide, 251
crisis situations, 109, 235, 238
cultural: attitudes, 142, 194, 199; differences, 109, 189; orientation, 190; shift, 83, 222; values, 190, 192
culture, 3–4, 70–71, 76, 79–81, 87–88, 116–18, 179–80, 191, 193, 198; competitive, 15, 65, 88; data-led, 194; diverse, 198; institutional, 198; organizational, 90, 107, 110, 211, 268; popular, 35; professional, 6; public, 6, 19, 35; publish-or-perish, 142; supportive, 19

degree program, professional, 121, 124, 131
degrees: academic, xxi; advanced, 124; bachelor's, 123–25
departmental politics, 57–58, 60, 64
department chairs, 8, 62, 263, 280
depression, 6–7, 9, 11–12, 48, 54, 70–71, 85–86, 127–29, 207, 266–67; increased, 9, 39; severe, 73
destigmatization, 46, 75, 90, 231, 240
diagnoses, 7–9, 193, 218, 263; common mental health, 10
diagnostic criteria, 210
disabilities, 18, 177, 179, 207–9, 215, 218, 221; coordinator, 220; invisible, 177, 218; psychological, 171, 176–77, 179–80; services, 44–45, 210, 218
Disability Access Information and Support (DAIS), 221
disability student services (DSSs), 207, 221
disclosure, 8, 139, 141–43, 145–48, 151, 154–55, 163, 239; chronic illness, 144; friend's, 148, 155; sexual assault, 232
discrimination, 8, 16, 59, 62, 171, 199, 246; behavioral, 107; systemic racial, 106
disorders, 170, 174, 180, 207, 209, 218–19, 228, 231, 240, 257; cardiovascular, 70; eating, 3, 9, 234; emotional, 6
dissertation, 41, 43, 54, 86–87
distress, xxi, xxiii, 9–10, 12, 86, 180, 197, 215, 230, 266, 268; emotional, 86, 229, 231, 236; psychological, 73
diversity, 57, 63, 113, 116, 118, 190, 194, 200; ethnic, 198; valorized, 57
dogs, 41, 210, 212–21; therapy, 207, 210, 212, 222

education, post-secondary, 121, 228
educational success, 125, 127
emotional exhaustion, 69–70, 109, 191, 232
emotional support animals (ESAs), 207–22
employee assistance program (EAP), 5, 191, 196–97, 261
employers, 7, 245, 248, 251, 253, 256–58, 260, 267, 270, 272
employment, 4, 19, 71, 124, 195, 199, 252, 256
environments, 16, 56, 60, 106, 117–18, 228, 239; antagonistic, 228; competitive, 12, 58; discriminatory, 247; healthy, 198; healthy work, 41; hierarchical, 115; hostile, 56; neoliberal, 87; occupational, 106; organizational, 109; political, 178; positive classroom, 153; safe working, 246; social, 15, 107, 109, 126; stressful work, 54; toxic, 64; unsupportive institutional, 53
epidemic, opioid, 240
epileptic seizures, 207, 218
evaluations, xxii, 80, 230
exhaustion, 73

expectations, xxiv, 17, 19, 81–84, 89, 149, 155, 157, 230, 235–36, 238–39; academic, 69, 116; cultural, 150; government, 240; high, 15, 38, 74; meritocratic, 233; performance/productivity, 251; professional, 53, 56, 233–34; reasonable, 65; unclear, 114; unrealistic, 72, 246
experiential learning, 284

factors: aggravating, 258; common, 130; economic, 121; institutional, 4, 271–72; organizational, 112, 271; psychosocial work, 245; sociocultural, 126–27, 129, 132; structural, 262; triggering, 73
faculty, 5–6, 10–11, 13, 15–19, 38–39, 46, 60–62, 64–65, 75–76, 83–84, 90, 108, 210, 212–13, 238–40, 277–78; adjunct, 15–16; benefits, 179; contingent, 38, 90; diverse, 238; full-time, 238; negative-minded, 75; non-tenured, 16; pre-tenured, 16; senior, 112; specialized, 112; supportive, 59
family, xxi, 7, 14, 39, 41, 126, 130, 139, 140, 146, 148, 233
fear, 42, 71, 81–83, 88–89, 128, 131, 234–35, 239, 261, 271
fellowships, 84
first-generation college students (FGCS), xxiii, 10, 12–13, 16, 18, 121–23, 125–28, 130, 132
first-generation graduate students, 65, 122–23, 125, 127, 129–32
freedom, academic, 228
friends: examined, 143; mutual, 150; particular, 163
funding: inadequate, 59, 61; models, 240; post-secondary, 238

gaps, cognitive, 106, 109, 112, 114
gender: designated, 173; feminine, 171; identity, 77; stereotypes, 16
graduate school, 12–13, 40–43, 54–56, 58, 60–61, 64, 69, 72–74, 77–78, 80

graduate students: current, 65; eligible, 69; female, 13, 128; first-generation, 129; impacts, 82; male, 128; overstressed, 64; queer, 12; studies on, 9, 12–13; successful, 60; supervise, 81; support for, 69, 83; thesis-based, 233
groups: cultural, 117; ethnic minority, 106; marginalized, 132; privileged demographic, 233; racial, 113, 117
guilt, academic, 41, 47

happiness, 221; long-term, 81
harassment, xxiii, 14, 19, 62–63, 87, 260; ongoing, xxii; sexual, 174
health: emotional, 85, 240; physical, 252–53, 263, 265; social, 115
hierarchy, 59, 114, 178; academic, 74, 114
higher education, 8–9, 17–18, 37–41, 89–90, 121, 125–27, 132, 170–73, 178–79, 181, 201
higher education institutions (HEIs), 9, 13, 19, 190, 192, 194–201
Hispanic, 77, 108, 144
horses, 208, 219–20
housing, 193, 209, 214, 218, 222

identities, 74–76, 80, 85, 123, 126–27, 132, 170–71, 177, 180, 259, 262–63, 279–80; cultural, 109; intersecting, 12–13, 122–23, 129, 181; intersectional, 122; marginalized, 123, 179; racial, 172; stigmatized, 46
illness, chronic, 17–18
imposter syndrome, 37, 40, 79, 128–29, 131; color experience, 40
incidents, critical, 252–53, 258, 261, 264, 266, 268
injuries: brain, 207; severe, 70
institutional policies, xxiii, 13, 18, 64, 75, 151, 187, 209
intercultural theory, 60
interventions, 10, 65, 125, 127, 129, 132, 156, 285; animal-assisted, 207; individual-level, 46

Index

interview guide, 143; semi-structured, 144
interview prompts, 110
isolation, social, 9, 12, 15–16, 248

job insecurity, 15, 17, 178, 180, 260
job market, academic, 12, 41, 54, 83
job satisfaction, 87–88, 269
justice, social, xxiii, 65, 79, 125, 221

language: inclusive, 179; insensitive, 189; sensitive, 190
life: academic, 6, 177, 233–34; balance, 12, 14, 71, 73, 80, 82–83, 85, 90, 127, 232; boundaries, 84; challenges, 233; decisions, 234; events, 258

management actions, reasonable, 256–57, 266–67
media, social, 86, 144
mental disability, 177, 179, 208
mental distress, xxi, 1, 10, 12–16, 18–19, 75, 82, 85–86, 280; experiencing, 277; frequent, 6; long-term, 73; severe, 9
mental health, xxiii–xxiv, 5–7, 9–14, 16–19, 35–40, 42–48, 69–72, 80, 83–90, 127–32, 179–81, 191–201, 228–32, 234–36, 238–39, 268–72, 277–80, 285–87; acute, 7; challenges, xxiv, 8, 10, 15–16, 18–19, 54, 228, 230–31, 237, 239; disclosures, 8, 141, 147, 151, 165; discussing, 149; disorders, 9, 231; diverse, 199; hotlines, 152; injuries, 264–65; multinational, 14; poor, 75, 85, 89, 125–28, 193, 269; resources, 13, 43, 86–87, 142, 179–80, 198–99, 229, 238, 280, 283, 286; stigma, 76, 153, 279; training, 86
mental illness, xxi, xxiv, 5–11, 13, 15–19, 35, 44–46, 48, 86, 280; common, 6; disclosing, 6, 8, 141; episodes of, 194; examined, 11; rates of, 6
mental injuries, 245–48, 251–53, 255–62, 264–66, 268–72; academic, 272;
cause of, 260–61; pre-existing, 258; secondary, 260–61; work-related, 257
mental injury claims, academic, 248
mentors, 65, 69, 81–84, 86, 89, 129–30, 227, 229, 239; close, 84; compassionate, 59; dedicated, 83
mentorship, 57, 59, 61, 65, 83–84, 177, 239–40
microaggression concept, 105
military combat, 170, 173, 175
minority, 16, 80, 107, 118, 123, 125, 129, 176, 190–91; ethnic, 175; racial, 12–13, 18, 175, 190
multiculturalism, 57

natural disasters, 169, 174
norms, 39, 54, 60, 79, 109, 117, 179–80, 193; cultural, 81, 83; institutional, 54; social, 46, 181, 189

outcomes: academic, 126; improved mental health, 130; negative mental health, 106; suicide-related, 73

panic disorder, xxi–xxiii, 41
parents, 121–24, 148–49, 234
patients, 155, 193–94
peers, 15, 54, 56, 60, 62–63, 65, 74, 122, 124, 127, 227–28, 230, 235–36, 238
perceptions, 55, 59, 74, 77, 81, 175, 181, 219, 222; idealized, 15; mixed, 212; popular, 14; positive, 8; public, 219; unfavorable, 83
perfectionism, xxi–xxii, 15, 72, 74
performance: academic, 229; faculty member's job, 88; management, 194; metrics, 88; monitoring, 259, 269
perspectives, 19, 110, 115, 229, 280–84, 287; confidant's, 141, 143; counseling staff member's, 221; critical, 245; personal, 36; public relations, 211
pets, 209, 214–16, 218–20, 222

policies, 58, 60, 64–66, 190, 195, 197, 208, 210–17, 219, 221–22, 248, 250–53, 258, 261–62, 270; academic promotion, 264; accessible, 239; accommodation, 46; departmental, 63; effective, 11, 19; government, 189; institution-wide mental health, 199; mandated, 270; no-pets, 209; robust mental health support, 192; sensitive, 194; streamlining, 65; working, 215

post-traumatic stress disorder (PTSD), xxi, 108, 169–78, 180–81, 220, 257

Preparing Future Faculty (PFF), 64

pressures, 6, 12, 14–15, 38, 73–75, 87–88, 114, 194, 228–29, 233; complex, 191; constant, 38, 43, 78; excessive, 199; extreme, 80; intense, 122; internal, 238; social, 180

primarily White institutions (PWIs), 106, 113–14, 116, 156

processes, 41, 108–9, 165, 211–12, 216, 219, 221, 239, 248, 251, 260–61, 265–67, 272; communicative, 157; decision-making, 216; formal, 4, 267; hiring, 190; informal, 211; institutional, 267; joint work, 211; transactional, 139; transcription, 144–45

productivity, 18, 70–71, 80, 85, 87–88, 178, 250; academic, 228; cognitive, 170; enhanced, 200; scholarly, 238

programs, 42, 54, 56–57, 84–87, 129–30, 219, 221, 227, 232, 234–35, 248, 251; academic, 219; doctoral, 39–40, 43, 89, 121; employee assistance, 5, 191, 196, 261; graduate healthcare, 73; institutional, 215; intervention, 130; mandatory faculty-student mentoring, 130; professional training, 126; stress relief, 219

promotion, 19, 82, 106, 109, 229, 237, 254, 257, 266–68, 271

psychologist, 261, 263, 265

race, 10, 16, 64–65, 107–8, 113, 117, 125, 130, 171, 174–75

racism, 62, 105, 116; perpetuating, 117; systemic, 105

rape, 169, 174–76

relationships, 12, 14, 45, 65, 109, 111, 145, 154, 157, 163, 211; destructive, 55; non-service-animal, 208; pivotal, 141; professional, 232; social, 191, 193; supportive, 130; toxic, 54; unconstructive, 57; unhealthy, 12

research: academic, 9, 18–19, 153; current, xxii, 128, 191; early, 17; emerging, 19; international, 10, 193; public-facing, 234; publishing, 73

researchers: female, 90

resilience, 55, 130, 238

resources, 13–14, 18, 59, 61–62, 64, 84–88, 152, 155–56, 193, 198–99, 229–30, 277–78, 283–84, 286; community-based, 194; disability, 177; inadequate, 57, 62; institutional, 211, 232; professional, 65; scarce, 60; web-based, 277

risks, 8, 37, 106, 110, 112, 115–17, 199

sabbatical, xxii, 264
safety, psychological, 109
schizophrenia, xxi, 5
self-disclosure, 147, 180
self-efficacy, 81, 129–30
self-esteem, 106, 129–30
self-mutilation, 3, 9, 208
sensemaking, 74–75, 84, 105–6, 109–10, 112–16; collaborative, 106
sex, 143, 163; assault, 174; intimacy, 140; orientation, 107, 171, 236
silence, xxiii–xxiv, 6, 19, 42, 61, 109, 281; culture of, 6, 43, 46
skills: administrative, 266; emotional, 248; problem-solving, 54; suicide intervention, 232

socialization, 65–66, 106, 110, 116, 207; academic, 115
socioeconomic status, 89–90, 127
staff: adjunct, 17; administrative, 222; casual, 195, 197, 201; departmental, 61; diverse, 191–92, 194–95; managing, 260; migrant, 200–201; occupational mental health, 75
stereotypes: common, 190; negative, 17, 113; racial, 59; rampant, 57
stigma, 8, 17–19, 37, 48, 69, 71, 74–76, 85–86, 131, 140–42, 171–72, 177–78, 189–90, 231, 279–80; cultural, 177; invisible, 153; label-related, 70; negative, 71; professional, 177; societal, 141
stress, 3, 7, 14–17, 38–39, 43, 53–55, 63–65, 75–76, 78, 83–86, 89–90, 256–57, 266, 268; academic workplace, 255; chronic, 82; decreased student, 207; emotional, 266; financial, 12; graduate student, 64; managing, 231; post-traumatic, 207; workload, 191; work-related, 14, 253, 255, 267
stressors: academic, 128; institutional-specific, 64
structuration theory, 53–54
students: Asian, 13; blind, 210; college-age, 152; competent, 41; disabled, 209; diverse, 65; doctoral, 55–56, 61, 63, 73, 128–30, 286; female, 62; gay, 57; graduate and professional, 128, 131–32; graduating, 58; impacted, 81, 279; international, 10, 12–13, 59–60, 62, 178, 198; non-ANZ, 217; post-secondary, 229; queer, 10; struggling, 18; traumatized, 176, 181; working-class, 178
success, 61–62, 72, 75, 84–85, 88, 128–30, 132, 228, 233, 239
suicide, 3, 70–71, 73, 85, 154, 272, 279; completion, 128, 251

support, xxiv, 18–19, 59, 64–65, 79–80, 83, 85–86, 129–31, 139–40, 178–79, 189–91, 195–201, 228–30, 232, 236, 238–39, 261–63, 266–69, 286–87; available, 189, 199, 201; caregiver, 230; emotional, 130, 191, 209, 212; familial, 127; institutional administration, 235; lack of, 55, 62, 69, 89; post-departure, 195; professional, 227; providing, 84, 125, 200; sensitive forms of, 199–200
syndrome, chronic fatigue, 263

teaching: evaluations, 54; excellence, 180, 227; obligations, 73; staff, 191–92
Teaching Assistants (TAs), 170, 176, 181, 237
tenure, xxii–xxiii, 3–4, 36, 38, 40, 43–44, 174, 177–78, 229–30, 235, 237; processes, 4–6
Theory of Planned Behavior (TPB), 170, 180–81
therapy, xxiii, 170, 208
training: intercultural, 237; mental health-related, 205; pedagogical, 59; professional, 10, 122, 125, 128; theoretical, xxiii
transgender, 128, 173
trauma, xxiv, 7, 169–70, 172, 174–76, 178; acute, 170; emotional, xxiii; vicarious, 232

undergraduates, 5–6, 9–13, 16, 38, 42–43, 46, 54, 56, 87, 89, 128, 131, 176–77, 234, 237
universities: competitive, 194; major, 112; neoliberal, 38, 46; research-intensive, 190, 227

veterans, 172; undergraduates, 180–81
violence, sexual, 174–76, 181
vulnerabilities, 128, 228, 230

weakness, 5, 88, 231; professional, 70
wellness, 17–18, 192, 229–30, 233, 239
women, 10, 12–13, 16–18, 40, 77, 90, 124, 172–75, 179; Black, 114
workers, injured, 248, 253, 269
work hours, 177; flexible, 71; long, 16; sociable, 245; strenuous, 72
workloads, 14, 82, 178, 192, 230, 245–47, 255; increased, 71, 246; never-ending, 15, 35; unmanageable, 194, 260
workplace: cultures, 70, 83, 270; emotionality of, 271; injuries, 248, 253, 258, 269; non-academic, 7

About the Editor and Contributors

ABOUT THE EDITOR

Teresa Heinz Housel
Teresa Heinz Housel is a senior tutor in the School of Journalism, Communication and Marketing at Massey University of New Zealand. She received her PhD in communication and culture from Indiana University. Her research has appeared in *Education + Training, Critical Studies in Media Communication, Journal of Critical Inquiry,* and *Information, Communication & Society.* Her co-edited publication with Vickie L. Harvey, "Impact of Technology on Interpersonal Relationships," was published as a special edition of the *Electronic Journal of Communication* in 2016. She has co-edited three books with Vickie L. Harvey: *Left Out: Health Care Issues Facing LGBT People* (Lexington Books, 2014); *Faculty and First-Generation College Students: Bridging the Classroom Gap Together* (2011); and *The Invisibility Factor: Administrators and Faculty Reach Out to First-Generation College Students* (2010). She has written about her experiences of being a first-generation college student for *The Chronicle of Higher Education* and *Inside Higher Ed.* Her most recent edited book is *First-Generation College Student Experiences of Intersecting Marginalities* (2019). Websites: www.teresaheinzhousel.com and www.ourmindstogether.com.

ABOUT THE CONTRIBUTORS

Nike Bahr
Born and raised in Germany, Nike Bahr completed her BA at the University of Mannheim. Seeking to further her education, she moved to the United States in 2016 to study professional communication at the University of Alaska, Fairbanks. During her graduate studies, Nike experienced and observed the mentally straining factors of academia in tenured professors, fellow graduate students, and herself. Nike's interest in studying the impacts of mental health was born from the lack of available support for faculty and staff in academia despite its ever-present impact. With a research focus in mass communication and social media, Nike has immersed herself in studies of negative body image and its portrayal on Instagram, the portrayal of Millennials in the media, as well as public speaking anxiety. After graduating, Nike continues to be an instructor for communication classes, a researcher, and lends her skills to local non-profit organizations.

Nubia Brewster
Nubia Brewster is an MA student in the Department of Communication at Wayne State University.

Patrice M. Buzzanell
Patrice M. Buzzanell (PhD, Purdue) is chair and professor of the Department of Communication at the University of South Florida and endowed visiting professor for the School of Media and Design at Shanghai Jiaotong University. A fellow and past president of the International Communication Association, she also has served as president of the Council of Communication Associations and the Organization for the Study of Communication, Language and Gender. She became a distinguished scholar of the National Communication Association (NCA) in 2017. Her research focuses on career, work-life policy, resilience, gender, and engineering design in micro-macro contexts. She has published four edited books; more than 200 journal articles, chapters, and encyclopedia entries; and numerous engineering education and other proceedings.

Erinn C. Cameron
Erinn Cameron is currently working on a PhD in clinical psychology with a specialization in neuropsychology and social justice. Her undergraduate degrees are in biology and chemistry, and she has also studied Latin, Greek, Hebrew, Spanish, Portuguese, and French. She is also a certified ESL instructor. Erinn currently serves as the research and publications coordinator for the Association for Trauma Outreach and Prevention, an affiliate of the United

Nations. She is also an international graduate fellow in the Ambassador for Humanitarian Service and Peacekeeping program and is an active researcher and member of the International Council of Psychologists. Her most recent talk at the 2019 American Psychological Association Conference was entitled, "Global Systemic Violence and Human Rights Violations: Empowering Women." She has ongoing research projects and clinical work in the areas of gender inequality, women's health, human trafficking, trauma, and global mental health. Having lived in several countries and participated in academic and humanitarian work across the globe, Erinn brings a wealth of international and cultural experience to her research and writing.

Nicole Campbell
Dr. Campbell received her undergraduate and graduate degrees from the University of Guelph in biomedical sciences. Throughout her graduate studies, she obtained numerous teaching experiences, including distance education instruction, course development, and course coordination. After completing her PhD, Dr. Campbell was an instructor at various institutions, teaching courses in physiology, pharmacology, pathophysiology, and research methodology. Dr. Campbell is responsible for the Year 4 Medical Science courses and the co-development and teaching of a Year 3 interdisciplinary lab course for students in the Honors Specialization Interdisciplinary Medical Sciences (IMS) at Western University. In addition to serving as a teaching fellow, she recently received the Marilyn Robinson Teaching Award for outstanding excellence in teaching.

Philip Dearman
Philip Dearman is a senior researcher in the Research Branch of the Parliamentary Library, Australian Parliament House, Canberra. At the time of writing, he was a lecturer and researcher in media and politics in the School of Media and Communications, RMIT University, Melbourne. His research explores the application of a range of communication technologies in modern liberal programs of governing, focusing on histories of educational technologies in education, the digitalization of information systems used in professional work, and the potential for citizen science in negotiating the politics of air quality.

Ursula Edgington
Ursula Edgington is an independent scholar, specializing in international sociological research into the development of tertiary teaching and learning. Her specialist areas are founded on the transformative nature of learning and issues of social justice. Ursula's investigations are situated within diverse educational settings including inner-city community projects, experiential

learning interventions for vulnerable young people, and vocational subjects in the workplace. Ursula completed her PhD in Education in Britain and moved to New Zealand in 2013. She was awarded the Fellowship of the Higher Education Research and Development Society of Australasia (HERDSA) in 2017, in recognition of her commitment to quality in teaching and learning and professional development. Ursula's published academic work ranges from aspects of emotional labor in teaching and learning, to the use of innovative research methodologies.

Beth Edmondson
Beth Edmondson is a senior lecturer in the School of Arts at Federation University Australia. She has long-standing interests in Australian health and employment policies, industrial relations, and university management practices. She is actively involved in research focused on the impacts of work-related trauma for human services workers in regional Victoria. She has personal and professional experience of navigating the complexities of workplace mental health injuries, and of managing staff who have made claims for workers' compensation.

Julia Grzywinski
Julia Grzywinski is an MA student in the Department of Communication at Wayne State University.

Susan Hafen
Dr. Susan Hafen is a full professor who joined the Department of Communication at Weber State University in 2003. Besides teaching and research, she is the department internship coordinator and honors adviser. Dr. Hafen previously taught at the University of Wisconsin for eight years. Prior to receiving her PhD, Dr. Hafen worked in the business world for a dozen years: In Ogden, Utah, at Kimberly-Clark Corporation as a human resource manager; in Gillette, Wyoming, at Mobil Oil as a training/employment relations advisor; and in Washington, D.C., at Potomac Electric Power Company as a communication trainer. Her first career, however, was in education: First, as a fashion merchandising/communication teacher at Brighton High School in Salt Lake City; next, as a curriculum specialist at the University of Maryland. Outside of work, she enjoys the outdoors with her Australian cattle dogs, hiking, and cross-country skiing.

Robert D. Hall
Robert D. Hall, MA, is an interpersonal, family, and health communication doctoral candidate at the University of Nebraska-Lincoln. He researches disclosure processes regarding mental and chronic invisible illnesses in close

and personal relationships. Currently, he focuses on qualitative and arts-based methodologies to develop translational materials for those affected by invisible illnesses. Throughout his career, he has won several awards for his research and teaching at the university, regional, and national levels.

Erica Knotts
Erica Knotts is a lecturer in the Department of Communication at Southern Oregon University in Ashland, Oregon. Previously, she worked as a public and academic librarian and recently co-authored (with Ma & Stahl) an article for the *Journal of the Medical Library Association* (2018). Erica's academic areas of interest include health and crisis communication, conflict resolution, mediation, and non-verbal communication. She has a particular interest in the effects of activity- based learning in the classroom. Erica holds an Interdisciplinary MA in crisis and health communication from Southern Oregon University and an MLIS from Emporia State University.

Victoria McDermott
Victoria McDermott is a doctoral student and graduate assistant at the University of Maryland. She was formerly science communication lead for Toolik Field Station and adjunct instructor at the University of Alaska Fairbanks in the Department of Communication and Journalism. She has an interest in gender communication, the communication of power in traditionally masculine environments, and organizational communication. Previous research projects have included the clash of the academy and the military, the communication of college students' understanding of consent, and the communication of power in field stations and marine laboratories. Victoria has an express interest in understanding the narratives of her peers as the value of academia comes under scrutiny. As an aspiring professor, she has recently watched her mentor experience the effects of academic burnout, ultimately inspiring this research. With a keen interest in research and adding to the discipline, Victoria looks forward to continuing her education by completing a PhD in communication.

Andrea L. Meluch
Andrea L. Meluch (PhD, Kent State University, 2016) is an assistant professor of business and organizational communication in the School of Communication and Department of Management at The University of Akron. Her research focuses on the intersections of health, organizational, and instructional communication. Specifically, she is interested in issues of organizational culture, mental health, and social support. She has published in *Communication Education, Southern Communication Journal, Qualitative Research in Medicine & Healthcare, Journal of Communication*

in *Healthcare*, and the *Journal of Communication Pedagogy*. She has also authored/co-authored more than a dozen book chapters and encyclopedia entries.

Rahul Mitra
Rahul Mitra is an associate professor, whose research is at the intersection of organizational and environmental communication. Prior to obtaining his PhD from Purdue University, he worked in the news broadcast and public relations fields in India for three and a half years. His scholarship focuses on environmental organizing, sustainability and corporate social responsibility (CSR), and meaningful work discourses. He is a critical-interpretive scholar, and uses primarily qualitative methods, such as ethnography, interviews, focus groups, discourse analysis, and arts-based research. His work has appeared in numerous peer-reviewed publications such as *Environmental Communication, Management Communication Quarterly, Human Relations, Communication Theory, International Journal of Business Communication, Public Relations Review*, and *Journal of Business Ethics*. At Wayne State, he directs the Resilient Institutions & Sustainable Environments (R.I.S.E.) Lab, which examines how communicative practices enable resilience and sustainability in a variety of organizations.

Jessica Wendorf Muhamad
Jessica Wendorf Muhamad, PhD, is an assistant professor of communication and associate director of the Center for Hispanic Communication in the School of Communication at Florida State University. Dr. Wendorf Muhamad is also the director of PEAKS laboratory (Participatory, Experientially based Applied Knowledge for Social Change), which focuses on developing— through action research—evidence-based interventions for complex social issues. Dr. Wendorf Muhamad's research focuses on understanding how and why enacted, entertainment-educational experiences (e.g., game-based interventions) influence individuals. Her primary line of research focuses on (1) the development of culturally relevant, experientially based health interventions constructed through a participatory and engaged approach; (2) examines how prosocial, persuasive narratives embedded within experiential learning opportunities influences individuals' attitudes and behaviors regarding health and social issues; and (3) extends beyond active entertainment-education mechanisms to a holistic understanding of intervention adoptability through an examination of implementation climate pre- and post-development. Her research has been published in *Journal of Health Communication, Health Communication, Computers in Human Behavior*, and *Journal of Industrial Medicine*, among others, as well as book chapters on serious games and communication engagement.

Juan S. Muhamad

Juan S. Muhamad is an engaged researcher whose primary research interest focuses on investigating the effects of participatory intervention design, implementation, and application of information systems (i.e., platforms, interfaces, assistive technology) to music therapy-based interventions centered on mental health. More precisely, his research examines how vulnerable and disenfranchised populations engage with assistive technologies for health outcomes, as well as prosocial attitudinal and behavioral outcomes. His background includes training and more than ten years of experience working with underserved communities. His advanced training in group and community facilitation as a mental health professional has allowed him to assist in translating health campaigns to communities through the localization of campaign materials, including cultural and contextual translation. Muhamad has worked providing direct service to clients and families (direct care) and consulting with service providing organizations (referral and service design). In this capacity, he has worked on both federally funded projects (e.g., United Way Early Head Start Childcare Partnerships), as well as foundational, federal, and university sponsored activities. He is a doctoral student in the School of Information at Florida State University's College of Communication and Information.

Elizabeth-Ann Pandzich

Elizabeth-Ann Pandzich is an MA student in the Department of Communication at Wayne State University.

Katie Rose Guest Pryal

Katie Rose Guest Pryal, JD, PhD, is a best-selling author, speaker, and law and creative writing professor. She is the author of *Life of the Mind Interrupted: Essays on Mental Health and Disability in Higher Education* (2017), #1 Amazon bestseller; *The Freelance Academic: Transform Your Creative Life and Career* (2019), winner of a Gold INDIE award; and *Even If You're Broken: Essays on Sexual Assault and #MeToo* (2019), winner of a Gold IPPY award. She has also written three novels, *Entanglement, Chasing Chaos,* and *Fallout Girl,* and many textbooks on law and writing. She is a columnist for *Women in Higher Education,* where she covers gender issues, labor, and academia. Her popular column for *Catapult* magazine, "Mom, Interrupted," is about family life, mental illness, and raising disabled kids as a disabled parent. Her column "Public Writing Life" for *The Chronicle of Higher Education* advises academics who wish to transition to writing for public audiences. She speaks frequently about mental health and disability, writing and publishing, gender issues, and higher education. Website: https://katieroseguestpryal.com/.

Alena Amato Ruggerio

Alena Amato Ruggerio is professor of communication and former interim coordinator of women's studies at Southern Oregon University in Ashland, Oregon. The editor of *Media Depictions of Brides, Wives, and Mothers* (2012), her work has appeared in *Feminist Media Studies, Great Ideas for Teaching Students (G.I.F.T.S.) in Communication* (2017), and *Talking Taboo: American Christian Women Get Frank About Faith* (2013). For her classroom work in feminist rhetorical theory, rhetorical criticism, persuasion, argumentation, and advanced public speaking, Dr. Ruggerio received the Distinguished Teaching Award from SOU in 2017. She holds a PhD in communication and culture from Indiana University.

Sandra Smeltzer

Dr. Smeltzer's areas of research and publication include critical pedagogy, experiential learning, communication in transitioning and developing countries (particularly in Southeast Asia), the ethics of activist research, ICTs for social justice, and the scholar-activist dialectic. She is a teaching fellow at Western, with a focus on experiential learning; a Moore Institute Fellow at the National University of Ireland, Galway; and the co-coordinator of the Media and the Public Interest program at Western. She has been awarded the University Students' Council Teaching Honour Roll Award of Excellence for every year she has taught full time at Western; is the recipient of the Faculty of Information and Media Studies Undergraduate Teaching Award; and holds a three-year Social Sciences and Humanities Research Council of Canada (SSHRC) Insight Grant to study experiential learning in Canada.

Vanessa R. Sperduti

Vanessa R. Sperduti is a PhD candidate of education at Western University in London, Canada. Her work focuses broadly on international education, and specifically on better understanding the impact of service learning on host communities. She has been the co-chair (2018–2021) of the New Scholars Committee of the Comparative International Education Society (CIES) and was the former editorial assistant of its newsletter, "Perspectives." She was also the Graduate Student Representative (2018–2020) on the Comparative International Education Society of Canada (CIESC).

Lukasz Swiatek

Lukasz Swiatek is lecturer in public relations and advertising in the Faculty of Arts and Social Sciences at the University of New South Wales, in Sydney, Australia. He has taught a range of undergraduate and postgraduate courses in universities in Aotearoa New Zealand and Australia. His research interests focus on multiple aspects of the future of strategic communication in a digital world, as well as effective higher education institutional policy and teaching development. He has co-organized and co-run Aotearoa New Zealand's annual Academic Development Symposia, which have helped educationalists (including academic developers and academics) build stronger academic institutions, better support part-time and full-time staff, and enhance teaching practice.

Maria Elena Villar
María Elena Villar is associate professor and chair of the Department of Communication at the School of Communication + Journalism at Florida International University. Her research focuses on culturally competent communication for social and behavioral change, and on strategic communication for diverse audiences. In her career as a researcher, Dr. Villar has focused on diverse topics that range from culture and communication, social determinants of disease and health, domestic and sexual violence prevention, stigma related to HIV, mental health and drug abuse, evaluation of program outcomes, and communication for social change. She has dozens of publications based on her research, including peer-reviewed journal articles, conference proceedings, a book chapter and many conference presentations, and several technical reports. Dr. Villar is also heavily involved in the community. She served as social marketing director to federally funded FACES (Families and Communities Empowered for Success), a community initiative to improve behavioral health services for youth and ensure that family voices are heard. In that role she oversaw all social marketing, branding, stigma reduction, and internal communication activities. For her work, she received various ECCO (Excellence in Communication and Community Outreach) Award from the Substance Abuse and Mental Health Services Administration. Based on this work, she was recognized by Florida International University as a 2012 Top Scholar for her scholarly contributions.

David M. Walton
Dr. Walton is a physiotherapist and associate professor with the School of Physical Therapy at Western University, an associate scientist with the Lawson Health Research Institute, and director of the Pain and Quality of Life Integrative Research Lab. His teaching duties are in the pain elective and professional consolidation courses in the Master's of Physical Therapy (MPT) program and he contributes as assistant and sessional lecturer in the Master's of Clinical Science (Manipulative Therapy) program. His research interests are focused on assessment and prognosis in acute and chronic pain, especially in pain arising from musculoskeletal trauma such as whiplash, sporting, or work injuries. Dr. Walton is de facto chair of two interdisciplinary research

groups at Western: the Collaboration for the Integration of Rehabilitation with Consumer Electronic (CIRCLE) and the Solving Traumatic Pain and Disability through Advanced Research Translation (START) groups. Significant awards include two faculty Teaching Awards of Excellence, the 2014 Canadian Physiotherapy Association National Mentorship Award, and Early Career Investigator Awards from the Canadian Pain Society (2015) and the Ontario Ministry of Research and Innovation (2016), and a nominee for the university-wide teaching (Marilyn Robinson Teaching Award). He is the only person in Western's history to simultaneously hold both a Western Faculty Scholar award (for scholarly productivity) and a Western Teaching Fellowship.

www.ingramcontent.com/pod-product-compliance
Lightning Source LLC
Chambersburg PA
CBHW021343300426
44114CB00012B/1059